Seminars in
the Psychotherapies

DATE DUE

19/2			
7/7/16			

PROPERTY OF LIBRARY SERVICE
Tees, Esk & Wear Valleys NHS Foundation **Trust**
IF FOUND, PLEASE RETURN TO: Inglewood Library,
Appletree Inglewood Unit. Lanchester Road Hospital
Lanchester Road. DURHAM. DH1 5RD

Seminars in
the Psychotherapies

Edited by
Jane Naismith & Sandra Grant

Gaskell

© The Royal College of Psychiatrists 2007

Gaskell is an imprint of the Royal College of Psychiatrists
17 Belgrave Square, London SW1X 8PG
http://www.rcpsych.ac.uk

All rights reserved. No part of this book may be reprinted or reproduced or utilised in any
form or by any electronic, mechanical, or other means, now known or hereafter invented,
including photocopying and recording, or in any information storage or retrieval system, without
permission in writing from the publishers.

British Library Cataloguing-in-Publication Data.
A catalogue record for this book is available from the British Library.
ISBN   9781904671459

Distributed in North America by Balogh International Inc.

The views presented in this book do not necessarily reflect those of the Royal College
of Psychiatrists, and the publishers are not responsible for any error of omission or fact.

The Royal College of Psychiatrists is a registered charity (no. 228636).
Printed by Bell & Bain Limited, Glasgow, UK.

Contents

Tables, boxes and figures

Contributors

Anthony Bateman, Consultant Psychiatrist in Psychotherapy, Halliwick Unit, Barnet, Enfield, and Haringey Mental Health Trust, St Ann's Hospital, St Ann's Road, London N15 3TH

Phil Brown, Consultant Psychotherapist, Lancashire Care NHS Trust, Psychotherapy Service, 1 Albert Road, Fulwood, Preston PR2 8PJ

Graham Bryce, Consultant Child and Adolescent Psychiatrist, Specialist Children's Services, 62 Templeton Street, Glasgow G40 1DW

Lynne M. Drummond, Consultant Psychiatrist, Senior Lecturer in Behavioural and Cognitive Psychotherapy, St George's, University of London, Division of Mental Health, Cranmer Terrace, London SW17 0RE

Sandra Grant, retired Consultant Psychotherapist, Glasgow

John Hook, Consultant Psychiatrist in Psychotherapy, Farnham Road Hospital, Guildford GU2 7LX

Susan Llewelyn, Director, Oxford Doctoral Course in Clinical Psychology, Warneford Hospital, Univesrity of Oxford, Oxford OX3 7JX

Frank Margison, Consultant Psychiatrist in Psychotherapy, Manchester Mental Health and Social Care Trust, Chorlton House, 70 Manchester Road, Chorlton Cum Hardy, Manchester M21 9UN

Tom Murphy, Consultant Psychiatrist in Psychotherapy, Royal Edinburgh Hospital, 40 Colinton Road, Edinburgh EH10 5BT

Jane Naismith, Consultant Psychiatrist in Psychotherapy, South Glasgow Psychotherapy Service, Ferguson Rodger Psychotherapy Clinic, Department of Psychiatry, Southern General Hospital, Glasgow G51 4TF

Jean Robinson, Child Psychotherapist and Consultant Child and Adolescent Psychiatrist, Department of Child and Family Mental Health, Royal Aberdeen Children's Hospital, Westburn Drive, Aberdeen AB25 2ZG

Jan Scott, Professor of Psychological Treatments Research, Institute of Psychiatry, De Crespigny Park, Denmark Hill, London SE5 8AF

John Shemilt, Psychoanalyst, 12 Wykeham Road, Glasgow G13 3YT; formerly Consultant Child and Adolescent Psychiatrist, Yorkhill Hospital, Glasgow and Consultant Psychotherapist, Stobhill Hospital, Glasgow

Hilary Warwick, Senior Lecturer in Behavioural and Cognitive Psychotherapy, St George's, Univerity of London, Department of Psychiatry, London SW17 0RE

Preface

Over the past decade the psychosocial components of psychiatric treatment and care have gained greater prominence and acceptance than for any time since the 1960s. There are a number of reasons for this, first, the ideological conflict between radical behaviourism and psychoanalytic psychotherapy has been replaced by more sophisticated and informed debate about what constitutes effective and acceptable treatment, for what kind of person, with what condition and in what context. This has led to innovative and shorter treatments, strongly endorsed by an increasing evidence-base. At the same time research has also demonstrated that in certain circumstances long-term psychodynamic psychotherapy is the treatment of choice.

There is increasing interest not only in the differences between therapies but also in finding common ground. There is recognition that different therapies are available and that they can complement one another; it is not necessary to be in competition for funding or recognition. An increasing evidence-base now exists for all the therapeutic modalities presented in *Seminars in the Psychotherapies*. There are significant overlaps, but also clear distinctions in the types of therapies that are suitable for different kinds of problem. Patients will have their individual preferences, and therapists too, as individuals will vary in the training they feel drawn to undertake.

The second sterile ideological battle was between biologically oriented psychiatrists and psychotherapists, many of whom are non-medical (adding to the tension). At the same time, as advances in pharmacology and neuroscience clearly demonstrate a central place for biological approaches for most severe mental illnesses, the brain damage inflicted by severe emotional trauma has been recognised and has led, for example, to therapeutic work based on attachment theory. There is common ground. The myth that psychotherapists deal only with the 'worried well', sadly fostered by stringent selection criteria, has been replaced with recognition that psychotherapeutic skills and understanding are needed when working with people with all kinds of disorder. This includes psychotic illnesses, learning difficulties, forensic patients and severe personality disorder. A developing role for the consultant psychotherapist is to provide specialist supervision for people working in a wide range of settings.

The final significant factor leading to the shift in attitude to psychotherapy has been the increased power of service users and their carers, who consistently request 'talking treatments', leading to the exponential increase in the numbers of psychologists and counsellors. There is a danger that what usually gets called the 'medical model' is perceived negatively as being only about drug treatments. While it is true that only doctors can prescribe psychotropic drugs, the attitude that this is all we do is seriously mistaken and belies the biopsychosocial model that underpins all medical training. Every psychiatrist must have skills in all modalities.

An overview of the major established psychotherapies is given. Although far from comprehensive, it is a starting point appropriate for trainees in psychiatry, but it also explores more complex areas. While trainees will constitute the main readership, *Seminars in the Psychotherapies* is also relevant for people from different professional backgrounds working as psychotherapists and also for psychiatrists in other specialties who wish to keep up-to-date.

The three main psychotherapy modalities required for trainees in general psychiatry and for psychiatrists training in psychotherapy are emphasised: systemic therapy, cognitive–behavioural psychotherapy and dynamic psychotherapy. *Seminars in the Psychotherapies* is not designed as an examination aid but it will cover relevant concepts, some in depth. A balance was aimed for between theory and practice and clinical examples have been used to portray, at times quite complex, theoretical concepts.

The editors are aware that this volume is not comprehensive. Some areas are covered in greater depth than others, there are gaps and there are biases in theoretical emphasis. Its limitations have to be acknowledged and recognised. We hope that by emphasising and identifying these, we will stimulate further thought for others to comment on and material for later editions. There are several newer brief therapies that we have not included, for example, interpersonal therapy and dialectical behaviour therapy.

Finally, readers may notice the relative Scottishness of this book. Scotland has a long established tradition in psychotherapy linked initially to the Scottish Institute of Human Relations, which contributed to the training of a number of consultant psychotherapists who became a 'critical mass' for the development of services.

As part of the College Seminars series, the aim of this book is to provide some background knowledge for psychiatrists who are developing their psychotherapeutic skills. The underlying objective, however, is to make a contribution to helping us deliver better services for our patients.

Jane Naismith
Sandra Grant

Acknowledgements

We are indebted to all the contributors for their encouragement and for their forebearance as this book as been long in the making. Many thanks also to those who contributed to earlier versions. We thank the staff of the Royal College of Psychiatrists for their encouragement, patience and for not giving up on us. We would also like to thank Dr Siobhan Murphy for reading earlier drafts of the book and most of all to thank Mrs Caroline Nimmo for her support, efficiency and perseverance throughout the whole process.

CHAPTER 1

Assessment in psychotherapy

Frank Margison & Phil Brown

What is psychotherapy assessment for?

Assessing a patient for psychotherapy is often seen as mystifying. This is not surprising given the diversity of opinion, even among experienced clinicians. In this chapter we will outline some of the basic concepts and skills and aim to provide a framework. This framework can be summarised as two main decisions: first, the appropriateness of any psychological treatment approach; and second, the choice of which particular psychological treatment method. These decisions involve knowledge gained from research (evidence-based practice) and views based on systematic clinical experience (practice-based evidence).

There are two distinct processes occurring during assessment. The first is idiographic; a unique formulation is being drawn that captures the essential features relevant to this person. The second, nomothetic, process draws inferences relevant to this individual from good quality research with similar subjects. Evidence-based medicine (Sackett *et al*, 1998) is one attempt to bring these processes closer together (Margison, 2001). The clinician tries to construct a well-designed question that is relevant, and perhaps unique, to an individual and then uses strategies to search the literature for information relevant to that question. The knowledge-base for answering questions with regard to psychotherapy assessment is far from ideal, but is more extensive than some critics would allow (for a detailed review see Roth & Fonagy, 2005).

In an ideal world there would be simple tools for carrying out an assessment. The tools would be accurate in predicting both positive and negative effects of therapy. Despite many attempts there has been little progress in developing an assessment tool able to make accurate predictions across a range of patients and conditions (Mace, 1995). Tools have been of little use, perhaps because they are often used 'without conceptual or logical justification' (see Bloch, 1979). Evidence-based guidelines are a sophisticated attempt to draw on the best available literature and to use 'expert consensus' methods (such as Delphi techniques) to synthesise the best way to tackle a clinical problem. These approaches have been difficult to implement and are expensive and time-consuming to produce. Critics have also pointed out that bad guidelines may be worse than having no guidelines at all (Woolf *et al*, 1999). Despite the limitations of the subject areas covered by good quality guidelines, they need to be considered as an integral part of assessment when they are available.

In reading this chapter, it is assumed that the description of assessment will supplement other methods of evidence-based medicine such as literature searches and evidence-based guidelines. The essence of assessment is in evaluating a person's strengths, weaknesses, desires and motivation. The skill in carrying out an assessment is in balancing all of these elements, while considering the best of several approaches to therapy. Doing this within a conversation that is both personally engaged and professionally detached is demanding. Assessors may believe that their approach is the best approach. Their assessment of a new patient may therefore focus on establishing whether the individual is suitable for treatment by their own approach, rather than on considering which approach of the many available would be best for that individual.

This chapter deals with a wide range of psychotherapeutic approaches. First, underlying principles relevant to any interview are detailed. Second, some of the strategies that are specific to the main modalities are considered briefly: cognitive–behavioural, systemic and psychodynamic–interpersonal. Integrative approaches that draw on several traditions to tailor an approach that is designed for a particular individual are also discussed.

To do this, the strategies used in an assessment interview have been summarised. We then discuss assessment in relation to formulation skills. Finally, a simplified decision model that summarises the main points is presented.

How to do an assessment interview: conflicting roles and expectations

It is crucial to distinguish between two quite different purposes of an assessment. The first has sometimes been called 'brokerage'. Here the therapist is acting as a guide, helping the patient come to the best decision about whether to undertake therapy and, if so, which approach might be most suitable. This requires the assessing therapist to know a fair amount about the range of therapies and their indications, and something of the local situation (for example, where to find different types of therapy, or in some cases, alternative approaches, including social and psychopharmacological). This process requires different skills from the second type of interview, where the therapist is assessing for a particular type of therapy.

A psychotherapy interview needs to provide structure within a freely flowing conversation. Such a narrative allows connections to become apparent. The interviewer may, however, need to deal with a relatively high level of uncertainty and anxiety. Finding out whether the patient can tolerate this ambiguity while exploring painful areas is in fact one of the issues being assessed. In a single interview the assessing therapist is trying to balance the need to take a social and psychiatric history while also modelling something of the actual therapeutic experience. Sometimes the interviewer manages to get to the heart of the patient's distress remarkably quickly. Paradoxically, this can make the subsequent task of the therapist more difficult because the patient has unrealistic expectations of being 'understood' to an almost magical degree.

Malan (1979) gave a succinct account of the main points to bear in mind throughout the assessment interview. These have been rephrased to highlight some key points that apply across different modes of therapy (see Box 1.1).

Assessment before the interview

Even before the assessor meets the patient a lot has happened. There is often a substantial therapeutic effect from just making contact. The need to maintain this initial 'mobilisation of hope' leads to the first conflict for the assessor. Should the therapist make contact as soon as possible, even if there is then a delay before the definitive therapy is offered? Or, should the therapist wait until the initial interview can be followed by therapy with no further delay.

One possible compromise is to have an initial few meetings as a form of very brief therapy, leading to a formulation and advice, while waiting for the definitive therapy, if that is still needed (Aveline, 1995).

Many departments send a preliminary questionnaire for the patient to complete before the interview, which typically covers similar ground to the interview, sometimes supplemented by standardised measures of symptoms and interpersonal problems. The Symptom Check List–90 Revised (SCL–90R; Derogatis, 1983) and the Inventory of Interpersonal Problems (Horowitz *et al*, 1988) are commonly used, and recently there has been the development of

---

Box 1.1 Checklist of tasks to consider in any assessment (after Malan, 1979)

Think psychiatrically:	Diagnosis, symptoms, medication
Think psychodynamically:	Triangles of conflict and person
Think psychotherapeutically:	Make forecasts and predictions
Think practically:	What is possible even if the ideal is unavailable?
Take care of the session:	Create and maintain rapport
Take care of the patient:	Avoid pointless anxiety
Be wary about your impact:	Watch the effect of your interventions, now and for the future

---

Box 1.2   Pros and cons of using a questionnaire

Advantages

- Extra detailed factual information available
- To understand the patient's hopes and expectations before meeting
- Style of filling-in reflects the patient's defence style
- Initial information is free of the interviewer's own bias
- Questions reflect the importance given to feelings, relationships, hopes and expectations
- To some extent, motivation and commitment can be checked

Disadvantages

- Questionnaire feels impersonal
- Patients feel uncomfortable writing down very sensitive information, for example, about abuse
- Postal security may not be perfect
- Written format tends to compound the existing bias against some patients with learning difficulties, who are not fluent in writing, where English is not the first language and in those with visual disability
- Savings in establishing motivation have to be offset against patients who are alienated by the questionnaire and do not respond

---

the Clinical Outcomes in Routine Evaluation (CORE) assessment instrument (Barkham *et al*, 1998). The use of initial questionnaires has been summarised by Mace (1995), and some key issues in using questionnaires are given in Box 1.2.

Some of the problems can be reduced by stating that the patient can still be seen if they cannot complete the questionnaire, having a space where the patient can say 'there is something I cannot put in writing', and by careful phrasing of sensitive questions.

Opening the interview

Presenting problem

The presenting problem can sometimes be specific, but may be much more diffuse (for example, a loss of direction, poor or unstable sense of self), masking other psychiatric difficulties.

Example

A 35-year-old woman, working as a successful computer analyst, started the interview by describing how she had been feeling empty, despondent and lacking direction about her future. She had not felt herself to be depressed but the interview helped her to trace the vague feelings of unease back to an earlier point in her life when she had been less successful than her sister who it turns out had just had a child, while the patient remained childless.

This highlighted for the patient that she faced a difficult choice between her role as a woman gaining self-esteem from her job, in conflict with a possible role as mother. She was then able to talk about episodes when she would feel hopeless and worthless and had considered suicide. She had felt ashamed to admit these feelings just as she had been unable to tell her parents how desolate she felt as a child.

This brief account shows how a vague presenting problem can be transformed into a much clearer area of conflict within the assessment itself. Sometimes the problem remains diffuse until much later and the assessment will then focus on the patient's capacity to engage in exploring the symptom.

Expectations

It is important to grasp the patient's understanding of the interview purpose and any areas of hopeful or negative expectations. 'I just want to be happy' is one of the least useful responses as it implies a positive expectation but a passive approach to the treatment.

Feelings about the interview

This leads on to the way the patient feels about the assessment, for example feeling exposed or anxious.

Example

A 36-year-old man started the interview looking particularly anxious even though a pre-treatment questionnaire had not suggested that he was prone to anxiety. When asked he commented that he had felt anxious in the waiting room and connected this feeling with a habit his father had of keeping him waiting before beating him with a steel ruler.

This exploration would have been useful simply to put the anxiety in context so that the patient can turn to the ostensible problem. However, as is often the case, the anxiety could be linked to the presenting problem. Here, the problem was of angry outbursts at work. The assessment led to a focus on rage towards junior colleagues at work being a replay of earlier relationships, with him unwittingly taking on the role of 'father'. Different approaches to therapy might highlight different aspects of this scenario: unwanted thoughts and actions, awareness of role conflict, managing a demanding job with insufficient support, making links between past and present. So, even in a generic interview, the strategy the assessor adopts may subtly lead to particular recommendations.

Gathering information

Presenting problem

As discussed above, it is often possible to move from the patient's feelings about the interview to the current difficulties they are experiencing. Why has the patient come for help? Why at this point? Are there any recent precipitants?

Historical factors

These are 'woven' into a personal narrative that can focus on anecdotes, which are then linked into themes. This section of the interview needs a careful balance between being comprehensive and structured on the one hand, while allowing the patient's own links to emerge naturally.

The main headings are the same as in a psychiatric history. For early life cover, as a minimum, family atmosphere, family history, separations and illnesses, school adjustment, friendships and experiences of bullying or abuse.

From adolescence there are the themes of sexual development, risk-taking and eventual separation. In adult life there are the themes of sustained sexual relationships, children, work, leisure and dealing with the ageing process in oneself and the ageing and death of parents. 'Mid-life' is a developmental point rather than a chronological one, when successes are re-evaluated and failures seen either as irrecoverable or assimilated.

In late life there are often themes of separation, illness and loss, either experienced personally or vicariously, or there might be themes of new-found creativity, independence and wisdom. This assumes that there are developmental themes in every individual's life, which are, in turn, linked to family themes, and to the broader culture in which the person lives.

A common error is to take a history assuming that developmental hurdles are locked to particular ages. It is common to face rivalry issues in adolescence during examinations, but these are often replaying themes from the time of starting school. A different opportunity for this theme to be played out might be the time of becoming a grandparent, which may lead to rivalry with one's own child. Although the history may emerge in a chronological sequence, the key task is to form themes from the relationship anecdotes. As will be discussed later, the different modes of therapy require somewhat different approaches to these themes, but in the assessment phase it is generally useful to gather a number of anecdotes and suggest linking themes.

It is best to see which themes emerge naturally, although there are traps related to our own prejudices, for example, reluctance to see someone from an ethnic minority as having to deal with envious attacks on their career success, or reluctance to see a male patient struggling with conflicts about how to nurture a child. Resisting stereotyping is always difficult, but perhaps especially so if the assessor is trying to form a 'story' of the patient's life. Patient and assessor are subject to a series of 'plots' (i.e. presumptive beliefs about the meaning of situations), which are especially subject to cultural bias.

Relationship history

The previous narrative will have covered various relationships in passing. In this section it is helpful to gain a detailed account of several key figures, again by getting the patient to recall significant stories about important people.

The quality and duration of the relationships, and ways of dealing with loss should be covered. Examples need to cover prototypes of relationships, for example, authority, peer, sexual, care-giving, and even 'casual' acquaintances.

Types of attachment pattern

Bowlby's work highlighted the importance of attachment types. In adult life these early patterns persist and can be brought out through the anecdotes mentioned earlier, particularly of parents and close family members. Abnormal relationship patterns are either intense, clingy and dependent; aloof and disconnected; or alternations between these two. In contrast a mature style can tolerate separation and ambiguity (see Holmes, 1996; Bartholomew, 1997; Mace & Margison, 1997). The research on attachment, through the introduction of the Adult Attachment Interview (Main & Goldwyn, 1995) led to the observation that the narrative style of the patient's accounts (rather than the content) was the most important information in assessing attachment style. Further studies (Sachse & Strauss, 2002) of attachment type (using a different taxonomy of avoidant, ambivalent, mixed insecure) in group therapy show less powerful predictions based on the attachment type, but meaningful links between therapeutic factors and attachment type. For example, avoidant patients rated group-linked change factors such as cohesion as least helpful, although the overall effectiveness of the group was not markedly less. This is an example of research evidence being consistent with, and supportive of, an underlying theoretical model, but of little value in helping a patient to make a choice about treatment.

The interview itself will display many of the key elements of relationship style through tone of voice, posture and gesture. This can be merely noted or brought into the discussion (although this needs tact as it can be intrusive and even persecutory to draw attention to your observations). The ability to experience 'basic trust' is fundamental in relationships and the patient's difficulty with this may become obvious in the interview.

Psychological mindedness and capacity for symbolism

There are several ways in which this appears in the interview, for example, the patient may talk about a dream and the dream may be seen to connect with the relationship themes already touched upon. The patient may use metaphor (with a greater or lesser degree of awareness of its multiple meanings) (Guthrie, 1999).

With some patients, exploring personal connections with characters from plays, films, television or books can carry the links further.

Coltart (1988a,b) suggests that psychological mindedness can be identified through the following factors:

- a history that deepens and becomes more coherent
- needing little prompting to give a story the patient seems able to relate to

7

- bringing up memories with appropriate affect
- awareness of an unconscious mental life
- a capacity to step back and observe reflectively
- a wish to take more responsibility for the self
- imagination
- capacity for achievement and some realistic self-esteem.

It will be clear from this list that suitability for psychotherapy is often taken to mean conditions predicting success in psychoanalytic psychotherapy specifically. It might be more accurate to see the absence of these predictive factors as indicators that other forms of therapy might be more appropriate. Recent studies on psychodynamic interpersonal psychotherapy suggest that the therapy might be beneficial even when the person is not psychologically minded (Guthrie, 1999).

McCallum, Piper and colleagues have investigated the relationship of psychological mindedness and alexithymia with therapy outcome in interpretive and supportive group and individual therapies. Both features do predict outcome (McCallum *et al*, 2003).

Assessing motivation

Motivation is notoriously difficult to assess (Bloch, 1979). Without at least a minimal agreement to attend sessions, therapy is clearly impossible. Beyond this, it seems that motivation may be as much a function of social compliance as a rational statement of intent.

Example

A 45-year-old man with a history of alcohol misuse and violence to women was denigrating the female therapist by calling her 'chick' and dismissing her suggestions, and by saying that 'therapy was for dickheads'.

The therapist felt the urge to make a 'clever' interpretation about his fear of his own sexuality (which would have been justified by the content of the interview). Instead she realised that this would have had the effect of merely making him look stupid (a 'dickhead') and instead chose to focus on how strange and even frightening the situation was for him. Eventually he talked about his need for alcohol to feel in control and accepted the suggestion of a support group to help with his violence to women and a planned detoxification from alcohol.

Therapists might be inadvertently biased towards accepting patients for therapy who are submissive and dependent, rather than dominant and assertive. This is to confuse motivation with compliance. This may lead to a refusal to take on apparently 'difficult' patients who are opinionated, dismissive or contemptuous of the therapist. In theory, therapists might acknowledge that being disdainful is a defensive manoeuvre to protect self-esteem, but it is still used as a reason for patients to be judged beyond therapeutic help.

Sometimes it is not possible to have a 'trial of therapy' to assess motivation because the patient may need several months to develop even basic trust, but it is sometimes possible to make a judgement based on previous commitment to therapy, and the ability to talk about the therapist as a separate person, whether the therapy was helpful or not.

Understanding problems and expectations of change

This section picks up whatever the patient had said at the opening of the interview and extends it in the light of what has been discussed so far. It is essential to explore the patient's model of what is wrong. Sometimes there is a natural style of thinking that favours either practical problem-solving or the exploration of an event's meaning.

Sometimes it is appropriate to agree with the patient's view, for example, by suggesting a rational and practical way of tackling phobic anxiety by exposure treatment. Alternatively, the patient may welcome the opportunity to explore the meaning behind a particular symptom. This might be the case for a patient coming for therapy at a point where those habitual ways of coping have collapsed and an alternative model is welcomed.

The assimilation model (Stiles *et al*, 1988) suggests that problem domains move through a fairly predictable sequence, from 'warded off' through 'painful' to 'problematic' to merely 'puzzling' and finally, 'mastered'. There is some support for the belief that psychodynamic therapies tend to be strongest at the unassimilated end of the spectrum, where the patient may only know in vague terms what is wrong. Further along the spectrum cognitive–behavioural techniques are powerful, as they are focusing on solutions to problems that are already clear and relatively circumscribed.

One of the most difficult problem areas to tackle is the belief that symptoms are caused by a physical illness. Here the problem may be clear to the patient, but its underlying nature and origin may be stereotyped within a disease model, despite repeated failure. Somatisation is amenable to various psychotherapeutic approaches (Guthrie, 1999) but the clash of models needs careful negotiation.

Example

A patient referred from the gastrointestinal clinic with irritable bowel syndrome was insistent that her abdominal pain and swelling was proof that there was a physical cause. The engagement in therapy was reliant on the therapist meeting the patient for a long first interview, where links, expressed in bodily metaphors like 'full up to here' and 'gutted', were explored. She seemed to give the therapist the benefit of the doubt and attended sessions and continued to explore the links between her bodily and psychological distress.

Resilience and robustness of defences

Throughout the interview the patient will have been displaying a characteristic defensive style and describing it in the anecdotes elicited earlier. Asking about times when the patient felt overwhelmed and how they then coped can develop this. The therapist may need to prompt with suggestions about previous defensive strategies such as cutting off from people, drinking more, working too hard and turning against friends.

9

In the patient's story there will usually be a good indication of the ability to tolerate change and there may also be clues to particularly difficult defensive strategies, such as the tendency to see the responsibility for problems in the other person. Maturity of defences is somewhat similar to 'ego strength', although it has been hard for clinicians to agree on its meaning (Lake, 1985).

Dealing with significant loss and the ability to mourn should be a specific focus. The pattern of a person's coping with issues of separation and loss can help the therapist predict how these themes will emerge, and be managed, in the therapy.

A hierarchy of defence and regression

There have been several attempts to categorise defence from the early clinical descriptions of Anna Freud to more recent questionnaire and standardised interview methods. One of the most useful is the model developed by Vaillant (1986), summarised below. One of the strengths of this model is that it was linked with a large follow-up of college students and the predominant defence was clearly linked to the subject's life adjustment.

Vaillant makes the important point that defence can be clearly constructed as a hierarchy, but that there is usually overlap in any particular person, and the person's defences might shift depending on the current life stresses. This tendency to 'regress' to coping strategies that originate at an earlier point in life can be 'regression in the service of defence', or a 'malignant' state that can lead to prolonged dysfunction. The proneness to malignant regression is sometimes picked up in the history from an account of the patient worsening and increasing self-harm after admission, when the removal of responsibility pushes towards a regressed state.

Vaillant's hierarchy (Box 1.3) is a helpful framework to understand the level of avoidance of feelings. However, it is meant as a guide and the assessor needs to look for the overall style and avoid simply trying to find examples of each.

Sedlak (1989) has illustrated the importance of a particular defence called disavowal, which means an ability to tell the therapist that something desperate has happened, without the ability to connect with the affects that belong to this experience. Patients with this difficulty have been dismissed in the past as 'hysterical' and manipulative.

Sifneos described an important state that may be either a defence or represent a developmental block in his concept of 'alexithymia' (Nemiah & Sifneos, 1970), which means literally having no words for feelings. On first sight it appears that this state must preclude any attempt at exploratory work. Some patients can learn to develop a 'feeling language' (Hobson, 1985) if the assessing therapist tries to model the use of metaphor in a sensitive way.

Box 1.3 Vaillant's hierarchy of defences

Mature defence
- Anticipation and objectivity — planning ahead for painful times
- Suppression — 'getting on' without denying the difficulty
- Altruism — meeting needs through service to others
- Sublimation — accepting difficulty but focusing on another activity as a substitute
- Humour — expressing distress in an oblique way to 'see the funny side'

Intermediate defence
- Repression — memory lapses, inexplicable naivety
- Reaction formation — feelings or behaviour diametrically opposed to an unacceptable impulse or feeling
- Displacement — avoiding conflict by expression towards a 'substitute'

Immature defence
- Passive aggression — ineffective expression of anger to others or directed against the self
- Hypochondriasis — somatisation of feelings and conflict
- 'Acting out' — allowing an unconscious impulse to be expressed to avoid the associated feelings
- Dissociation — a temporary and drastic loss of identity or personal action, e.g. conversion symptoms, fugues
- Projection — attributing unacknowledged feelings to others
- Schizoid fantasy — avoiding relating and substituting gratifying fantasy

Primitive defences
- Splitting, delusional projection, denial — distortions of reality which are psychotic or bordering on psychosis

Coming to a decision
The patient's own preferences

Some patients may have quite explicit requests (such as wanting 'psychoanalysis') that may be carefully thought through or may be based on misconceptions. The patient may also have strong feelings about the possibility of working in a group, or working in a structured way (for example, keeping diaries and reviewing homework). These beliefs and prejudices need to be disentangled and put in the context of the rest of the interview and the resources actually on offer. There have been systematic attempts in research to look at the interaction between patient 'aptitude', type of therapy, and outcome (Aptitude Treatment Interaction (ATI) paradigm: Shoham & Rohrbaugh, 1995). As Shoham points out, the paradigm has been used extensively but the results are still ambiguous. She suggested that the most important area to explore in 'aptitude' might be relationship style, rather than the demographic and personality variables studied in most research to date (Garfield, 1994)

One particular aptitude, or sometimes preference, is the ability to work in a group setting (Knowles, 1995). Dealing with the fantasy that group therapy is a diluted form of therapy rather than a different method of exploring needs careful handling so that the patient can see what the option actually involves.

Preferences about the gender, age, or ethnic origin of the therapist are sometimes difficult to clarify. They may be expressions of social preference, or they may reflect a carefully considered position, or they may be part of a defensive stance. The evidence is equivocal about the impact of social similarity on outcome but the preferences may at least need discussion if mismatches are not to interfere with the development of the therapeutic alliance. However, the balance of evidence suggests that ethnic origin and similarity between patient and therapist in ethnicity do not have a powerful effect in predicting therapy outcome (Maramba & Hall, 2002).

Double-checking for problems

Psychotherapy assessments run the risk of overemphasising psychological and relational issues. Part of the argument for maintaining the role of the medical psychotherapist is to pick up medical and psychiatric complications. Almost as a routine, the usual screening questions for the main psychiatric syndromes need to be followed.

This can lead to a sudden shift for the therapist, when the attempt to understand an odd experience becomes suddenly reframed as a possible physical illness such as epilepsy. Experienced assessors seem to have a capacity to be attending closely to the patient's immediate experience while at the same time monitoring and sifting the evidence. Box 1.4 suggests some key issues to consider when weighing up the risks of therapy.

Assessment for specific forms of psychotherapy

The account of assessment given above is drawn strongly from the psychodynamic–interpersonal approaches. Some of the points are specifically relevant to psychodynamic therapy, but many are relevant to any form of assessment. However, there are additional factors that need to be taken into account when assessing with a view to other models of therapy.

Family therapy

Therapists use methods that assess typical communication patterns and, through analysing these, develop strategies to encourage more adaptive

---

Box 1.4 Checklist for assessing the risk of therapy

- Is there any history of alcohol or drug misuse?
- Is there any history of impulsive behaviour (overdoses, self-harm, violence, sudden avoidance by moving away)?
- Find out the point of maximum disturbance in the person's life (as the therapy might reactivate comparable levels of difficulty)
- Were there any problems in a previous therapy?
- Who is responsible for prescribing and monitoring any concurrent medication?

---

family function (see also Lieberman, 1995). (Family therapy is covered in Chapter 11.)

Behavioural therapy

In behavioural therapy a formal approach known as behavioural analysis describes the antecedents, behaviours and consequences (ABC) under study and identifies target behaviours whose frequency is to be increased or decreased, and assessment may involve specialised observational techniques. (See also Chapters 6 & 7.)

Cognitive therapy

Cognitive therapy takes a broadly similar approach (including diary keeping) but focuses on dysfunctional cognitions and uses homework tasks to assess the conditions that alter the intensity and frequency of these dysfunctional beliefs. The assessment interview might include many of the features described earlier, particularly the development of good therapeutic alliance, but the focus in the assessment is on errors of thinking, as originally outlined by Beck *et al* (1979). (This is covered in more detail in Chapters 6, 7 & 8.)

An interesting synthesis of cognitive and interpersonal approaches from Safran and colleagues (Safran *et al*, 1993) has led to an empirical approach to selection for cognitive therapy with an interpersonal focus. Although this work was originally focused on cognitive–interpersonal approaches, the principles are, again, of wider applicability. They listed 9 areas (summarised in Box 1.5) to be explored and then rated in order to predict whether brief cognitive therapy might be an appropriate treatment. It will be apparent that many of the themes are variations on the approaches outlined earlier, but focused on the factors that have been shown to predict outcome in brief cognitive therapy. It could be argued that they are primarily a list of good prognostic features for any therapy, but the method uses particular ways to probe in the interview to gain maximal information about specifically cognitive aspects.

Box 1.5   Assessment of suitability for brief cognitive therapy

Accessibility of automatic thoughts	Enquire about thoughts and also images; try 'here and now' assessment of negative thoughts with therapist; attempt to distinguish thoughts from feelings
Awareness and differentiation of emotions	Probe a particular episode for quality and intensity of feelings; ask the individual to describe as if 'here and now' the detail of what happened
Compatibility with cognitive rationale	How far can the patient see and accept the cognitive conceptualisation of distress? Is it compatible with their health beliefs?
Acceptance of personal responsibility for change	Can the patient take responsibility, within a collaborative alliance, for homework tasks, monitoring progress and carrying out suggested procedures between sessions?
Alliance potential (in session evidence)	Openness in the interview, and ability to stay with uncomfortable material with the therapist
Alliance potential (out of session evidence)	Ability to confide, and develop meaningful relationships
Chronicity of problems	How long the problem has been present
Security operations	These are strategies to 'ward off' anxiety with habitual strategies (e.g. controlling the interview, changing topic, being vague or even evasive, intellectualising). Continue despite being drawn to the patient's attention
Focality	How circumscribed is the problem?

Psychodynamic psychotherapy

Many of the general points raised earlier about assessment in general are drawn from psychodynamic thinking. Coltart's views (see above; Coltart, 1988*a*, *b*) summarise the features that are associated with psychological-mindedness of a sort which is conducive to psychodynamic work. Garelick (1994) and Milton (1997) have presented views about the essential features of an assessment for psychodynamic therapy. Milton makes the point that 'consultation' is a better word because the potential patient is being given an indication of the nature of the therapeutic experience. Hobson and colleagues showed that an unstructured interview with little prompting or reassurance from the assessor brought out the characteristic communication patterns that allowed reliable distinction between depressive and paranoid–schizoid functioning (Hobson *et al*, 1998). Some psychodynamic approaches use a formulation to focus the therapy (for example, see Guthrie, 1999) and are particularly relevant for brief approaches (Marmor, 1979; Hoglend *et al*, 1992). Box 1.6 lists the advantages and disadvantages of psychodynamic psychotherapy.

Group therapy

A significant difference in assessing for any type of group approach is that the impact of the patient on the rest of the group must be considered. For example, a patient with antisocial personality traits might make positive changes in a group setting where there is the possibility of confronting some exploitative strategies. However, this could be at a considerable cost to the other group members and the group as a whole (Knowles, 1995). Similarly, patients who attend while intoxicated may significantly disrupt the work of the group and may need to be excluded. However, problems that can be played out and understood in a group setting might be amenable to change within a 'social microcosm'. Mild social inhibition and anxiety are positive indications, whereas extreme social anxiety makes this approach impractical. Sometimes a resistance to see problems can be challenged by confrontation within the group. A trial of suitability has been developed by setting up group interviews, although this has not been used extensively. The assessment usually involves a preparatory stage of a 'role induction' interview.

Knowles (1995) suggests that the emotional level of functioning of the individual is crucial. This is distinct from the level or intensity of disturbance. She gives an example of a patient who was unable to tolerate the affront of having to share in a group, and that this led to a regression to a developmental level when he was narcissistically wounded by a badly-handled late adoption.

Therapeutic community

The assessment for in-patient and therapeutic community programmes is another highly specialised form that typically draws on a wider range

Box 1.6 Factors for and against psychodynamic psychotherapy

Pros	Cons
Patient factors	
• Able to express feelings verbally	• Uncontrolled 'acting out' (e.g. alcohol or drug misuse, repeated self-harm)
• Able to tolerate a range of feelings	
• Wanting change rather than symptom relief	• Previous maximum level of disturbance very severe (e.g. psychosis or past history of severe regression or 'acting out')
• Psychologically minded; introspection, curiosity, and reflection	
• Ego strength; consistent, tolerance of stress, flexible range of defences	• Insufficient environmental support
• Able to carry on life out of therapy	• Firmly held non-psychological theory of causation
• Basic object relatedness; basic trust and at least one meaningful relationship	• Previous evidence of dependency in therapy
Psychodynamic formulation	
• The central problem can be understood in psychological terms	• Marked schizoid or paranoid elements in personality
	• Marked passivity
	• Circumscribed symptoms seen as stable derivatives of conflict
	• Severe resistance including denial and evasion
The interview	
• Can see relationships in feeling terms	• Patient looking for an intellectual understanding of conflict
• Some link between key outside relationships mirrored in sessions	• Unrealistic expectations of therapy as a 'magical answer'
• Reasonable level of rapport maintained	• Difficulty with basic trust
• Some ability to explore early transference links and trial interpretations	• Rapport difficult to develop
Symbols	
• Can work with dreams and fantasy	• Unable to see things in 'as if' way
• Can link historical and personal material to dreams and fantasy images	• Blurring of fantasy and reality
• Not over-reliant on fantasy and able to keep reality of interview in mind, as well as fantasy	• Cannot see the point of links between past present outside and 'here and now'
Therapist factors	
• Therapist able to cope with the degree of disturbance expected and countertransference aroused by the interview	• Therapist feels overwhelmed by material

of assessors, including patient members of the community, as well as the therapeutic team (Denford, 1995). Essentially, Denford suggests that the criteria for an in-patient community are broadly the same as those for out-patient settings. As for group therapy as an out-patient, there are some patterns of behaviour that are so disruptive to the structure of therapy that the patient cannot use this type of therapy. The threshold may vary between units, but the exclusion is primarily based on the expected risk of harm, physical and emotional, to other members of the community. Clearly, the issue of resources plays a part in assessment for a very intensive programme. There is likely to be an implicit or explicit 'filter' so that referrals tend towards the more severe, treatment-resistant end of the continuum. Many in-patient units have very detailed assessments to check whether the huge investment of time involved in an admission is worthwhile (Dolan *et al*, 1990). This might involve an initial screening interview with completion of several assessment schedules followed by meetings with residents and the community as a whole.

The above comments should be seen as no more than a brief note about some of the additional approaches and strategies that may be appropriate for particular modes of therapy. For fuller consideration of the particular strategies used see the references and the relevant chapters in this volume.

Assessment in relation to formulation

Whatever the type of therapy, there is an argument that the assessment needs to be linked to a case formulation. There are a number of advantages of incorporating a formulation as the basis of a treatment plan (Aveline, 1980; Perry, 1987; Hinshelwood, 1991; Crits Cristoph, 1992; Tillett, 1993). There has been a substantial body of recent research showing that case formulation can be reliable, and that there are advantages in maintaining a focus. However, slavish adherence to a formulation, particularly where the therapist has a rigid, self-critical personal style, has been shown to be associated with poorer outcomes (Strupp, 1993). Accurate and timely interpretations, however, in the context of a stable alliance and linked to an agreed formulation result in better outcomes (Joyce & Piper, 1993).

The advantages of a formulation stated in Box 1.7 mainly refer to brief therapies where the goals can be agreed and made explicit. Malan (1979) pointed out that some goals could not be made consciously available until the therapy had taken place. He suggested that an alternative in psychoanalytic therapy is for the therapist to set goals (the psychodynamic significance of which need not be made explicit to the patient). The goals should have a specific relationship with the underlying unconscious theme leading to the main symptoms.

Example
A 21-year-old man had experienced difficulty with a male supervisor. The assessment led to an understanding that the man was seeing the boss as a

---

Box 1.7 Advantages of a formulation

Conceptualisation
A formulation draws together descriptive, evaluative, causative and predictive factors. The information from the assessment interview is sorted under different headings that allow a conceptual overview, leading to recommendations about the optimal treatment.

Stable focus
It is very easy to lose sight of the main therapeutic focus; in brief therapy by moving onto different themes without resolving any, and in longer therapy by losing sight of any therapeutic goal.

Sets limits
The therapist may come under immense pressure to meet unrealisable dependency needs and an agreed formulation helps as a reference point to avoid extending the therapy in response to countertransference pressures.

Predicts blocks, resistance and likely transference.
The therapist can easily feel at sea in the middle of a therapy and a formulation can help by predicting likely areas of difficulty.

Sets goals
The formulation process can help to specify goals in advance. In focal therapy these are usually explicit goals agreed between therapist and patient.

---

father-like rival, which is characteristic of unresolved Oedipal issues. Most models of therapy would set a goal of better work adjustment, but a specific dynamic goal might be derived from an understanding of the conflict. So, a goal might be set of being able to collaborate with the boss and to feel admiration and identification with him, reflecting what is expected in successful resolution of the Oedipal phase.

A formulation can function, then, as an 'anchor point' for the therapy. From this anchorage it is possible to work in two complementary ways. First, it is possible to keep the formulation in the back of one's mind while attending to the free flow of conversation. Second, it is possible to review progress periodically to check that the conversation is still focused on the agreed goals.

A good example of the use of formulation as a main element of a therapy is cognitive analytic therapy (Ryle, 1990) (see also Chapter 5). This uses particular concepts such as the target problem procedure, traps, snags and dilemmas, reciprocal role procedures and systematic diagrammatic reformulation as tools to keep focus on the main, recurrent issues that cause difficulties. The structure involves four initial sessions leading to a narrative and/or diagrammatic reformulation. This then provides a framework (with therapeutic opportunities described as 'exits') for the remaining sessions of work (typically 8–20), ending with 'goodbye' letters that summarise and consolidate change.

Working from a cognitive analytic therapy perspective, Denman (1995) summarises the key issues in making a formulation. She suggests that they help in initial management (overall suitability and type of therapy), but also have a function later in the therapy to 'guide the treatment plan, focus interventions [and] help predict the evolution of treatment' (Denman, 1995: p. 169).

There are other comparable approaches including the core conflictual relationship theme approach of Luborsky (Luborsky, 1990). This delineates a central wish/fear theme from the patient's account of typical relationships. There is also the Weiss and Sampson's plan diagnosis system from the Mount Zion group (see Silbershatz *et al*, 1989). Although working from a psychodynamic perspective, their model of formulation has some similarity with cognitive interpersonal therapy, in that there are 'irrational pathogenic beliefs' that hinder the realisation of goals. In the cognitive–behavioural tradition, Persons (1991) described 'schema focused cognitive therapy', which has many elements in common with Safran's approach (Safran *et al*, 1993) to predicting the effects of cognitive therapy. Persons' view was that the correct unit of analysis in reviewing outcomes of therapy should be the assessment plus the therapy, and that diagnostic groups are of little value, or are actually misleading to practitioners.

Elements of a formulation

A formulation pulls together the information from the interview into a coherent form. The goals can be specified in a hierarchical way. Early goals include amelioration of distress and the restoration of hope; intermediate goals involve symptom improvement, then improved social and occupational functioning, improved relationships; and finally, long-term goals include evidence of enduring change in the sense of self and 'being in the world'. As far as possible, the formulation should state explicitly the goals in practical and unambiguous terms, focused on what would be different in their every-day interactions, rather than vague hopes for change such as 'feeling better'. Questions for the formulation are shown in Box 1.8.

A simple guide to assessment

The patient will often fulfil the 'criteria' for several approaches. In this situation the assessor will draw out the patient's preferences and link them with therapy availability. The simplest algorithm has considerable merit.

Always try to recommend:
* short before long
* safe before risky
* inexpensive before costly
* effective before unproven before discredited
* patient-chosen before imposed.

Box 1.8 Questions for the formulation (after Aveline, 1980)

Causes and effects

- Which stresses and why the reaction? (Recent precipitants such as losses?)
- Are there any re-activating factors? (Current stress that links to early life experience?)
- Meaning of symptoms? (How does the person make sense of their predicament, for example with spiritual values?)
- How are the symptoms handled? (Coping and defence style?)
- What is the biological and social substrate? (Early and late predisposing factors?)

Maintaining factors

- Are there advantages to keeping the symptoms?
- Are there any vulnerabilities of self in relation to others?

Factors promoting change

- Are there disadvantages and limitations from the symptoms?
- Is there an openness to change?
- Can the consequences of change be predicted?
- What is the individual's motivation and expectation of change?

Making predictions

- What is the likely outcome?
- How is the alliance likely to evolve?
- Are there potential threats to the alliance?
- What are the goals in different domains?
- What resources are needed (e.g. number of sessions)?

With such simple principles the task of assessment should be very simple. Even if assessment is, in practice, more complex, these simple 'rules of thumb' have surprising utility in managing a safe and effective service (see Fig. 1.1 and Box 1.9 for a more detailed expansion of these 'rules').

Below, in Tables 1.1*a* and *b* there is a more sophisticated model that attempts to look at factors which might maintain safe practice and also differentiate between indications for different types of therapy. It should be noted, however, that the summaries are based on very limited evidence. They should be seen as a summary of current practice rather than guidelines. Few of the statements made could be supported with the substantial body of evidence expected for a practice guideline.

For example, studies have shown that cognitive therapy and family interventions are highly effective in schizophrenia, but they have been slow to appear in routine practice (Margison & Mace, 1997). Many of the treatment decisions implied in Tables 1*a* and *b* are wrongly based on the

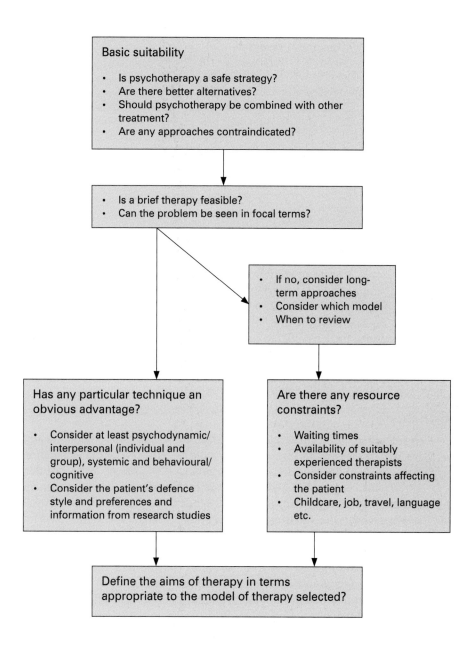

Fig. 1.1 An overview of the assessment process

Box 1.9 Key questions in assessment

- What format (group, individual, couple, family, other)?
- What depth/intensity?
- Which techniques (psychodynamic, behavioural/cognitive, systems)?
- What frequency of sessions?
- How many sessions expected? Open-ended or fixed?
- Balance of support versus exploration?

assumption that psychological treatments are relevant solely for neurotic illnesses and perhaps personality difficulties.

Moreover, studies of clinician behaviour suggest that decision-making about therapy is linked to allegiances and availability of preferred therapies in the clinician's department (Skynner & Brown, 1981; Margison *et al*, 1998).

The final point of the interview should be to check that the patient has followed what has been offered and knows what will happen next. Frequently the anxiety of the interview situation impairs the patient's ability to process this information. Some departments confirm in writing the main issues, the decision about therapy and the likely waiting time.

Conclusions

This chapter has focused on the clinical aspects of assessment. Ideally, this 'art' of assessment (Storr, 1979) would be balanced by the application of scientific knowledge (Svartberg & Stiles, 1991; Mace, 1995; Beutler, 2001). This chapter deals with the paucity of evidence about assessment by providing clinically-relevant guidance, but there is still a significant gap between what is derived from empirical studies and the knowledge base for clinical practice. For example, in a very large study of over 4000 patients using survival analysis and clinically significant change measurement, Hansen & Lambert (2003) showed that 15–19 sessions were needed to achieve a 50% recovery rate (across various therapies and various diagnoses), but this type of information, although valuable in planning services, is difficult to apply to individual patients.

The growth of evidence-based practice and the use of clinical guidelines may transform the way that assessments are carried out. Currently, integration of the clinical and research approaches to assessment requires particular commitment on behalf of the assessor. Recent advances such as those described earlier from Lambert and colleagues (Hansen & Lambert, 2003) and Beutler (2001) are coming to a new level of sophistication, although not yet in routine practice outside teaching centres. For example a group in Germany has established a computer-assisted feedback system to

Table 1.1a Summary of factors to consider in assessment where the individual therapy model is favoured

Factors favouring short-term therapy

Favouring short-term dynamic therapy	Favouring integrative, structured brief therapy (e.g. cognitive analytic therapy)	Favouring cognitive–behavioural therapy
Clear treatment goals which can be expressed as a focal conflict Patient active in establishing focus Acceptance of limited treatment goals Recent change rather than a chronic state Problems 'Oedipal' in type (competitiveness, anxiety in sexual relationships, conflicted triangular relationships and authority problems) Sufficient basic trust to tolerate frustration in therapy Ability to work with an explicit time limit	Need for concentrated work on an avoided theme (e.g. post-trauma, unresolved grief) Problem linked with typical stressors, characteristic patterns of relationships and repeated self-limiting themes Themes tend to be complex and interactive rather than discrete	Problem can readily be expressed in terms of abnormal cognitions and/or behaviours These maintain specific patterns of dysfunction (e.g. depression, anxiety, eating disorder) Problem already partly clarified Patient does not use defences to keep the problem out of awareness Absence of overwhelming relationship themes (e.g. dependency, control) that would prevent the development of a therapeutic relationship

Factors that may favour long-term therapy

Severe personality difficulty and early developmental failure
Lack of definable conflict area and problems difficult to clarify
Goals expressed in terms of general interpersonal function (e.g. problems with intimacy and control)

Table 1.1b Summary of factors to consider in assessment where the non-individual approach is favoured

Group analytic therapy	Family and marital therapy	Therapeutic community
Generally suitable for a dynamic approach	Problem can be seen to involve several family members (or couple)	Patient otherwise suitable for a dynamic approach, but where regression is likely
Conflict themes can be seen in interpersonal terms	Evidence of scapegoating or labelling of patient within family	Structured, stable boundaries cannot be maintained in individual or group therapy
Difficulties expressed in group settings	Patient and family (or couple) recognise a shared problem and wish to work collaboratively	Life circumstances make prolonged 'time-out' feasible
Tendency to avoid responsibility for change by trying to rely on others	Problem transcends the presenting patient and may involve systematic splitting within the family	Problem severe and disabling
Capacity to work with confrontation	Problem presented as a couple or family issue	
Ability to tolerate a group setting without severe anxiety	Presenting patient enmeshed in a complex system and vulnerable (e.g. a child patient or a patient with psychosis)	
Individual therapy difficult because of diffuse personal boundaries, or limited capacity to initiate exploration		

correct therapist errors at assessment and subsequently these models have been acceptable to patients and therapists (Kordy *et al*, 2001). The central part of the system is an 'alarm' function, signalling a possible deficit of the psychotherapy provided on the basis of the standard evaluation of treatment outcomes for large numbers of patients, against which this individual is measured. Such systems are currently experimental, and may go against the grain for many who see psychotherapy as an art. However, the weakness of our current methods of prediction needs to be acknowledged and, as yet, further evaluation of these emerging models is required.

To improve patient care clinicians may wish to revise the simplified models we have presented in the light of emerging research findings and also to challenge some of the assumptions we have made. However, the algorithm and boxes may be valuable in applying therapeutic knowledge to day-to-day practice.

Acknowledgement

We thank Graeme McGrath for his contribution to the research and audit of psychotherapy and for work on the 'guide to assessment' section.

References

Aveline, M. (1980) Making a psychodynamic formulation. *Bulletin of the Royal College of Psychiatrists*, (December), 192–193.

*Aveline, M. (1995) Assessing the value of brief intervention at the time of assessment for psychotherapy. In *Research Foundations for Psychotherapy Practice* (eds M. Aveline & D. A. Shapiro), pp. 129–149. Chichester: John Wiley and Sons.

Barkham, M., Evans, C., Margison, F., *et al* (1998) The rationale for developing and implementing core outcome batteries for routine use in service settings and psychotherapy outcome research. *Journal of Mental Health*, 7, 35–47.

Bartholomew, K. (1997) Adult attachment processes: individual and couple perspectives. *British Journal of Medical Psychology*, 70, 249–263.

Beck, A. T., Rush, A. J., Shaw, B. F., *et al* (1979) *Cognitive Therapy of Depression*. New York: Guilford.

Beutler, L. (2001) Comparisons among quality assurance systems: from outcome assessment to clinical utility. *Journal of Consulting and Clinical Psychology*, 69, 197–204.

Bloch, S. (1979) Assessment of patients for psychotherapy. *British Journal of Psychiatry*, 135, 191–208.

Coltart, N. (1988a) Diagnosis and assessment of suitability for psycho-analytical psychotherapy. *British Journal of Psychotherapy*, 4, 127–134.

*Coltart, N. (1988b) The assessment of psychological mindedness in the diagnostic interview. *British Journal of Psychiatry*, 153, 819–820.

Crits Cristoph, P. (1992) The efficacy of brief dynamic psychotherapy: a meta-analysis. *American Journal of Psychiatry*, 149, 151–158.

Denford, J. (1995) How I assess for in-patient psychotherapy. In *The Art and Science of Assessment in Psychotherapy* (ed. C. Mace), pp. 42–60. London: Routledge.

*Denman, C. (1995) What is the point of formulation? In *The Art and Science of Assessment in Psychotherapy* (ed. C. Mace), pp. 167–181. London: Routledge.

Derogatis, L. R. (1983) *SCL–90: Administration, Scoring and Procedures Manual for the Revised Version*. Baltimore: Clinical Psychometric Research.

* key references

Dolan, B. G., Morton, A. & Wilson, J. (1990) Selection of admissions to a therapeutic community using a group setting: association with degree and type of psychological stress. *International Journal of Social Psychiatry*, **36**, 265–271.

Garelick, A. (1994) Psychotherapy assessment: theory and practice. *Psychoanalytic Psychotherapy*, **8**, 101–116.

*Garfield, S. (1994) Research on client variables in psychotherapy. In *Handbook of Psychotherapy and Behaviour Change* (4th edn) (eds S. L. Garfield & A. E. Bergin), pp. 190–228. New York: John Wiley and Sons.

Guthrie, E. (1999) Psychodynamic interpersonal therapy. *Advances in Psychiatric Treatment*, **5**, 135–145.

Hansen, N. B. & Lambert, M. J. (2003) An evaluation of the dose–response relationship in naturalistic treatment settings using survival analysis. *Mental Health Services Research*, **5**, 1–12.

Hinshelwood, R. D. (1991) Psychodynamic formulation in assessment for psychotherapy. *British Journal of Psychotherapy*, **8**, 166–174.

Hobson, R. F. (1985) *Forms of Feeling: the Heart of Psychotherapy*. London: Tavistock.

Hobson, R. P., Patrick, M. P. H. & Valentine, J. D. (1998) Objectivity in psychoanalytic judgements. *British Journal of Psychiatry*, **173**, 172–177.

Hoglend, P., Srbye, O., Srlie, T., *et al* (1992) Selection criteria for brief dynamic psychotherapy: reliability, factor structure, and long-term predictive validity. *Psychotherapy and Psychosomatics*, **57**, 67–74.

Holmes, J. (1996) *Attachment, Intimacy, Autonomy: Using Attachment Theory in Adult Psychotherapy*. New York: Jason Aronson.

Horowitz, L., Rosenberg, S., Baer, B., *et al* (1988) The inventory of interpersonal problems: psychometric properties and clinical applications. *Journal of Consulting and Clinical Psychology*, **56**, 885–892.

Joyce, A. S. & Piper, W. E. (1993) The immediate impact of transference interpretation in short-term individual psychotherapy. *American Journal of Psychotherapy*, **47**, 508–526.

Kordy, H., Hannover, W. & Richard, M. (2001) Computer-assisted feedback-driven quality management for psychotherapy: the Stuttgart–Heidelberg model. *Journal of Consulting and Clinical Psychology*, **69**, 173–83.

Knowles, J. (1995) How I assess for group psychotherapy. In *The Art and Science of Assessment in Psychotherapy* (ed. C. Mace), pp. 78–89. London: Routledge.

Lake, B. (1985) The concept of ego-strength in psychotherapy. *British Journal of Psychiatry*, **147**, 471–478.

Lieberman, S. (1995) How I assess for family therapy. In *The Art and Science of Assessment in Psychotherapy* (ed. C. Mace), pp. 61–77. London: Routledge.

Luborsky, L. (1990) A guide to the CCRT method. In *Understanding Transference: the CCRT Method* (eds L. Luborsky & C. Crits-Cristoph), pp. 15–36. New York: Basic Books.

*Mace, C. (1995) When are questionnaires helpful? In *The Art and Science of Assessment in Psychotherapy* (ed. C. Mace), pp. 203–215. London: Routledge.

Mace, C. & Margison, F. (1997) Attachment and psychotherapy: an overview. *British Journal of Medical Psychology*, **70**, 209–215.

Main, M. & Goldwyn, S. (1995) Interview based adult attachment classification related to infant–mother and infant–father attachment. *Developmental Psychology*, **19**, 227–239.

Malan, D. (1979) *Individual Psychotherapy and the Science of Psychodynamics*. London: Butterworth.

Maramba, G. G. & Hall, G. C. (2002) Meta-analyses of ethnic match as a predictor of dropout, utilization, and level of functioning. *Cultural Diversity and Ethnic Minority Psychology*, **8**, 290–297.

Margison, F. (2001) Practice-based evidence in psychotherapy. In *Evidence in the Psychological Therapies: A Critical Guide for Practitioners* (eds C. Mace, S. Moorey & B. Roberts), pp. 174–198. London: Brunner-Routledge.

Margison, F. & Mace, C. (1997) Integration and psychosis. In *Psychotherapy of Psychosis* (eds C. Mace & F. Margison), pp. 199–204. London: Gaskell.

Margison, F., Loebl, R. & McGrath, G. (1998) The Manchester experience: audit and psychotherapy services in north-west England. In *Rethinking Clinical Audit: the Case of Psychotherapy Services in the NHS* (eds R. Davenhill & M. Patrick), pp. 76–110. London: Routledge.

Marmor, J. (1979) Short-term dynamic psychotherapy. *American Journal of Psychiatry*, **136**, 149–155.

McCallum, M., Piper, W. E., Ogrodniczuk, J. S., *et al* (2003) Relationships among psychological mindedness, alexithymia and outcome in four forms of short-term psychotherapy. *Psychology and Psychotherapy: Theory, Research and Practice*, **6**, 133–144.

Milton, J. (1997) Why assess? Psychoanalytical assessment in the NHS. *Psychoanalytic Psychotherapy*, **11**, 47–58.

Nemiah, J. & Sifneos, P. (1970) Psychosomatic illness: a problem of communication. *Psychotherapy and Psychosomatics*, **18**, 154–160.

Perry, S. (1987) The psychodynamic formulation: its purpose, structure and clinical application. *American Journal of Psychiatry*, **144**, 543–550.

Persons, J. B. (1991) Psychotherapy outcome studies do not accurately represent current models of psychotherapy: a proposed remedy. *American Psychologist*, **46**, 1348–1350.

Roth, A. & Fonagy, P. (2005) *What Works for Whom? A Critical Review of Psychotherapy Research* (2nd edn). New York: Guilford.

Ryle, A. (1990) *Cognitive Analytic Therapy: Active Participation in Change*. Chichester: John Wiley and Sons.

Sachse, J. & Strauss, B. (2002) Attachment characteristics and psychotherapy outcome following in-patient group psychotherapy treatment. *Psychotherapie, Psychosomatik, Medizinische Psychologie*, **52**, 134–140.

Sackett, D. L., Richardson, W. S., Rosenberg, W., *et al* (1998) *Evidence-based Medicine: How to Practice and Teach EBM*. London: Churchill Livingstone.

*Safran, J. D., Segal, Z. V., Vallis, T. M., *et al* (1993) Assessing patient suitability for short-term cognitive therapy with an interpersonal focus. *Cognitive Therapy and Research*, **17**, 23–38.

Sedlak, V. (1989) Disavowal and assessment for psychotherapy. *Psychoanalytic Psychotherapy* **4**, 97–107.

Shoham, V. & Rohrbaugh, M. (1995) Aptitude x treatment interaction (ATI) research: sharpening the focus, widening the lens. In *Research Foundations for Psychotherapy Practice* (eds M. Aveline & D. A. Shapiro), pp. 73–95. Chichester: John Wiley and Sons.

Silbershatz, G., Curtis, J. & Nathans, S. (1989) Using the patient's plan to assess progress in psychotherapy. *Psychotherapy*, **26**, 41–46.

Stiles, W. B., Elliott, R., Llewelyn, S., *et al* (1988) Assimilation of problematic experiences by clients in psychotherapy. *Psychotherapy*, **27**, 411–420.

Skynner, A. C. R. & Brown, D. G. (1981) Referral of patients for psychotherapy. *BMJ*, **282**, 1952–1955.

Storr, A. (1979) *The Art of Psychotherapy*. London: Secker and Warburg/Heinemann.

Strupp, H. H. (1993) The Vanderbilt psychotherapy studies: synopsis. *Journal of Consulting and Clinical Psychology*, **61**, 431–433.

Svartberg, M. & Stiles, T. (1991) Comparative effects of short-term psychodynamic psychotherapy: a meta-analysis. *Journal of Consulting and Clinical Psychology*, **59**, 704–714.

Tillett, R. (1993) Assessment and outcome in psychotherapy. *Current Opinion in Psychiatry*, **6**, 353–357.

Vaillant, G. E. (1986) An empirically derived hierarchy of defence mechanisms. *Archives of General Psychiatry*, **43**, 786–794.

Woolf, S. H., Grod, R., Hutchinson, A., *et al* (1999) Potential benefits, limitations and harm of clinical guidelines. *BMJ*, **318**, 527–530.

CHAPTER 2

Psychodynamic theories I

John Shemilt & Jane Naismith

Psychodynamic theories centre on the use of transference to study unconscious and conscious aspects of the mind. This and the following chapter will describe the meaning of terms such as 'transference relationships' and how 'conscious' and 'unconscious' mental processes interact to shape personality.

The term psychodynamic is used as a general term for all forms of psychoanalysis and psychoanalytically derived psychotherapy. Psychoanalysis began in Vienna over a century ago when Sigmund Freud (1856–1939) observed basic unconscious mental forces in his patients and described how these unconscious factors motivate and shape perceptions and behaviour.

Unconscious motivating forces, called instincts or 'instinctual drives', or just 'drives', were defined in terms of their aim: sexual (or libidinal), life (or self-preservative) and aggressive (or death). As well as an aim, there is an object, meaning a person, or part of a person, through whom that aim is sought. For example, in infancy the mother's breast may be the object through which oral drive pursues the aim of oral gratification. Controversy has continued over the nature of drives and the concept is much more complicated than Freud thought in the beginning. Nevertheless, the fundamental idea of the unconscious as an active or dynamic (driving) system has survived.

The roots of modern psychoanalysis lie in the observation that in a psychoanalytic setting a person's unconscious motives and personality structure are expressed in the relationship they make with their analyst. Freud called this relationship the transference. Transference may also be defined as a re-enacted memory of earlier situations, developmental stages and relationships. Unconscious traces of these memories and associated ideas and feelings shape the patient's perception of the analyst and his behaviour towards him or her. The concept of transference paved the way for recognition that the analyst also has a relationship with the patient. This two-way interaction is called the transference/countertransference relationship.

In summary, two basic ideas are central to all psychodynamic theories:
- the dynamic unconscious
- transference and the transference/countertransference relationship.

Over time psychodynamics became the science of how the unconscious and conscious minds of two people interact and is now much less preoccupied with describing and interpreting abstract instinctual patterns as occurred in the beginning. Out of this trend, the idea of object relations emerged. The relation between subject and object as unconsciously perceived by the subject is referred to as an 'object relation'.

Following Freud, many diverging psychodynamic theories were developed, but in recent years a 'quiet revolution' has reshaped mainstream psychoanalysis, bringing back together ideas from seemingly irreconcilable schools (Ogden, 1992; Wallerstein, 1999). Mainstream psychoanalysis now:

- places the analytic relationship alongside interpretation and insight as the major agents of psychological change
- challenges many classical concepts from an object relations perspective
- recognises that in any clinical interaction analyst/therapist and patient will be simultaneously interpreting one another's behaviour.

In this and the following chapter, the main theories behind this reconciliation within mainstream psychoanalysis will be described. As a rough guide, these theories fall under the following headings:

- core aspects of classical Freudian psychoanalytical theory
- ego and self psychologies
- object relations theories.

This chapter describes the work of Freud, Anna Freud, Klein, Fairbairn, Winnicott and Balint. In Chapter 3 (Psychodynamic theories II), the work of American ego psychologists and Bowlby's attachment theory will be followed by more complex material, potentially more demanding for those not already familiar with basic concepts. These sections describe the work of Kernberg and Kohut in the USA, the British post-Kleinians, and the British independent group of psychoanalysts.

Theoretical schools that diverged from the mainstream and have not participated to such a degree in any process of re-integration will be omitted. Although of interest and significance, they are beyond the scope of these chapters. These include Rank's absolute will, Sullivan's interpersonal relations, R. D. Laing's existentialism and Lacan's linguistic reworking of the Freudian text.

Psychoanalysis in the UK

The broad groups that now form mainstream British psychoanalysis (with a degree of overlap) are:

- contemporary Freudian
- Kleinian (including modern post-Kleinian theories)
- independent (characterised by object relations theory).

Divisions have always existed in British psychoanalysis, but have also stimulated creative debate. Freud's theories of personality have been clarified and updated. British psychoanalysis is probably best known internationally for the object relation theories, which have been widely applied, not only to intensive individual psychotherapy, but also to marital and family therapy, group therapy and child and adolescent psychotherapy.

Psychoanalysis has never been widely popular in the British Isles, even in intellectual and academic circles. The few hundred psychoanalysts working in Britain during the past century have nevertheless made a disproportionately large contribution within psychoanalysis worldwide. This has been recognised to a greater degree in the Arts in Britain and among psychiatrists and psychoanalysts in other countries (Rayner, 1991).

Freudian psychoanalysis and its critics

In contrast to a mixed reception for Freudian ideas in Britain and many parts of Europe, the second half of the twentieth century began with widespread acceptance of psychoanalysis in North America, followed later by the rapid spread of Kleinian psychoanalysis from the British Isles to South America. Freud was hailed as one of the great thinkers of all time and as a key influence in twentieth century Western culture. It has probably been unhelpful that one man has held such a prominent position because the standing of psychodynamic theory and practice has often been confused with Freud's personal life and cultural outlook.

In the 1960s and 1970s, Freud and his theories became the subject of intense criticism. The feminist critique was aimed at weaknesses in Freud's theory of sexual development in women. In agreement, many analysts were by this time only too relieved to abandon at least some of Freud's ideas on women that seemed culture-bound in European society's attitude towards women at the end of the 19th century.

This feminist critique of Freud began in 1949 with an assault by Simone de Beauvoir in *The Second Sex* (de Beauvoir, 1953). Then Betty Friedan in *The Feminine Mystique* (Friedan, 1963), Kate Millett in *Sexual Politics* (Millett, 1970) and Germaine Greer in *The Female Eunuch* (Greer, 1970) all attacked Freud as a source of modern misogyny. Fiercest vilification was reserved for Freud's theory of penis envy. Despite the fact that this aspect of Freud's theory had been supported and expanded, most prominently by the psychoanalyst psychiatrist Helene Deutsch, in other psychoanalytic quarters it had already been modified or rejected. Nevertheless, the fundamental feminist objection remained that a core part of the original Freudian approach to women's psychology, which includes concepts such as women's natural passivity, narcissism and masochism, had been founded on a mistaken idea that feelings of genital inferiority are at some level a universal experience in women (Robinson, 1993). This contrasted with the new emphasis on the reality of power differentials and social structures within patriarchal society.

Further criticism of Freud emerged from new directions in the 1980s. Among those who approached their subject from a position well-versed in psychoanalysis and its philosophical basis were Jeffrey Masson and Adolf Grünbaum.

In 1984, the psychoanalyst and Sanskrit scholar, Masson, published *The Assault on Truth: Freud's Suppression of the Seduction Theory*, contradicting the view that Freud was a great twentieth century thinker and scientist of integrity. In this high profile book, Masson argued that cowardice led Freud and the analysts who followed him to excuse or ignore adult sexual abuse of children by attributing psychological disorders to childish erotic imagination. Masson, having made a personal break from psychoanalysis, had become one of its fiercest critics thereafter.

In contrast to Masson, Grünbaum is not a psychoanalyst. *The Foundations of Psychoanalysis* (Grünbaum, 1984) is the response of an academic philosopher of science looking in on psychoanalysis from the outside. Grünbaum argued that Freud's theories were not as adequately supported by the evidence as Freud believed and that Freud was impressively resourceful, but ultimately a failure, in his quest for scientific credibility.

Why have psychodynamic psychotherapies of all kinds continued to flourish despite these withering attacks? Paul Robinson argues that a period of excessive uncritical acceptance and adulation would always be followed by reappraisal (Robinson, 1993). He concludes that Masson and Grünbaum are representatives of an intellectual backlash against ambiguity and against recognition that human knowledge is subjective and not always based on 'objective' reality. They refuse to engage scientifically with ambiguity and subjectivity. Psychoanalysis does engage with these areas of human experience. In so doing it is in keeping with a modern view of the relativity of knowledge that has become familiar as a cutting edge in contemporary academic, scientific and literary thought if not yet in establishment psychiatry.

The development of Freudian psychoanalysis: Sigmund Freud and Anna Freud

Sigmund Freud initially used hypnosis to access his patient's unconscious. He then realised that this method relied on the therapist's power of suggestion rather than on both patient and therapist working actively together to try and uncover the patient's resistances to conscious understanding. From the 1890s onwards he abandoned hypnosis and encouraged his patients to participate by free association.

Free association is sometimes called the 'fundamental rule of psychoanalysis'. Patients try to say out loud everything they spontaneously think of, including ideas that appear, at first sight, trivial, irrelevant, nonsensical, or embarrassing. This replaced 'directed association' in which Freud would press on the patient's forehead and direct the patient to say the first thing that came to mind (Gill, 1994). Free association follows from Freud's theory of resistance and conflict, i.e. conflict between desire to remember and desire to forget (Etchegoyen, 1991). The desire to forget forces memories to remain unconscious, i.e. repressed, producing resistance to analysis; complete free association is an unattainable ideal. Even at the end of a lengthy analysis, resistance or repression will continue, interrupting the stream of conscious thoughts and associations.

When Freud first observed his patients' transference he regarded it as unwelcome resistance. The conceptual leap in which transference became the major focus of interpretation further underlined the patient's active role in the analytic process.

Freud continually modified his theories. For example, in the earlier topographical model the driving force of the mind is the id, an amorphous collection of unconscious instinctual drives and fantasies. In *The Ego and the Id* (Freud, 1923) he described his last major revision, the structural model. The unconscious forces of the id, ego and superego were now seen as a tripartite system and in analytic work equal attention would be paid by the analyst to all three:

- id; unconscious, relatively unstructured collection of sexual and aggressive drives and fantasies
- ego; capacity of the mind to mediate between internal need or desire and the demands of the external environment. This not only includes skills and coping strategies that are more logical and rational, but also coping strategies in the form of defences that distort perception of reality instead of dealing with reality more directly. Ego is partly conscious and partly unconscious
- superego; roughly equivalent to conscience, can be encouraging as well as critical and is partly unconscious and partly conscious.

Freud had moved psychoanalysis from mainly studying id processes to being a more ego-oriented psychology. This new structural model was then refined and developed by Anna Freud (1895–1982), Freud's younger daughter, who was both a pioneer in child psychoanalysis and a major figure in her own right in adult psychoanalysis.

When Anna Freud summarised new developments within 'classical' psychoanalysis in the 1930s, analysis of transference and resistance was well established at the centre of technique, but only as one source of information about the patient's unconscious (A. Freud, 1966). Free associations, dreams, memories and fantasies were all used as the patient (i.e. the patient's ego) actively participated in what was seen as uncovering layer by layer down towards the depths of the unconscious, perhaps somewhat like peeling an onion.

Freud and Anna Freud's emphasis on this therapeutic alliance between patient and analyst, along with their personal styles of working, led to a more 'natural' approach. They might discuss any subject of mutual interest within the session, including the analyst's opinion on concerns, predicaments, or successes, in the patient's life. Perhaps Freud and his daughter felt more confident than most others that they could allow this apparent relaxation of analytic 'rules' without losing track of strict boundaries and a total analytic attitude? In contrast, Freud's writings on clinical technique have been interpreted by 'orthodox' psychoanalysts, particularly in North America, as meaning strict adherence without any such informality or temporary deviation to principles of anonymity, neutrality, mirror-like opaqueness, relative unresponsiveness, surgeon-like detachment, impersonality and blank screen passivity (Couch, 1995).

In the extreme, this model of Freudian analysis is a rigid stereotype much caricatured in cinema and television. The orthodox approach is probably best known for its connection with North American psychoanalysis, one influential branch of which is the school of ego psychology. When balanced with humanity, a spirit of benevolent inquiry and personal adaptation to each patient's situation, the orthodox method is a refined discipline of observation to guide the clinician. This issue is discussed in relation to psychodynamic psychotherapy in Chapter 3.

Analysts within the British 'contemporary Freudian' school and many like-minded American analysts have taken a different direction and incorporated aspects of Kleinian and British independent object relations theory. These developments have also widened the scope of Freudian psychodynamic therapy to include the treatment not only of neurotic patients but also patients with narcissistic, borderline, perverse or psychotic personalities.

Unconscious motivation

Psychodynamic theory includes a working assumption that nothing somebody does happens by chance and that there is a potential hidden motive behind every thought, feeling, dream or fantasy. This is called psychic determinism. Unconscious motives lie beyond the conscious surface of mental life. How one chooses to earn a living, whom to love and to marry, whom to hate and the kinds of attachments to make, are all determined by unconscious drives, not merely rational thinking. Many different unconscious factors may combine in the ways a person reacts to their circumstances, including personal history, fantasy and dream life, self image and other ego functions, superego or conscience and 'transferences' towards seniors and peers (Strean, 1994).

The conscious, unconscious and preconscious

Unconscious memories, thoughts, feelings, perceptions and impulses accompany and interact with conscious thoughts and feelings, which are more immediately evident. Freud recognised that other memories may not be fully conscious but are easily recalled once attention is focused onto them, or they transiently escape from conscious recall (as in the feeling that something is 'on the tip of the tongue'). He referred to these as preconscious.

Freud's revisions of his own theories of personality

Freud regarded psychodynamics as a science because his theories were open to modification in the light of observation. He made repeated amendments in the light of clinical experience and by the end of his life he had outlined five major theories of personality, each building on what had gone before but radically different, these theories are:

- economic
- dynamic
- genetic
- topographical
- structural.

The economic model, the most outdated, introduced a quantitative factor with the idea of mental energy that the individual constantly strives to dispose of through cathexes. An individual cathects another person or thing when they attribute some emotional significance to that person or thing. The dynamic model describes Freud's theory of instinctual drive, originally that the main instincts are libidinal (sexual) and self-preservative and later that the main instincts are life (libidinal) and death (aggressive and destructive). The genetic model refers to the way that each individual's past history participates in and shapes their present state of mind. States of mind in the topographical model are conscious, preconscious, or unconscious. In the structural model the mind is composed of the id, ego and superego.

Defence mechanisms and pleasure and reality principles

The theory of defences in Freud's psychodynamic theory closely relates to the idea of the unconscious. Thoughts and feelings that cannot be tolerated in conscious thinking are actively made unconscious and this process is called repression, as already described. The various ways in which the mind modifies emotionally intolerable ideas and removes them by repression from conscious thought are collectively called defence mechanisms.

Defence mechanisms operate through the interplay of drives with the pleasure principle. The pleasure principle is the rule that the mind naturally seeks pleasure. Freud suggested that the dynamic unconscious is mostly oriented towards experiencing pleasure and avoiding pain. In contrast the ego is predominantly reality oriented. The ego is partly unconscious and partly conscious and is motivated by trying to adapt to deal effectively with reality rather than always being dominated by pleasurable wish fulfilment in itself; this is termed the reality principle. Loss of the ego's capacity to test reality reasonably effectively is one of the hallmarks of psychosis.

Body ego

Freud conceived the reality of bodily sensation to be the first and dominant reality with which the ego is engaged and structured. He famously wrote 'The ego is first and foremost a bodily ego'. In other words the experience of the body (and in particular sensations from the surfaces of the body) is the foundation from which the ego then develops its capacity to deal effectively with the reality of the external world. The ego, initially oriented to the body, then has to mediate the developmental process by which the infant having emerged into the outside world following birth, grows up through childhood and eventually, in health, achieves the capacity for an adult perspective on both the body that the person inhabits and the external world in which the body exists.

Many aspects of perceptual and emotional experience are best understood in terms of the ego operating as a 'go between' reconciling the demands of 'internal reality' and 'external reality'. The ego uses both defence mechanisms and practical coping strategies to deal with the competing demands of bodily needs and sensations versus the practical outside world and moral imperatives located in the superego. There is a need to make the internal (often unconscious) desires fit in better with the outside world. The practical action adopted by the individual may cover the full range from what is ultimately effective to what is in some way ineffective or maladaptive. This reflects the capacity of the ego to serve the reality principle in the face of internal drives towards wish fulfilment and the pleasure principle.

The mechanisms that the ego uses to deal with demands and conflicts tend towards patterns associated with core bodily functions, whether bodily sensations or expressed indirectly in symbolic form. These also correspond to the major instinctual drives and bodily pleasures, focused around erogenous zones: oral bodily functions such as sucking, biting and spitting out; anal and urethral functions, including both the capacity to expel and excrete and to hold in and retain; and the genital regions and functions, starting with childhood masturbation and leading to a mature shared sexual relationship.

Clinical evaluation commonly includes some implicit or explicit assessment of the strength, range and flexibility of the ego capacities available to the individual in dealing with different aspects of reality in a more or less effective way.

Denial and projection

Projection is the term used to describe the way a person can avoid feeling an emotion or wish in themselves, but instead feels that the emotion or wish is in someone else. The concept of projection as a form of defence mechanism occupies a prominent place in psychodynamic theory. Projection was already a familiar concept in philosophical debates about perception when it was first described in a psychoanalytical sense by Freud in 1911 (in his notes on Dr Schreber's autobiography, Freud, 1911). Freud's theory was that delusions of persecution in a paranoid patient could arise from denial and projection of homosexual feelings. After being denied and projected into the other, these feelings could then be subjected to another defence, that of reversal so that the love and sexual desire attributed to the other person was reversed into hatred. In other words, the subject denied that he loved (or hated) the other male in the first place, but ended up with the opposite persecuted feeling that the other male hated him all along. Because of its significance, projection will be discussed again in relation to the Kleinian formulation of introjection, projection and projective identification in Chapter 3.

Conflict

Conflict is another psychodynamic term that has such widespread relevance that it has entered everyday language. It can be used both as a more abstract and more practical way of describing mental tension. In the abstract it refers to conflict between opposing instincts or opposing parts of the mind. In more directly practical terms it refers to conflict between groups of ideas, feelings and motives that may work against one another to produce symptoms. It also refers to conflict between emotionally significant figures and as with any internalised relationship within the mind this conflict would be thought of as an 'object relationship'. All these variations on conflict are different ways of describing the same things.

Freud's theory of conflict changed three times. At first Freud included sexuality (reproduction, 'sex' and 'sexual' activity) in a general instinctual drive, libido, that aims to pull together living beings and living matter. In this model, basic conflict is libido versus self-preservative instincts (which can also be called ego instincts). In his theory of narcissism (self-oriented gratification) Freud recognised that some self-directed ego instincts in narcissism are libidinal ('self loving') and not inherently in conflict at all. Freud then observed the compulsion to repeat, a general tendency for each individual to try to return to former states through death or by destroying anything new. This drive seemed to oppose any creative urge or wish to grow through life and sexuality. Freud reframed basic conflict in this view as life instinct versus death instinct.

These changes have divided psychoanalytical therapists and analysts into those who accept Freud's theory of innate destructiveness and aggression and those who have continued to regard libido as the primary instinct, and aggression as a secondary reaction to frustration of libido or as a reaction to threats against self-preservation.

The Oedipus complex

When Freud used the notion of conflict, sexual drive was always involved on at least one side of the conflict. Freud's classical description of the Oedipal complex is a description of conflict between desire and prohibition, i.e. sexual desire for one parent balanced by the other parent's prohibition of incestuous desire. Freud always regarded the Oedipal conflict as central in all emotional life and development. The Freudian Oedipus complex, Kleinian treatment of Oedipal situations and departures from both of these, such as Fairbairn's critical account, occupy a central position in the development of psychodynamic theory and will be described later in more detail.

Clinical implications

What are the implications of the theory outlined so far for the actual practice of psychoanalytic therapy? As therapy proceeds the patient usually develops a preoccupied interest and emotional investment in the clinician and this transference takes on the same qualities as the patient's inner mental life. It is therefore shaped into the form of the patient's neurotic conflicts that now engulf the figure of the clinician in the patient's fantasy life and behaviour (transference neurosis).

Those who follow Freud's approach emphasise analysis of the transference neurosis, but regard this as only one of several significant factors, therefore paying attention to all of the following with any one patient:

- transference neurosis
- dreams
- childhood memories and reconstruction of the patient's history
- analysis of resistances and defence mechanisms
- other aspects of a patient's life that may not belong predominantly to the transference.

Early dissenters from the Freudian movement: Adler and Jung

Alfred Adler (1870–1937) and Carl Jung (1875–1961) were early pioneers of Freudian psychoanalysis who left after acrimonious disagreements with Freud. Adler severed relations with psychoanalysis in 1911 and Jung in 1913 (Roazen, 1976). Adler founded individual psychology. Jungian psychotherapy and psychological theory are known as analytical psychology. Although now outside the mainstream psychoanalytic movement, both Adler's and Jung's ideas continue to exert influence on many psychodynamic counsellors and psychotherapists. Both foreshadowed the critique made from within psychoanalysis leading to object relations theory, by disagreeing with Freud's central emphasis on sexuality.

Adler's individual psychology

Adler's most famous contribution was the concept of the inferiority complex. Instead of Freud's theory of infantile sexuality as the source of neurosis, Adler suggested that infancy is dominated by feelings of inferiority and the urge to overcome or compensate for this. What form this compensation takes depends on relationships in the family, from which a person acquires their own life style. The inferiority complex is the uncompensated experience of inferiority and is countered by attempts to become more competent in those skills felt to be inferior. Examples are the child with a speech defect who becomes a great orator, the bully or fascist who is concealing underlying cowardice, or neurotic behaviour that is a retreat into illness as a kind of excuse for failure.

Adlerian psychotherapy is based on revealing these strategies and allowing more realistic adaptations to develop. Adler was also a pioneer of treating children in child guidance clinics, opening the first in Vienna in 1921.

Jung's analytical psychology

Jung kept his distance even when Klein, Fairbairn, Winnicott, Balint and others were broadening the scope of psychoanalytic theory from within the Freudian psychoanalytic establishment. Instead of Freud's libido theory of sexual drive, Jung divided individual experience and behaviour into three areas:

- conflicts in personal history; the personal unconscious
- conflicts in racial history; the collective unconscious
- personal aims and aspirations.

The collective unconscious is central in the theory. Each individual has memories of ancestral history and traces of ancient ways of thought inherited over long periods of time. These are known as archetypes and can be studied through myths and through dreams. Jung believed that dreams are less to do with past conflicts and wish fulfilment as in Freud's theory and more to do with the dreamer's state of mind at the time of dreaming.

Jung's two basic personality types, extroversion and introversion, have entered common use far beyond the confines of psychotherapy practice. In contrast, Jung's system of personality subtypes based on sensing, feeling, thinking and intuiting, has not been widely accepted nor applied, at least until more recently when it has achieved some recognition as a useful approach to personal coaching and management training.

Jung concluded that neurosis arises not so much in the past as in the present moment. Whereas Freud believed that patients are disabled in the present because they cannot free themselves from fixations that occurred in the past, Jung thought that the emergence of this kind of material from the past happens only when there is something wrong in the present.

Individuation is central in Jung's system of child development and also a prime aim of Jungian therapy. It is the search for creative development, wholeness and a sense of completion and continues throughout all stages of childhood and adult life. In the treatment of neurosis Jung, like Adler, emphasised the present situation a patient refuses to face through illness, as well as the traditional psychodynamic aim of bringing together and integrating conscious and unconscious mental life.

Many of Jung's ideas anticipate modern cultural and social concerns. Examples are theories about the function of symbols; decentred selves, multiple realities, the necessity of multicultural perspectives and the role of adult development and spiritual self discovery. Yet at a personal level he has been accused of cultish mysticism, sexism, racism, anti-Semitism and professional misconduct. Jung used an antiquated and hazy intellectual approach, entrenched, rather like some of Freud's writing, in culturally biased concepts such as 'masculine versus feminine' and nebulous ideas such as the 'shadow' and the 'wise old man'. According to his critics this produced a type of elitism, extreme individualism, biological reductionism and naive views on gender, race and culture (Young-Eisendrath & Dawson, 1997).

Revision of Freudian theory from within psychoanalysis

Klein

Under the influence of Melanie Klein (1882–1960), a broad group of British object relations oriented practitioners shifted from classical Freudian reconstruction of the patient's past history to focus on the here-and-now interaction between patient and clinician. In this approach everything that the patient says and does in the consulting room, whether it refers to the present or to the past, is regarded as transference. Everything that the clinician experiences with respect to the patient is the countertransference. There is less emphasis on reconstruction of past history or on interpretation of events in the patient's life outside of the consulting room.

Further far reaching implications of this Kleinian development in psychoanalytic theory and practice will be detailed later in this chapter and in Chapter 3.

Contemporary Freudians

The contemporary Freudians have also incorporated many aspects of the object relations approach into their development and revision of earlier Freudian theory. They too place greater emphasis on the interpretation of here-and-now communication between patient and clinician and emphasise how this, from the perspective of the transference, gives a window into the unconscious inner fantasy life and emotional structure of a patient's mental life. In Britain, the contemporary Freudians Anne-Marie Sandler and Joseph Sandler (1927–1998) have been especially associated with this rapprochement between Freudian and Kleinian approaches to the theme of object relationship.

British independents, Kleinians and Freud's instinctual drives

While some Freudian analysts adopted Freud's concept of a death instinct, it was especially Melanie Klein who adopted the death instinct wholeheartedly in her theory. Kleinians combine an object relations approach with Freud's later model in which the dominant instinctual conflict is between libido and death instinct expressed through so called 'good' and 'bad' objects.

In Britain the independent group of object relation analysts, especially Ronald Fairbairn, felt that instincts can have no separate existence except when channelled through a framework of relationships. Instinct without structure, i.e. without relating to somebody or something, is a nonsense. Because this placed object relationships at the heart of things instead of trying to reduce mental life to abstract instinctual drives, it is often simply referred to as object relations theory, to distinguish it from Freudian and Kleinian approaches. While it is in the nature of psychodynamic instincts to seek an object, i.e. another person or part of a person, object relations theory specifically emphasises that 'object seeking' is the primary organised motivation within the human psyche.

Challenging these views: here-and-now or 'you mean me' techniques

Emphasising the here-and-now interaction between patient and clinician, even from the perspective of a patient's fantasy life, could lead to a technique of interpretation criticised as a 'you mean me' method. Taken to an extreme it could lead to a mechanical interpretation of everything the patient says as referring to the clinician ('you mean me') irrespective of the significance of what the patient is saying about other aspects of their life. On the other side of the argument in defence of here-and-now interpretation, whatever a patient says about events in life outside the session, everything that is said is said to the clinician. Communication from patient to clinician can only be fully understood within context; which is within a consulting room within a session and whatever other external events to which the patient may also have referred.

Summary: the main trends in psychoanalytic theory

First there was the line of practice formed by classical psychoanalysis initiated by Sigmund Freud. Then some people who had followed Freud to begin with, notably Adler and Jung, broke away to form separate psychodynamic movements. Freud's work was supported and developed within the Freudian movement by Anna Freud, whose own work was closely linked both with the branch of Freudian psychoanalysis represented by ego psychology (in the USA) and with the contemporary Freudians (in the UK). The earliest stages of human development were described as self-directed sexuality and love, called autoerotism or narcissism. Rather than emphasising the role of object relations in early infancy, attention was drawn to the function of instinctual drives in self maintenance. This approach later led to the development of self psychology in North America.

In the UK, Melanie Klein and the Kleinian group, as well as others, collectively known as the British independents departed from this position. The focus was on the earliest relation of the infant with the mother. At the core was the idea that instinctual drives are object seeking from the start.

Object relations theory itself is a loose term used to include practitioners who on one side of a divide, have emphasised the relationship to the internal object (especially the Kleinian school, not only Klein herself but also other post-Kleinians such as Wilfred Bion, Herbert Rosenfeld and more recently Donald Meltzer, John Steiner and Ron Britton). On the other side of this divide within object relations theory are those who have emphasised the external relationship to a 'real' mother as forming the patient's inner mental life and fantasy (prominent examples are John Bowlby and attachment theory and other independents such as Michael Balint, Ronald Fairbairn and Donald Winnicott).

Transference and object relationships within Freudian theory and links with object relations theory

Another way of defining transference relationship is as an expression of the patient's previously repressed unconscious memories, impulses and desires. As one part of a transference/countertransference relationship, transference provides an arena to study a patient's personality in live personal interaction, not simply in a distant or abstract way. In this sense psychoanalytic therapy is a two-person psychology rather than the study of one person in isolation.

Transference reflects basic forms of unconscious object relationship that can be categorised as arising from one ('part object'), two and three person situations.

- Part object relations could figuratively be called 'one' person relationships. Emotionally the other person in a relationship is made to disappear as if it were too difficult to relate to another person as they are. In part object relations a patient's emotions and underlying drives are directed towards parts of themselves or towards parts of the analyst emotionally disembodied and incompletely distinguished from the patient's own self. Part objects are disembodied from the other person (the analyst) instead of being experienced as part of a separate complete human being, or whole object. To treat a person as though they were a breast or a penis or any other part of the body are examples of part object relationship; in ordinary terms these are usually disturbing ways for people to relate to one another.
- Two person relationships are characterised by mother and child. This relationship has a basic biological primacy in human development, whatever the practical arrangements actually are for child care in infancy

41

after the physical separation of birth. It is also a pivotal psychological unit of relationship.

- Three person situations have a special place in the history of psychoanalytic ideas. Freud based a theory of neurosis on types of anxiety inherent in a child's unconscious object relationship with two parents and called this the Oedipus complex. The child, mother and father family constellation is another basic unit of relationship. It introduces sharing and more sophisticated forms of parent/child boundaries and can be regarded as the prototype for group relationships as well as more mature forms of gender identity.

Freud has been much criticised for attributing to the Oedipus complex the development of morality, that kind of self-monitoring he called superego and also the development of basic male or female gender identity. In this theory superego and gender identity are formed by a child's identification with his or her parents within the Oedipus complex. The child wishes to replace the parent of the same gender and is sexually attracted to the parent of the opposite gender. Developmental resolution involves identifying with, and unconsciously, as well as consciously, wishing to emulate rather than replace the same gender parent. Freud felt that what his patients reported suggested that children expect to be punished for their incestuous wishes and rivalry. Yet, as a child learns to monitor and control incestuous wishes, this self-control is incorporated in the child's identification with the parent as the basis of moral sense, i.e. the superego.

Further implications of Oedipal or triangular relationships

In Oedipal situations, either the constellation of child and two parents or equivalent triangular relationships, the child is faced with inevitable 'facts of life'. If they are not excessively distorted or denied using defence mechanisms, these require the child to significantly alter an internal view of where the child stands in relation to the rest of the world. The child is faced with the knowledge:

- of being separate from parents
- that parents have attributes that a child does not yet have, such as the capacity for genital relationship and the ability to create children
- that there are differences between the sexes.

Even partial acceptance of such external conditions of life promotes internal developments in the child, for example, greater tolerance of emotions such as competitiveness, jealousy or envy that probably are an inevitable consequence of seeing life as it is. In healthy development these kinds of feelings become bearable and less likely to cause maladaptive and destructive mechanisms such as denial and avoidance.

The psychodynamic model of human development is one in which developmental tasks are repeatedly worked through each time internal emotional pressures and external reality demands threaten to overwhelm and undo maturational achievements. For example issues of ageing in middle and later adult life characteristically rekindle Oedipal emotional conflicts. In therapy, Oedipal conflicts appear in the transference as present moment, live experiences, not merely as developmental history.

One of the central features of 'classical' Freudian theory, as developed by Freud himself, is that the Oedipus complex is the most important developmental stage a child must negotiate in order to achieve emotional fluency and the capacity for mature relationships. Freud regarded the Oedipus complex as belonging to the ages of 3 to 5 years. Others, particularly Klein, have accepted the basic theory, but disputed the developmental timing while also emphasising that the Oedipus complex rests on the developmentally earlier resolution, successful or otherwise, of conflicts in part object relations and two person relations. Fairbairn and Independent object relations theorists have specifically criticised Freud over the Oedipus complex, feeling that earlier developmental stages are more significant because of the importance of the primary mother–child relationship. Some of these disputes can seem like arguing about whether the right or the left leg is more important for normal walking while obviously both sides are necessary and interdependent.

Childhood sexuality: normal and abnormal perverse sexuality

Freud linked all pleasurable bodily activities with sexual satisfaction. When he said that an infant is polymorphous perverse he meant that early childhood 'infantile' sexual wishes are not directed only to the genitals, but invested in any bodily function. He expected criticism for this view, but it stems from the theory of an underlying unconscious pleasure principle governing all bodily functions. This broad sexual motivation is what is meant by the term libido. Nowadays more criticism is directed at Freud's extension of the theory of infantile sexuality to suggest that the newborn infant is auto-erotic and approaches mother solely to gratify self-loving need, implying primary narcissism rather than a primary desire to relate 'socially' to the mother. Freud regarded adult perversion as a developmental arrestment, or fixation, at an earlier childhood stage when sexuality was naturally expressed through many different body functions. Adult perversion therefore represents a pathological failure of the genitals to develop a primary role during the transition through Oedipal resolution to adult genital sexuality. (See also Chapter 3.)

Anxiety associated with different types of object relationships

Freud revised his theory of anxiety in the light of clinical experience. At first he regarded anxiety as the experience of repressed libido. In order to understand the development of Freud's thinking it is helpful to remember that the Freudian concept of libido is rooted in bodily experience; libido arises from the pleasurable (erotogenic) zones of the body, however much it may be secondarily displaced to other parts of the body or to objects and aims in the external world.

Subsequently Freud thought of anxiety as repeating the experience of birth. This idea was then superseded in Freud's thinking by a third theory of anxiety. He now proposed that two basic forms of anxiety exist; primary anxiety and signal anxiety.

Primary anxiety is the emotion associated with disintegration of the ego. Signal anxiety guards and warns against primary anxiety, stimulating defences to avoid primary anxiety when it threatens.

If it is remembered that the Freudian ego is first of all a body ego, then the relationship of the later theory of anxiety to the earlier one is easier to understand. Frustration and repression of the pleasurable expression of libido, in Freud's earlier theory, is intimately related to anxiety about the integrity of the body, the threat of loss of bodily functions or, more concretely, the loss of body parts (in particular giving rise to castration anxiety). In Freud's later theory primary anxiety is focused on the integrity of the ego and the threat of disintegration of the ego. The threat of disintegration of the ego and of the body are intimately bound together. How this is negotiated psychologically by a patient in analysis is affected by their individual pattern of ego strengths and defence mechanisms, physical health, body strengths or weaknesses and emotional experience of body function. This theme is central to the clinical practice of Freudian psychoanalysis, alongside the patient's relationship and developmental profile.

Within this model different types of relationship also produce characteristic qualities of anxiety:

- the 'one' person, auto-erotic or narcissistic type of relating produces fear of disintegration of the ego or self through paranoid and persecutory anxiety, fear of attack by what are experienced as bad objects
- the two person, or mother and infant dyad type of relationship produces separation anxiety
- the three person or Oedipal situation produces fear of censorship by a parent, castration anxiety and guilt.

Kleinian theory, instinctual drives and object relations

To begin with Melanie Klein seemed to accept Freud's instinctual drives, but her views gradually changed. Freud's instincts were constitutional and initially directed to the body of the infant in an auto-erotic way, becoming attached to objects only through experience. Klein began to feel that drives are inherently attached to objects and cannot exist without an object. Although regarded as innate, the basic drives of love and hate were seen as more psychological than strictly biological forces. Her theory is arguably both an instinctual drive based theory and an object relations theory. For this reason her theory is usually distinguished from other purely 'object relations' theories.

The Kleinian concept of unconscious fantasy

Freud used the concept of fantasy in different ways but mainly to refer to the way that retreat into fantasy occurs when instincts are frustrated. In contrast, for Klein unconscious fantasy is the basis of mental life and is the internal mental representation of instincts. Instinctual representation of love and hate are innate in unconscious fantasy. Unconscious fantasy continues whether external conditions are gratifying or frustrating, unconscious fantasy is not just a way of dealing with a frustrating object. Klein also believed that an infant has innate unconscious knowledge of objects such as the breast, mother, womb, sexual intercourse, penis, birth and babies.

In this theory, at all times in life unconscious fantasy is operating, representing objects, their relationships and their fate at the hands of circumstances. Unconscious fantasy, although unconscious, is always influencing how a person thinks, feels and is motivated.

Direct observation of children was at the centre of Melanie Klein's original psychoanalytic theories. She developed a method for analysing children as young as 3-years or less. She used the narrative and symbolic content of play as the equivalent of the adult's spoken free associations. As a communication of conscious and unconscious preoccupations, play can be used to supplement a young child's limited verbal capacity.

Klein uncovered a world of ideas and fantasies that can seem startling at first, until it is remembered that similar ideas remain in unconscious fantasy in the adult (note, it is adults who make these observations on children). Many thoughts, emotions and impulses are normally disowned by the social and developmental demand to be 'adult', to relinquish childish preoccupations and adapt to adult reality. There is a convention that the spelling 'phantasy' refers to the unconscious, whilst 'fantasy' refers to conscious daydreaming, conscious imagination and other everyday meanings of fantasy. This chapter for clarity uses the alternative term 'unconscious fantasy', not 'phantasy'.

Kleinian views on introjection and projection and the Oedipal situation

Klein placed great emphasis on detecting the constant operation of introjection and projection during treatment.

- Introjection is when aspects of the external person (object) are taken into mental representation, forming a mental structure variously called the introject, introjected object, or internal object.
- Projection is the opposite process of attributing mental contents to an external object.

Klein specifically related the superego to internal objects within the infant during the first year of life (in contrast to Freud's timing of the Oedipus complex and superego at about 3-years-of-age). These internal objects are figures, or parts of figures, that were external and have been introjected. In this way Klein, like Freud, regarded the Oedipus complex as central to the development of the individual, but she adopted the term Oedipal situation and included in it what Freud had referred to as the primal scene, the sexual relations of the parents both as perceived and as imagined (Britton, 1989).

In the Kleinian version, a child's recognition of a parental relationship begins the Oedipal situation and is critical to the development of the child's desire to learn about the external world into which she or he has been born. This desire to learn is sometimes called the epistemophilic impulse.

As in Freudian theory, each stage in this developmental process is associated with characteristic anxieties, but Klein added an emphasis on earlier phases that have similar qualities to aspects of adulthood psychosis. Psychotic anxiety generally means anxiety from threats to a person's identity or integrated experience of self. Paranoid or persecutory anxiety arises from fear of being attacked by bad objects. Depressive anxiety is stimulated by fear of one's own aggressive attitude towards good objects.

The later phases have the quality of neurotic anxiety. Separation anxiety arises from separation from, or the threat of separation from, objects that are felt to be essential for the survival of the subject. Castration anxiety is stimulated by fear of threats to the subject's sexual function (often represented by the idea of any bodily mutilation).

Kleinian positions

Klein observed two kinds of state of mind characterised by different types of anxiety representing particular attitudes towards objects. She called these states of mind positions:

- paranoid–schizoid position
- depressive position.

The paranoid–schizoid position was originally called the paranoid position, but renamed in recognition of Fairbairn's work on splitting and schizoid states. In Klein's view the paranoid–schizoid position characterises the first 3 months of infancy and at this time persecutory anxiety, the fear of annihilation from within, predominates. In unconscious fantasy the feared malignancy is characteristically projected outwards, but then what follows is the experience of fear of annihilation from outside as well. Concern is with oneself and not yet for the object. Anxiety is dealt with by splitting and projection. The infant splits bad from good in his/her own feelings and in unconscious fantasy projects these into objects that are felt to be 'not self'. Then the self and its ego and the object are experienced as split into extremes of bad and good. Emotions are strongly on one side or another, with no initial recognition that bad and good objects are the same person. This is a world of part objects that the infant is living in, in which Klein assumes that the infant experiences sensations as caused by benevolent or malevolent objects, for example, hunger is not just experienced as lack of food, but 'that something is attacking and starving me'. Similarly, comforting feelings are felt to emanate from the loving motives of a good object.

Example

A patient who always came to his session with a newspaper under his arm arrived outside his psychotherapist's consulting room earlier than usual and met his therapist in the street with a newspaper under his arm. The patient thought this was most likely a chance event but couldn't get out of his mind for several days the idea that his psychotherapist had deliberately arranged this encounter in order to make a friendly gesture.

The patient, experiencing his therapist as a good object, had projected loving feelings into the therapist so that the therapist was felt to have loving feelings towards the patient. This was on the basis of an unconnected piece of reality that the therapist happened to have a newspaper.

The depressive position arises as the infant's object relations change from part-object relationships into relating to a whole object, normally according to Klein at about 3–6-months-of-age. Now the good and the bad 'mother' are seen to be the same person. With this realisation comes the painful appreciation that the good mother the infant loves has been damaged by attacks made on the bad mother, who is after all one and the same person. This pain gives rise to depressive anxiety rather than persecutory anxiety. In the depressive position, depressive anxiety is a mixture of concern for the object (as well as for one's self), guilt, fear of the object being damaged beyond repair and a sense of responsibility for the damage that has been done. The depressive position is marked by fear of losing the object and the experience, in healthy developmental progress, of a strong impulse to repair this damage.

Kleinian notions of progression through the paranoid–schizoid and depressive positions and the strong emphasis on guilt and reparation can be criticised for being overprescriptive and for introducing a particular ethic into infantile development, a judgement that depressive concern is a more desirable quality than other states of mind. The latter, despite its sophistication as a theory, may be as culture bound as Freud's earlier views on female sexuality. Klein has also been criticised for placing too little emphasis on external reality. Whether this is a justified criticism of Klein herself has always been a matter of controversy, but in clinical practice it should be noted that in the depressive position, the actual state of the external object is of great importance. If the mother (or therapist) appears to be damaged, the child's guilt and despair are increased. If she appears well, or at least able to empathise with her child's problems about her state, the child's fear of the child's own destructiveness is decreased and trust in reparative wishes is increased.

Klein herself did not explicitly refer to separation anxiety. The treatment of psychotic, borderline and very envious patients using Klein's conceptual framework has, however, led to recognition of separation anxiety as a hallmark of the depressive position. The depressive position is typified by realisation not only that the object is an integrated whole but also that the object must, therefore, be separate (and can leave) (Quinodoz, 1991).

Reparation

Reparation is a key concept in the Kleinian view of healthy development. The depressive position involves integration of good and bad objects, which means affection and hatred for a person being held together in the same state of mind. This can be so painful that it stimulates defences against the depressive position such as manic and obsessional reparation, denial, triumph and contempt. When these defences fail, the person (of any age) retreats to the paranoid–schizoid position or to the kind of idiosyncratic intermediate position referred to by post-Kleinian analysts as pathological organisations (these are discussed in more detail in the section on post-Kleinian developments in Chapter 3). When healthy integration of good and bad objects takes place in the depressive position the development of a wish to restore the object, which is now recognised in unconscious fantasy as damaged, offers a creative solution to guilt and concern. The other person in a relationship can now be felt to be the object and reparative responses can be made.

Projection and projective identification

Klein had misgivings when she introduced the concept of projective identification because of the potential for analysts and therapists to misuse it to attribute too many of their own feelings to their patients. Despite these doubts it has become her most widely used concept. In keeping with her fears this has included applications that are not necessarily compatible with the rest of her theory, but which have been of practical clinical value. An example would be projective identification as a form of unconscious communication during family therapy.

Projective identification is normal in the paranoid–schizoid position. It is a way of acquiring new internal objects. Parts of the self or ego, with associated impulses and wishes, are projected into the object. These parts of the self are then taken back in, or introjected, to form new internal objects in the self. These are new internal objects because they have been altered by being passed through the external object that may typically be the analyst representing some aspect of mother in the transference. The new object will have acquired some of the characteristics of the external object as well as what remains of the original projected part of the self. Another way of describing projective identification is that it is the recruitment of the object to participate in the projective process as well as the projecting self.

Example

A patient complained endlessly about the lack of guidance and practical advice that her analyst provided for her in long-term psychoanalytical therapy, as the analyst's method was based on listening patiently and offering relatively brief comments mainly referring to the transference. This made the analyst doubt her own way of working was suitable for this patient. After some time and self-reflection by the analyst about her own responses, the analyst called to mind that the patient described listening patiently to colleagues at work and being appreciated for this and noticed the significance of her own self-doubt. At this moment she became consciously aware that she, the analyst, had become filled with feelings of inadequacy and doubt that had previously belonged to the patient, while the patient, without expressing any conscious awareness of where this had come from, had acquired the analyst's ability to listen patiently.

Klein and envy

In her later work Klein introduced a refinement of the theory of death instinct (Klein, 1957). This was to conceive of primary envy as the principal expression of this destructive force and as the archetypal attempt to destroy the good object. An infant with excessive envy is predisposed to develop pathology associated with the triumph of the bad object relation over the good object relation and in unconscious fantasy this is experienced as the tyrannical triumph of the bad object over the good. This is the antithesis of the developmentally creative mobilisation of guilt in the form of concern for the other and desire to make reparation that occurs in the depressive position.

Fairbairn

Ronald Fairbairn (1889–1964) produced theories that interweave with those of Klein and in many clinical situations lead to a similar practical clinical method. While based originally in classical Freudian analysis, there is more emphasis on interpretation of the earliest infantile object relationship as it comes into the here-and-now transference between patient and analyst. Nevertheless, Fairbairn radically departed from both Freud and Klein when he postulated that schizoid states of mind arise from the child's failed love relationship with an object (namely, the mother) and that schizoid states developmentally underpin most, if not all, psychopathology.

Along with Wilfred Bion perhaps, Fairbairn is regarded by some as one of the most revolutionary thinkers in psychoanalysis since Freud, and as laying a foundation for many modern developments (Symington, 1994). He is also regarded by others as eccentric and unnecessarily difficult, especially in the use of idiosyncratic terminology in his scheme for ego development. In later life Fairbairn also experimented with face-to-face seated sessions with his patients without feeling he was departing from psychoanalysis. This further alienated sections of the psychoanalytic 'establishment', but is in keeping with much modern psychoanalytic psychotherapy practice. Yet in practical application, Fairbairn's clinical technique generally followed Freud. When relevant he would painstakingly interpret both the negative (hostile) transference and castration anxiety in the Oedipus complex.

Fairbairn, drives and the Oedipus complex

Fairbairn was sharply critical of how the concept of instinctual drive had been used, but he did not completely reject Freud's theory of instincts. He disagreed with Freud that the Oedipus complex (and infantile sexuality within it) is universally central to every child's development.

Fairbairn's approach to the Oedipal situation as a pattern of object relations can be summarised as follows (Sutherland, 1989):

- the Oedipus complex is a social situation, albeit a highly significant one, but not an internally driven state of mind
- the innate potential of the individual (including instinctual drives) is structured as a set of object relationships within the mind. Only through experience within relationships can instincts find any expression. Therefore instincts can be said to have no existence separate from the mental structures formed by the individual's experience in relationships
- for healthy growth the individual has to be loved for himself or herself from the start by the unconditional affectionate care of the mother (or whichever person the child experiences as mother)
- this loving care has then to be continued by the father as well, and from then on the interplay of maternal and paternal care (the Oedipal situation) adapts within the family at different stages under the influence of maturation and the wider social and cultural environment
- in all phases of development and maturity, satisfying relationships are necessary not only for the survival of the family or other group, but also for the emotional survival of the individual
- in earliest infancy it is not only self-directed sexuality or libido that ensures the physical survival of the infant, but the infant's predisposition to engage with parents who, being adults, can adapt to the infant's needs.

Fairbairn did believe that sexuality in the Freudian sense of libido played a key role in binding family relationships together, but disagreed with Freud's instinct-driven model of the Oedipal situation. Although libido contributes to relationships, Fairbairn believed that Freud was wrong to suggest that it did so simply in the service of pleasure and summed up his own view in the now famous dictum 'libido is not primarily pleasure-seeking, but object-seeking'. One patient illustrated this by saying to Fairbairn, 'you're always talking about my wanting this and that desire satisfied; but what I really want is a father' (Fairbairn, 1952).

Ego, self and the autonomous self

The early pioneering psychoanalysts, including Freud, assumed that at the start the infant does not have any ego (nowadays referred to as 'self'). The idea of the self or ego in a purely instinct-based approach is always likely to lead in any case to an impersonal, 'instinctual' kind of ego as the general organising principle of the mind, which cannot easily account for the holistic experience of existing as a personal self.

Fairbairn directs attention towards personal experience within relationships as the central organising principle in personality. Fairbairn's scheme bears the hallmark of 'object relations theory' because the first emotionally charged object relation is intimacy with mother. From that start, Fairbairn's ego develops as a self that in health is capable of autonomous experience and action and yet is dependent on being in relationship for its existence and effectiveness (Sutherland, 1980, 1989).

Fairbairn and schizoid states

Fairbairn believed that much of a person's behaviour and responses can be explained as a search throughout life for intimacy with mother or other substitute objects, even if this gives more pain than pleasure, or is sexualised or aggressive.

There are two ways that a child may feel responsible for a failure of this intimacy:

- in the depressive state: the child feels his hate has destroyed his mother's love for him
- in the schizoid state: the child feels his love has destroyed his mother's affection for him.

The latter (schizoid state) occurs when deprivation intensifies a feeling of need and imparts an aggressive quality, until the child, in oral terms, feels his need will consume not only the contents of the breast but everything – the breast itself and even the mother. In Fairbairn's view this is the way that emotional intimacy is lost and converted into part-object relating and into predomination of bodily function over emotional responsiveness.

Schizoid is a term used in more than one way in different branches of clinical psychiatry. In psychodynamic psychiatry, schizoid has been used to refer to a person who habitually withdraws from emotional aspects of relationships and hides their desire for intimacy. This characteristically involves introjecting, or keeping inside, good objects while denying bad objects by splitting them off from the rest and projecting them away. Fairbairn clarified the meaning of 'bad' object as desired but frustrating; both good and bad objects are desired. Internal objects are also parts of the self. Therefore denial, splitting and projection of objects means splitting the self (thus the term schizoid) and means denying and withdrawing from what is covertly and unconsciously desired. Fairbairn agreed with Klein's concept of psychic positions, but he felt that the most common, basic origin of psychopathology was brought about by environmental failure leading to schizoid states. In contrast, Klein saw the root of pathology in aggression and envy, which are internally driven expressions of the death instinct. Fairbairn did not feel that he needed the idea of innate death instinct. He felt the origin of aggression lies in the frustration and trauma of not feeling adequately loved.

Fairbairn's endopsychic structure

Fairbairn called the internal framework of the mind endopsychic structure. He thought that from the beginning of mental life there must be some central organising capacity in the mind to stop it disintegrating and he called this the central ego. Now it is recognised that Fairbairn was writing about the self. In the 'schizoid position' during the earliest stage of infantile dependence he suggested that the infantile ego splits into three parts and each of these parts means a different type of object relation. It is beyond the scope of these chapters to describe this splitting and associated object relations in detail, but writing before the growth of information control theory and the growth in applications of systems theory in family therapy and child psychiatry, Fairbairn had hit upon an information systems theory of mind to replace a mechanistic energy discharge model. Fairbairn felt that he had discovered an internal (or as he called it, 'endopsychic') structure in which each significant object relation forms an ego subsystem. Within each ego subsystem feelings and motives have their own feedback system, while also being dependent on their relationship to each other and to the central ego. The self, in turn, is dependent on external relationships to maintain the coherent integrity of the whole person.

The total structuring of these internal relations is characteristically complex, but some internal objects are relatively separate and more easily recognisable, for example, Freud's superego, which is an internalised object relationship.

In clinical practice this scheme leads to a new way of thinking. For example, dreaming is not so much wish fulfilment as the internal playing out of relations between objects within the geography of the mind. A dream reveals a multiplicity of selves and their adaptation to one another as the central self continuously tries to bind them together to prevent the psychological disintegration of the individual. In this respect Jung's theory of dreams is similar to Fairbairn's object relations theory of dreams. Fairbairn abandoned Freud's wish fulfilment theory in favour of seeing dreams as dramatisations of situations existing in the patient's inner world.

In summary (Sutherland, 1980, 1989):

- the mind that the individual experiences and knows as the self is not so much a closed system of energy exchanges as in Freud's original conception but is an open information control system
- this information control system deals with feelings and motives, as well as perceptions and actions
- it is this self that seeks intimate relationship from the beginning. If successful in this first venture it begins to develop a sense of agency, a sense of being a person who can act effectively in relationship with others
- it is an open system that maintains itself, as any sustainable biological system must do, by absorbing from outside
- the schizoid attempt to become a closed autonomous self cannot succeed and leads to neurotic restriction, existentially false positions and narcissistic responses, in contrast to the adaptability and development that is implied by self autonomy that is open within relationships.

Despite the foundation Fairbairn laid for much of modern self theory, he failed to provide a comprehensive scheme for mental function and personality development. He was not able adequately to clarify the nature of the initial relationship, or primary identification, that the infant makes with mother. When does the capacity to relate begin and what happens in the developing mind before that, even if this is before birth? He also had little to say about later stages of childhood development after the stage of dependence on which he had concentrated his attention.

Fairbairn's influence

Fairbairn's influence on others remains ambiguous. Although Fairbairn encapsulated revolutionary changes in psychoanalytic theory in a series of papers written in the early 1940s, he did not found a school and continued to work in relative isolation from other mainstream psychodynamic movements, while remaining within the broad psychoanalytic community. His theories were thought by most to represent an idiosyncratic side alley, but after a period of relative neglect, Fairbairn's ideas have attracted renewed interest on both sides of the Atlantic.

Fairbairn's theories were re-interpreted and modified in different ways by two of his analysands, Harry Guntrip (1901–1975) and John Sutherland (1905–1991). The contemporary sphere of Fairbairn's influence included the writing of John Padel in Britain and James Grotstein and Otto Kernberg in the USA. The clear influence of Fairbairnian concepts in the work of the founder of self psychology in the USA, Heinz Kohut, was not acknow ledged by Kohut himself, but was noted by Sutherland. The overlap between Fairbairn's work and the subsequent theories of Kohut have also been described from a Kohutian self psychology perspective by Howard Bacal and Kenneth Newman (Bacal & Newman, 1990). Fairbairn suggested that the personal relationship between analyst and patient is a factor for therapeutic change in addition to systematic analysis of the transference. Guntrip went further and changed the emphasis so that this personal relationship took precedence over all else in the development of a stronger self during therapy.

Although he gave no credit to the Scottish psychiatrist and psychotherapist Ian Suttie (1889–1935), it is inconceivable that Fairbairn was not influenced by Suttie's book *The Origins of Love and Hate* (Suttie, 1935; published the year Suttie died). Suttie knew the work of Freud's Hungarian disciple Sándor Ferenczi. Suttie's wife, Jane, translated some of Ferenczi's papers into English. Suttie is a link between Fairbairn's object relations theory and that of Ferenczi's influential pupil, Michael Balint. It was also Fairbairn and not Winnicott who first coined the term transitional stage, to refer to the phase between infantile dependence and mature dependence. It was Winnicott's recognition of the transitional object, the toddler's teddy bear or comfort blanket, which Fairbairn would have called a transitional technique, that became famous.

Winnicott's object relations theory

Donald Winnicott (1896–1971) was one of those leading British psychoanalysts, including Fairbairn, Bowlby and Balint, who felt that most psychopathology arises from relationship (i.e. 'environmental') failure and trauma during infancy. Winnicott's object relations theory has much in common with both Klein and Fairbairn, but it also has differences. He especially disagreed on schizoid positions, regarding them as deviations from normal development. Klein and Fairbairn both based their object relations theories on paranoid–schizoid (Klein) and schizoid (Fairbairn) states being part of normal infant development.

Winnicott's good-enough mother and holding

Winnicott realised that when an emphasis is given to environmental, relationship failure, there is greater potential for idealising the 'perfect parent' and that this can appear to set up impossible requirements for the achievement of ordinary developmental tasks. He coined the term good-enough mother. The good-enough mother provides holding.

Holding is a facilitative environment that puts the natural skill and constancy of the good-enough mother to use in helping the dependent infant organise, explore, satisfy and assimilate basic needs and also to tolerate their frustration. Holding by the good-enough mother is Winnicott's more elaborate equivalent of Fairbairn's concept of intimacy. It also shares many similarities with the post-Kleinian concept formulated by Bion as containment (see Chapter 3 on Psychodynamic theories II).

True self and false self

Winnicott used the terms true self and false self to signify the outcome of early environmental failure during infancy.

The true self, rather like the concept of the central ego in Fairbairn's structural scheme for the developing self that experiences intimacy, evolves from a relationship with a good-enough mother who provides satisfactory holding. This is the self that a person feels belongs uniquely to themselves. In existential terms it might be said that this is where the individual experiences authenticity in their life.

The false self is the person who collaborates with a parent, or later in life with their psychotherapist, while inwardly feeling somewhere else within themselves that this is futile. Winnicott pointed out that in this sense the patient's false self can be on the psychotherapist's side in a game of endless analysis of defences that cannot end until the psychotherapist recognises and interprets the patient's non-existence in this situation.

Winnicott's true and false self compared to other theories

Winnicott offered the true self as central agency in the mind of a different order from the classical Freudian concept of id. Freud had divided personality structurally into a part that is 'central' and internally powered by elementary instincts, the id and parts that are significantly turned outwards to the external world as well as having their own internal presence, the ego and superego. Winnicott distinguished 'ego-needs' from 'id-needs'. He suggested that only when the infant ego has built up sufficient strength to integrate psychic and somatic experience can the ego take in instinctual excitation, frustration and satisfaction as belonging to the true self. A patient said to Winnicott, 'Good management such as I have experienced during this hour is a feed'.

Winnicott understood this as meaning good management equals ego care, while 'such as I have experienced during this hour is a feed' equals id satisfaction (Winnicott, 1960).

The patient could not have said this the other way round, that a feed is good management. If Winnicott had actually or metaphorically fed him directly, the patient would either have been complying with Winnicott, which would have been to fit in using his false self, or instead would have had to react against and reject Winnicott's advances, maintaining his integrity but at the emotional cost of choosing isolation and frustration.

Winnicott's division of self into true and false is also an alternative way of describing what Klein called splitting of the ego and Fairbairn called splitting of the central ego or self. Kleinian theory suggests that such splitting results from excessive projection and envy, but Winnicott takes a typical object relations theory position that this splitting of the self results from early environmental relationship failure.

Winnicott and regression

Winnicott developed a sophisticated theory of regression in analysis and therapy that also illuminates the nature of antisocial or delinquent behaviour. (For further discussion of regression see both this chapter and Chapter 3, Psychodynamic theories II.) Regression can be easily misunderstood as advocating the kind of 'therapy' that slides into id instinctual satisfaction and passive tolerance of 'infantile' antisocial behaviour. Winnicott observed that the mother in the earliest stages and the father who acts during this phase as 'another mother', must inevitably fail to satisfy many of the instinctual demands of their infant. The good-enough mother (and in this special sense, father) can nevertheless completely succeed in 'not letting the infant down' by catering for ego needs through the way that she holds the infant.

This is what makes Winnicott's system a fully fledged object relations theory. By ego needs he means not mechanistic instinctual satisfactions, but psychological requirements between two or more people. The relationship between mother and child is an emotional environment in which learning and development can take place; a relationship between two persons or selves (egos), albeit one mature, adapted adult and one unadapted but nascent being.

Winnicott viewed regression in therapy not so much as a return to the past but as the past that is still within the patient coming into the present (and in a key sense it is also the past within the psychoanalyst or psychotherapist made available for the relationship with his or her patient).

The mother and infant and transitional phenomena and objects

In his theory of the mother–infant relationship, Winnicott extended Fairbairn's concept of the transitional phase to incorporate, rather than resolve, a paradox in early human development. That paradox is the way in which an infant requires to have an innate capacity for autonomous existence and at the same time requires to be created by its mother, not only in the womb but after birth, in the mind, emotions and expectations of the mother.

In other words, from before the baby is born and for several weeks afterwards in the healthy situation a parent exists in a state of primary maternal preoccupation with the baby. This fits with the baby's needs and emotional as well as physical dependence on the parents.

Winnicott startled colleagues by saying, 'There is no such thing as an infant' (Khan, 1975). He meant that there can be no infant without maternal care and therefore the infant only exists as part of an infant–mother relationship.

In order to move towards independence the infant and mother create between them what Winnicott called potential space within which transitional phenomena may happen. In this potential space the mother and infant can explore creatively through play. The transitional object, often a soft toy or cloth, allows a child to possess something that is ambiguous as being 'not me' or being 'part of me'. Yet the transitional object is not so much the teddy bear or cloth that the baby uses, but refers to the way that the baby makes use of the object (that is, both the object as mother and the object as the thing that is a teddy, say). The transitional nature of the object is the paradox that is to be accepted, tolerated and respected by both mother and child if it is to be successful.

Delinquency 'as a sign of hope', acting out and the false self

A false self may arise through over-stimulation of instinctual drives before the immature ego can integrate this experience. It may also arise from substantial deprivation. Winnicott believed that antisocial tendencies develop when a child is able to recognise deprivation as actually arising from the external environment (rather than depressively attributing failings to one's self). In this situation the child makes a nuisance of him or herself as a demand to the environment, as a demand to others to respond to this sense of deprivation. This carries forward directly into the therapeutic setting where the nuisance value of a behaviour can be linked with the patient's sense of deprivation expressed in the form of antisocial, anti-therapeutic, behaviour, known generally as acting out.

Winnicott, in characteristic form, recognised the paradox in this and saw such behaviour as a sign of hope. What he did regard as futile is the posturing compliance of the false self that does not protest. The antisocial tendency, as he called it, indicates that the infant, now the patient, did at some point in development reach the stage of being able to perceive that the cause of the disaster lies in an environmental failure outside himself.

Winnicott and psychoanalytic therapy

For psychotherapy (with all age groups) Winnicott believed:

- that the transitional object is the precursor of all creative activity, starting with play and going on to every kind of creative human activity from the most ordinary daily exchange through to the highest forms of art
- that the flight into split-off intellectual thinking, in an attempt to resolve the paradox of the transitional object, causes loss of the paradox itself along with loss of its potential for creative development.

Instead of regarding playing in psychotherapy as just a useful technique for children, Winnicott wrote about playing as part of the creative exchange between any therapist and patient, not only the child patient but also with adults. Although it may be harder to recognise playfulness in the interchange with an adult because the overt medium of communication is that of words, all psychotherapy and psychoanalysis can be viewed as taking place in the overlap between two areas of playing – that of the patient and that of the therapist. Art therapy and music therapy may also be thought of as approaching this area, and art and music are commonly thought of as 'therapeutic' in themselves.

Winnicott suggested that when creative playing in therapy is not possible the therapist aims to help the patient to begin to be able to play, thereby creating a developmentally useful space between patient and therapist. Then the patient, like the developing child, can begin to use fantasy and symbolic communication to explore creative being (true self relating to good enough therapist) and not so much as an escape from being (false self compliance). At this point in therapy Winnnicott believed that a patient may feel that their true self is taking enormous risks without the protection of the false self with which they are accustomed. At these times the patient may require other forms of practical management and caring support as well as psychotherapeutic interpretation. The skill of the psychoanalytical therapist is to understand these needs and to communicate that understanding, without being drawn out of her/his role as the patient's therapist, given that the patient also needs the psychoanalytic work to continue for their future progress and wellbeing.

Winnicott took a developmental approach to psychiatric classification. Three factors contribute to the emotional development of an individual:

- on one side there is heredity
- on the other side there is the environment

- in the middle is the individual 'living and defending and growing' (Winnicott, 1959).

Winnicott was interested in classification. In his view psychoanalytic psychotherapy deals with the individual living, defending and growing. Psychiatric classification at its best accounts for the total 'phenomenology'. The best way to classify from a psychodynamic point of view, according to Winnicott, is first to classify the environmental states involved; then to go on to classify the individual's defences; and finally to look at heredity. Winnicott, like Freud, recognised constitutional factors and anticipated recent developments in the genetics of mental illness that clearly establish a hereditary factor (for example, in schizophrenia), but also clearly establish that other factors are involved in the final expression of the illness. Winnicott suggests that these other factors can be grouped under environmental states, developmental growth and defences.

Winnicott believed:

- neurotic symptoms contain the conflict and this is all too apparent to the neurotic individual
- antisocial behaviour exteriorises and converts conflict into actions so that characteristically the disturbance is experienced by others more than the individual himself is capable of experiencing
- the psychodynamic aspect of psychotic illness is not in itself a breakdown, but it is a defensive organisation relative to what Winnicott calls a 'primitive' or 'original' agony.

In psychotic illness it is the fear of the original agony that produces the defensive organisation that forms an illness syndrome: self-defences work for the patient to protect the self from unthinkable anxieties. These defences typically also destroy the ability to enter the depressive position or the Oedipus complex. In clinical situations fear of breakdown does trouble patients. In typically poetic fashion, Winnicott noted that the patient who fears breakdown characteristically fails to recognise that the breakdown has already been experienced in the past. In the present, breakdown is defended against through illness and through non-existence as a person, generally achieved by denial and disavowal of reality and by projection.

Michael Balint

Best known for adapting psychoanalysis for the use of general practitioners, Michael Balint (1896–1970) gave his name to what became known as Balint Groups. These train general practitioners in a psychodynamic understanding of what happens within doctor–patient relationships. It is not so widely known that Balint also wrote on a broad range of subjects in psychoanalysis.

Balint based his work firmly on the premise that the infant is motivated from the start of life to form a personal relationship with the mother. He followed his fellow Hungarian psychoanalytic mentor Sándor Ferenczi

(1873–1933) and the British psychiatrist Ian Suttie (1889–1935) in their view that the basic motivation in children to relate to others is the desire for tenderness rather than sexuality. This concept of tenderness is close to Fairbairn's notion of intimacy.

Balint moved to Britain in 1939 to escape rising anti-semitism in Budapest and subsequently became firmly associated with the object relations theory that British independent group psychoanalysts were developing. Within object relations theories Balint's approach is at an extreme. He unambiguously attributed faulty development of the child's personality and failure in the capacity for satisfactory relationships later in adult life to real events and actual failures in the caring environment during very young infancy. Like Fairbairn, Balint had radical ideas but did not himself develop these into a comprehensive system. (For further discussion of the British independent group of psychoanalysts see also Chapter 3.)

Balint's relationship to classical Freudian and Kleinian instinct theory

During the 1950s, Fairbairn's collected papers had been published, Winnicott extended the idea of transitional phenomena and coined the term transitional object and Balint described the implications of a radical object relations approach for understanding ordinary patterns of character formation (Balint, 1959). His approach to character development was a reaction against classical Freudian and Kleinian theory.

Balint, Winnicott and Fairbairn all highlighted how socially significant instinctual drives operate in ordinary development through the medium of a family environment and relationships. They were critical of those branches of Freudian and Kleinian psychoanalysis that seem to attribute psychopathology solely to internal distortions of instinctual pattern. They were not against the idea of instinctual drives as such. They were against those who talk about drives as though instincts are enclosed within themselves and think that drives can express themselves in ways that are independent of what external conditions and relationships are actually available for a person to experience.

Balint regarded Freud's classical stages of pregenital sexuality as pathology rather than normal development because they imply that sexuality dominates and the desire for tenderness is denied. To him these sexual developmental distortions were not innate biological factors but more to do with a child's upbringing. In keeping with this, Balint believed that hate and aggression have their origin in the absence of adequately loving and understanding relationships between a child and significant adults around that child.

By the late 1950s Balint was unequivocal that the development of object relationships and the development of instinctual aims, although continuously influencing each other, are none the less fundamentally different processes. Freud had divided instinctual phases of development according to oral, anal, phallic, Oedipal and genital aims. From Balint's object relations perspective, this is not in itself wrong, just utterly inadequate. He felt that Freudian instinct theory can lead, for example, to the uncritical use of 'oral' to cover everything that is developmentally primitive. Concepts commonly used by Freudians and Kleinians to describe the early period of mental life based on the idea of orality include greed, incorporation, introjection, internalisation, part-objects, destruction by sucking, chewing or biting, projection in the pattern of spitting or vomiting. Balint felt that this approach ignores other primitive spheres of experience such as feeling warmth, rhythmic noises and movements, sounds of intonation and humming, tastes and smells, bodily contact, touching and muscle sensations especially of the hands and the power of any of these to evoke or allay anxiety and suspicion, blissful contentment, or desperate loneliness.

The concept of primary narcissism originated in classical instinct theory as the normal developmentally earliest state of mind. Balint also rejected this suggesting instead an early pre-ambivalent state in which the infant feels that the parent has identical wishes to those the infant is himself or herself experiencing. Balint used two terms for this state, primary object relationship or primary love.

Balint's approach to character development and therapeutic change

Given that it is inevitable that there are shortcomings in reality for sustaining unequivocal primary love, such shortcomings can lead to different kinds of reaction in the infant.

Balint coined the term basic fault for the patient who feels that the whole of development has been a faulty or false experience (Balint, 1968). He believed that this can only be overcome through regression to a state of dependence on the analyst. Balint called the start of therapeutic recovery after regression a new beginning. This corresponds closely to Winnicott's concept of the emergence of the 'true self' (Rycroft, 1972).

Balint noted the way that many people excitedly, or even feeling a little 'mad', seek pleasure in thrills. This is the basis of the funfare and many sports that involve voluntary exposure to fear, to pleasure and to the confident hope that all will be safe in the end. This is a person who confidently moves away from their safe objects, being potent through the thrill of moving into the friendly expanses between objects. He used the term philobat for this personality structure. He also noted that other people shy away in disgust or boredom from such activities; for this he used the term ocnophil.

Balint felt that the best way to help a patient to change these attitudes was to expose the patient in therapy to a 'calculated fraction' of whatever trauma was thought in the first place to have caused the encumbered frame of mind. To do this, in Balint's view, the analyst must constantly adjust the degree of exposure to traumatic ideas and feelings by observing the patient's capacity to maintain the analytic and other relationships throughout the whole process of therapy. The patient's personal skill in maintaining intimate, durable contact with other people gives a measure of both the patient's resilience and ability to change at any given moment.

References

Bacal, H. A. & Newman, K. M. (1990) *Theories of Object Relations: Bridges to Self Psychology*. New York: Columbia University Press.

Balint, M. (1959) *Thrills and Regressions*. London: Hogarth.

Balint, M. (1968) *The Basic Fault*. London: Tavistock.

Couch, A. S. (1995) Anna Freud's adult psychoanalytic technique: a defence of classical analysis. *International Journal of Psycho-analysis*, **76**, 153–171.

de Beauvoir, S. (1953) *The Second Sex*. London: Jonathan Cape.

Etchegoyen, R. H. (1991) *The Fundamentals of Psychoanalytic Technique*. London: Karnac Books.

Fairbairn, W. R. D. (1952) *Psychoanalytic Studies of the Personality*. London: Tavistock.

Freud, A. (1966) The ego and the mechanisms of defense. In *The Writings of Anna Freud*, Volume II, pp. 18–27. Madison: International Universities Press.

Freud, S. (1911) Psychoanalytic notes on an autobiographical account of a case of paranoia (dementia paranoides). In *The Standard Edition of the Complete Psychological Works of Sigmund Freud* (ed. J. Strachey), Vol XII, pp. 59–79. London: Hogarth.

Freud, S. (1923) The ego and the id. In *The Standard Edition of the Complete Psychological Works of Sigmund Freud* (ed. J. Strachey), pp. 3–66. London: Hogarth.

Friedan, B. (1963) *The Feminine Mystique*. London: Victor Gollancz.

Gill, M. M. (1994) *Psychoanalysis in Transition: a Personal View*. Hillsdale, New Jersey: The Analytic Press.

Greer, G. (1970) *The Female Eunuch*. London: MacGibbon & Kee.

Grünbaum, A. (1984) *The Foundations of Psychoanalysis: a Philosophical Critique*. Berkeley, Los Angeles & London: University of California Press.

Khan, M. M. R. (1975) Introduction. In *Through Paediatrics to Psychoanalysis* (D. W. Winnicott), pp. xx–xvii. London: Hogarth.

Klein, M. (1957) *Envy and Gratitude*. London: Tavistock.

Masson, J. M. (1984) *The Assault on Truth: Freud's Suppression of the Seduction Theory*. London: Faber and Faber.

Millett, K. (1970) *Sexual Politics*. New York: Doubleday.

Ogden, T. (1992) The dialectically constituted/decentred subject of psychoanalysis, II: the contributions of Klein and Winnicott. *International Journal of Psychoanalysis*, **73**, 613–626.

Quinodoz, J. -M. (1991) La Solitude Apprivoisée. Paris: Presses Universitaires de France. Reprinted in English translation (1993) as *The Taming of Solitude: Separation Anxiety in Psychoanalysis*. London: Routledge.

Rayner, E. (1991) *The Independent Mind in British Psychoanalysis*. London: Free Association Books.

Roazen, P. (1976) *Freud and His Followers*. Penguin: London.

Robinson, P. (1993) *Freud and His Critics*. Berkeley: University of California Press.

Rycroft, C. (1972) *A Critical Dictionary of Psychoanalysis*, p. 171. London: Penguin.

Strean, H. S. (1994) *Essentials of Psychoanalysis*. Berkeley: Brunner/Mazel.

Sutherland, J. D. (1980) The autonomous self. In *The Autonomous Self: The Work of John D. Sutherland* (ed. J. S. Scharff). Northvale, New Jersey & London: Jason Aronson.

Sutherland, J. D. (1989) *Fairbairn's Journey Into the Interior*. London: Free Association Books.

Suttie, I. D. (1935) *The Origins of Love and Hate*. London: Kegan Paul, Trench, Trubner.

Symington, N. (1994) The tradition of Fairbairn. In *Fairbairn and the Origins of Object Relations* (eds J. S. Grotstein & D. B. Rinsley), pp. 211–221. London: Free Association Books.

Wallerstein, R. S. (1999) A half-century perspective on psychoanalysis and psychotherapy: the historical context of Joseph Sandler's contributions. In *Psychoanalysis on the Move: The Work of Joseph Sandler* (ed. P. Fonagy, A. M. Cooper & R. S. Wallerstein), pp. 30–50. London: Routledge.

Winnicott, D. W. (1959) Classification: is there a psycho-analytic contribution to psychiatric classification? Reprinted (1965) in *Maturational Processes and the Facilitating Environment* (D. W. Winnicott), pp. 124–139. London: Hogarth Press.

Winnicott, D. W. (1960) Ego distortion in terms of true and false self. Reprinted (1965) in *Maturational Processes and the Facilitating Environment* (D. W. Winnicott), pp. 140–152. London: Hogarth Press.

Young-Eisendrath, P. & Dawson, T. (1997) *The Cambridge Companion to Jung*. Cambridge: Cambridge University Press.

CHAPTER 3

Psychodynamic theories II

John Shemilt & Jane Naismith

The new psychoanalytic language that has emerged in recent years may at first seem unfamiliar and difficult. The final sections of this chapter venture into some of these challenging areas and highlight current issues in clinical practice. Among the most striking changes in psychodynamic theory has been a far greater emphasis on the idea of psychic space replacing classical Freudian ideas of energy and instinct. Although energy is implicit in every mental activity, psychic energy is not a very practical clinical concept. Current debate in psychodynamic theory and practice concentrates more on the relative importance that should be given to the analysis of spatial experience rather than the classical style of analysis of unconscious instincts. Feelings of closeness and distance are involved in spatial experience and psychic space may be space between people as 'external objects', intrapsychic space between 'internal objects', or transitional space, in which what is internal and what is external are combined.

This chapter considers subsequent developments starting from the way that ego psychology took up Sigmund Freud's structural theory which is essentially a spatial metaphor. Ego psychology evolved predominantly in the USA, but with roots also in the work of Anna Freud. The work of Heinz Hartmann, Edith Jacobson, Margaret Mahler, Daniel Stern, Thomas Ogden and Eric Erikson will be described. The theoretical advances they represent prepared the way for two pre-eminent North American psychoanalysts, Heinz Kohut and Otto Kernberg. Kohut and Kernberg each provide their own distinct link from ego psychology and contemporary North American psychoanalysis back to contemporary British psychoanalysis. Distinct features of current British work will be described by looking at attachment theory in which Bowlby's emphasis on the biological basis of psychodynamics transformed the concept of instinct into that of attachment, and then by looking at how the post-Kleinians and independents have approached some of the same issues and their clinical application.

Anna Freud

Anna Freud occupies a prominent place in the history of psychodynamic thought in her own right (see also Chapter 2). In summary her most widely applied psychoanalytic ideas were:

- psychoanalysis with children and child development (see also Chapter 10)
- detailed account of the ego's defensive and adaptive role in reconciling the instinctual drives of the id, the demands and ideals of the superego, and the reality of the outside world
- practical clinical method in which she advocated that the analyst remains equidistant from the ego, id and superego. By this she meant that in classical psychoanalytic technique the analyst tries not to identify specially with or take an excessive interest in the aims of any one of these agencies of the mind, but has an equal and impartial interest in exposing the operation of all three.

Anna Freud moved with Sigmund Freud from Vienna to London in 1938, but travelled regularly to the USA and significantly influenced psychoanalytic developments in North America, where, by the late 1950s, the psychodynamic community came to be largely dominated by the school of ego psychology led by Heinz Hartmann.

Heinz Hartmann and ego psychology

For Heinz Hartmann (1894–1970) the ego of Freud's structural model was too weak (see also Chapter 2). Hartmann felt that the ego he observed in his patients had inborn elements, which he called apparatuses of primary autonomy and conflict-free ego spheres, including mental skills such as perception, memory, motility and association.

Hartmann noted that without possessing these capabilities the developing ego would not be able to relate to reality at all. He did not abandon classical drive theory for an object relations theory of early ego development like many European and Latin American analysts. Instead, he called the first developmental stage of infancy the undifferentiated matrix. Hartmann's ego, with its inborn abilities, and his id, with its inborn instinctual drives, develop from there in parallel. This means that in Hartmann's theory the ego will relate to reality whether or not instinct gratification (of the id) takes place. The infant has more channels to reality and the environment than Freud allowed for, yet in contrast to object relations theory, relationship is not a fundamental or primary source of motivation in itself.

For Hartmann, the aim of psychodynamic theory is primarily to describe the self-deceptions and misjudgements about the external world to which human beings are prone. The analyst interprets these self-deceptions and misjudgements to make new connections, rather than seeking experiential change based on the quality of relationship between patient and analyst.

In a sense ego psychology retains a Freudian theoretical framework, in that it agrees that personality and self development arise from abstract, irreducible biological instinct drives, while at the same time attempting to address the criticism that Freudian reductionism cannot explain the full complexity and subtlety of human experience (Greenberg & Mitchell, 1983).

Freud's theory and Hartmann's theory of narcissism: self as an internal representation

Classical Freudian theory equates 'self' with the experience of the ego exercising defensive functions in the face of internal conflict. Narcissism exists when libido is predominantly invested in the ego. Narcissism means self-loving (self-directed libido) that is directed to part of the mental structure itself, instead of towards mental representations of what is outside (external objects). In Freud's structural theory ego, id and superego are the three basic mental structures to which narcissistic emotional flow can be channelled, avoiding mature, non-narcissistic engagement with other people.

Hartmann's ego psychology extended the concept of self beyond the classical Freudian view based on conflict. It included what Hartmann called primary autonomous ego functions. These depend on the presence of an average expectable environment, meaning an environment that is not especially characterised by conflict between instinct and reality.

Hartmann also departed from Freud's views by defining self as a mental representation rather than a structure or agency in itself. This means that self is the construction within the ego, from experience, of one's whole existence. Hartmann saw narcissism as the channelling of libido into this self-representation.

Hartmann's ego psychology, cognitive–behavioural therapy and cognitive analytic therapy

Hartmann's ego psychology and its emphasis on replacing misjudgements and self-deceptions with new connections provides a point of contact between psychoanalytic psychotherapy and both cognitive–behavioural therapy and cognitive analytic therapy (see Chapter 5, Cognitive analytic therapy and Chapter 6, Behavioural and cognitive theories). Yet a distinction also exists between:

1. psychodynamic therapies based on mutual reflection and transference interpretation within the context of the transference/countertransference relationship
2. cognitive–behavioural therapy based on structured reflection on the patient's inward cognitive/affective experience combined with an educative relationship and cognitive theory, which in turn uses aspects of learning theory applied to emotional experience

3. cognitive analytic therapy that explicitly sets out to base clinical method on a combination of psychoanalytic object relations theory and cognitive theory (Ryle, 1995).

Edith Jacobson: ego, self and emotional experience

Edith Jacobson (1897–1978) highlighted the role of affect (i.e. emotion), while retaining Hartmann's concept of personality as a self-representation in relationship with object-representations.

In Jacobson's theory the first stage of development is a primal psychophysiological self, another version of what Hartmann had called the undifferentiated matrix. Not only libidinal and aggressive drives differentiate from this primal self (or matrix) but also self-representations and object-representations as well. Although she regarded libidinal and aggressive drives as innately programmed sources of biological energy, Jacobson did not believe that such instinct drives could explain the full spectrum of experience. She did not regard affects or emotions simply as the product of discharge of instinctual tensions, but saw them as including a quality of experience. It is useful to note that in practice this implicitly includes the factor added by a specific emotionally significant relationship to another person (Sutherland, 1980).

Jacobson thus prepared the way for others, particularly Otto Kernberg, to make a link between ego psychology and object relations theory, recognising that experience includes higher order relationship as well as narrowly defined instinctual satisfaction. For example, orality includes what the mother is for an infant in all ways and includes the infant being helped to organise that experience by the mother; it is not merely a process of instinctual satisfaction through feeding.

In summary, Jacobson followed Hartmann in regarding the ego as a system of functions and the self as a representation within the ego. Jacobson gave to the self greater power of autonomous influence than Hartmann with his vaguer notion of self.

Margaret Mahler: self, identity and separation–individuation

In contrast to both Hartmann and Jacobson, Margaret Mahler (1897–1985) conceived of self more clearly as the whole person. In Mahler's developmental theory, the beginning of life is a symbiotic matrix of mother and infant from which a self differentiates to form a coherent identity for the individual. The shadow of Freud's stage of autoerotism is essentially retained by Mahler in the first phase of this developmental sequence, which she called the autistic stage. In sequence the stages are:

- autistic phase
- symbiosis
- separation–individuation.

Mahler broke down the process of separation–individuation into sub-stages through which self-hood and 'individuated' identity emerge by about the end of the third year. The sub-stages of separation–individuation in developmental order are:

- differentiation
- practising
- rapprochement
- hatching.

As a child experiences the sense of being different from mother (differentiated), this experience is normally tested and consolidated by practising and by the exploration of independent action. Rapprochement refers to the need to be able to regress and reunite with mother in the face of frustration and anxiety while exploring the wider world. The final sub-stage of hatching is the acquisition of a firmly established identity as a separate and individual person.

Mahler presented her work as descriptive observations, but her notion of a normal initial autistic phase of development does not stand up in the light of evidence from early infant developmental research. In retrospect we can now see it more as a homage to classical Freudian instinctual drive theory than was apparent before the emergence of further research evidence on normal child development.

Daniel Stern and recent advances in developmental research

Daniel Stern, another North American psychoanalyst who is also a developmental research psychologist, reviewed psychodynamic theory in the light of more recent results that emerged from modern experimental methods of mother and baby observation. He concluded that there is no normal autistic phase after birth and that from birth the healthy human infant possesses independent resources and separateness (Stern, 1985). It is therefore also doubtful that the severe pathological developmental condition of childhood autism and the deficits observed in that condition can be adequately accounted for in terms of a return to any known phase of normal development.

Thomas Ogden and the autistic contiguous position

A similar criticism may apply to the concept of the autistic contiguous position, which Thomas Ogden, also from the USA, has described as a state of mind developmentally more primitive than both the paranoid– schizoid position and the depressive position (Ogden, 1989). In effect Ogden adds on another version of an autoerotic or undifferentiated (i.e. not object-relation-dominated) phase in this instance to the Kleinian system. Some post-Kleinians would, on observing the features in their patients that Ogden attributes to his autistic contiguous position, think of these as belonging to a pathological organisation. A pathological organisation is a defensive organisation between rather than before the paranoid–schizoid and depressive positions.

Erik Erikson, identity and culture

Erik Erikson (1902–1994) studied the interplay of developmental and cultural influences in identity formation. He extended the concept of ego identity forming in childhood developmental stages to include the entire life cycle from infancy through childhood, adolescence and adulthood to old age. Perhaps his most influential observations were on adolescent identity formation and the maturational function of identity crises at each stage (Erikson, 1968).

Otto Kernberg: American ego psychology encounters British object relations theory

Otto Kernberg has been writing prolifically since the 1960s on theory and practice. His views have been influential on both sides of the Atlantic especially on the treatment of patients with borderline disorders and narcissistic disorders.

While the origins of his approach are in Hartmann's and Jacobson's theories, he was the first prominent American psychoanalyst explicitly to take up British object relations theory. He was introduced to Fairbairn's work by Fairbairn's biographer, J. D. Sutherland, but disagreed with Fairbairn's view that classical instinctual drive theory is not compatible with a theory of dynamic structure based on internal object relations (see Chapter 2, Psychodynamic theories I). Kernberg suggested that self-representations and object-representations are developed into internalised relationships from instinctual drives. Like Jacobson, he emphasised the role of affect (emotion) in regulating this process.

By combining a form of instinct drive theory with a modified version of object relations theory, Kernberg produced a distinct theoretical position in which the role of instinctual drive is to provide the affects that organise a dynamic system of internalised images of self and object linked together (Greenberg & Mitchell, 1983). These can be thought of as child–parent relationships, internalised to form object relations, but referred to by Kernberg as internalised images.

In Kernberg's view, at the earliest stage of development self and object are poorly separated and affect is intense, including violently negative feelings. During later stages ego identity forms by identification with relationships that are linked by having similar emotional tone. The self is organised by the ego in these ways, but in Kernberg's view remains secondary to the experience of relationships. This brings his position closer to that of British object relations theory (Sutherland, 1980).

Kernberg, splitting and Kleinian theory

Kernberg's description of splitting has much in common with Kleinian theory. In his view splitting maintains developmentally early patterns in 'non-metabolised', (i.e. unprocessed) form. This follows from the developmental theories of Jacobson and Mahler that significant disturbance results from pathological fixation at a primitive stage of development when the early ego is cognitively too weak to integrate experience. According to Kernberg the early ego is influenced by the emotional tone, whether good or bad. The early ego constructs defences to keep good and bad experiences separate: it 'splits' to deal with intense affect. This use of the concept of splitting is similar to splitting in Kleinian theory. Some splitting is a common mental mechanism in health, but Kernberg went on to describe in detail how the experience of patients with severe personality disorders comes to be organised and maintained through profound and persistent patterns of splitting.

Kernberg and psychotherapy with narcissistic and borderline personality disorders

Kernberg has based much of his theory on his work in psychoanalytic psychotherapy with severely disturbed patients, diagnosed as having narcissistic and borderline personalities. In this context borderline refers to that type of character disorder in which psychotic mental processes are sufficiently close to the surface to predominate in the transference during psychotherapy, but the patient's ego is able to muster sufficient defences at other times to prevent this underlying psychosis from dominating the rest of their lives. These patients characteristically form chaotic transferences with violently contradictory feelings towards the therapist in which there are primitive defence mechanisms such as splitting, primitive idealisation or devaluation, projection and projective identification.

For Kernberg, interpretation during psychotherapy targets the patient's use of splitting and the existence of seemingly incompatible states of mind arising from it. The aim is to enable the patient to integrate split-off images of herself or himself into a less divided vision of self and others.

Heinz Kohut: self psychology

In the late 1950s, Heinz Kohut (1913–1981) re-defined the range and limits of psychoanalysis in terms of introspection and empathy (Kohut, 1959). He had been a prominent orthodox Freudian member of the psychoanalytic community in the USA, but after this the concept of empathy became central in his new radical theory of self-development. By the mid-1970s a recognisable school had been established known as self psychology.

Kohut saw self psychology as a distinct psychoanalytic theory, only declaring some common ground with Heinz Hartmann and ego psychology.

He did not acknowledge obvious similarities between aspects of his work and the North American interpersonal school of psychoanalysis of Harry Stack Sullivan (1899–1949), and with the British object relations theories of Fairbairn, Winnicott and Balint (Bacal & Newman, 1990; Greenberg & Mitchell, 1983; Sutherland, 1989).

For Hartmann the self was essentially an experience or representation. Kohut saw in the self a central and functional role in the mind, not just a representation of something without intrinsic functional powers of its own. This development had much in common with similar advances made in Britain by Fairbairn, Winnicott and Balint although expressed by them in the language of object relations theory.

Kohut and the treatment of narcissistic personality disorder

Unlike Kernberg, Kohut continued to regard both psychotic and borderline conditions as generally untreatable by psychodynamic methods. Nevertheless, like Kernberg, Kohut did take on for treatment a group of severely disturbed individuals with narcissistic personality disorder who had previously been regarded as unsuitable. Kohut now saw narcissism not as the opposite of object relations (being able to relate to another person), but as the 'opposite' of object love (being able to love another person) (Ornstein, 1978). He observed that his narcissistic patients formed transferences dominated by mirroring and by idealising. He felt that he had discovered a method for working with these kinds of reaction. Unfortunately he described all of this in difficult, idiosyncratic language.

Kohut's true object and selfobject

The notion of object relation was not explicitly used by Kohut. Instead he focused on the development of self. His pivotal concepts were the selfobject, and the self–selfobject relationship (the cumbersome term self–selfobject relationship is often abbreviated to selfobject relationship). Nevertheless, these clearly imply a type of object relation. In Kohut's system these relationships are the determinant of self-experience and the vehicle for self-development (Bacal & Newman, 1990).

Kohut used the new term selfobject with types of transference–countertransference in which there is a narcissistic (self-centred) lack of adequate differentiation between self and object and lack of separation in the infant and mother transference. As a result, the selfobject is related to only in terms of the specific needs of the developing self at each stage, without recognition of the object and without recognising that the object has its own centre of initiative as a distinct self. The selfobject is also referred to as archaic to indicate that it has persisted from a much earlier developmental stage. A true object grows from more mature differentiation between self and object (between infant and mother in the transference).

Kohut defined self as 'a unit, cohesive in space and enduring in time, which is a centre of initiative and a recipient of impressions'. The concept selfobject is similar to Balint's primary love and Fairbairn's intimacy. The selfobject is internal within the mind. In a sense Kohut also used the selfobject to retain a link with classical psychoanalytic intrapersonal theory, and to avoid his theory becoming an interpersonal theory.

The origin of narcissistic personality disorders

Kohut believed that narcissistic disorders are the result of the impact of parental pathology on the child. This is particularly likely with parents who themselves have narcissistic fixations that prevent them responding empathically. This is in contrast to elements of narcissism in healthy development, which, being more flexible and adaptable rather than rigidly defensive, do not prevent an individual from forming empathic, mutual relationships with others.

Kohut agreed with Freud that it is normal for narcissism to develop out of a phase of autoerotism, but Freud's developmental path was autoeroticism leading to narcissism leading to object love. Kohut replaced this with a new pathway in which autoeroticism leads to narcissism, but this earlier stage narcissism then leads to higher forms of narcissism. Kohut suggested that this narcissism pathway exists in two parallel lines, as:

- the grandiose–exhibitionistic self, (mirror transference)
- the idealised parent imago[1] (idealising transference).

Unlike Freud, Kohut separated developmental lines for narcissism from those for object love as though they are two entirely different processes.

Narcissism in the transference: mirror and idealising transferences

In mirror transference the grandiose self of the developing infant or individual in treatment passes through a stage when there is recognition of the object only as a replica of the grandiose self. The grandiose, narcissistic infant self recognises the existence of mother, but only feels the mother to be a replica of itself.

The idealised parent imago develops in parallel with the grandiose self (and the mirror transference in therapy) in stages beginning with the earliest infantile merging of the self with an omnipotent idealised object to make a barrier against narcissistic vulnerability and trauma. This barrier maintains the narcissistic perception of mother as a replica of the grandiose self. With greater developmental maturity, at a stage corresponding with the oedipal period, when in optimal conditions the parents are seen as mainly separate and are invested with both love and hate, the idealised parents are instead experienced as embodiments of power and perfection (Ornstein, 1978).

---

1. Imago is Freud's word for the unconscious representation of an object.

Shame, narcissistic rage and splitting

Kohut felt that shame and rage emerge clinically as typical reactions when the existing narcissistic equilibrium in a patient is disturbed. Shame follows the failure of selfobjects to provide mirroring, approval and admiration of the relentless exhibitionism of a grandiose self. In early childhood the expression of narcissistic rage is age appropriate. It is the forerunner of a myriad of forms that aggression can take in later life. Narcissistic rage indicates a grandiose self that responds in fury at the injury it feels when it perceives its own failure to control, either its own functions, or the functions of its omnipotent selfobjects. In the transference this means rage aimed at the therapist.

Working with transferences in adult psychoanalytic therapy, Kohut suggested that during treatment he had been able effectively to piece together or 'reconstruct' the traumatic experiences that caused splits in the self. These splits in effect are forms of emotional disavowal that correspond to the familiar defences of denial and repression.

Kohut's theory of therapeutic change: transmuting internalisation

According to Kohut the creation of new permanent psychic structures within the ego and superego in development and during treatment occurs through transmuting internalisation. This is the gradual, or at times more sudden, relinquishment of the functions of the archaic selfobjects, the idealised objects and the Oedipal objects (Fig. 3.1). To begin with these functions are performed by the object ('mother') on behalf of the child (or the adult patient). When that person's self is ready, Kohut believed that they can be internalised in transmuted forms by virtue of being broken up, and withdrawn from the object into a new intrapsychic structure in a similar manner to that of mourning. If the therapist can mobilise and maintain empathic attunement, a narcissistic patient can progress. Using these characteristic forms of regression and selfobject transferences, reflecting development failure during childhood, an adult can belatedly make use of transmuting internalisation to acquire new, more mature ego and superego structures, new self-formation and new capacity for relationship.

Kohut's theory of narcissistic development and transmuting internalisation evolved from work with severely narcissistic individuals, but can also be used to understand lesser degrees of personality disturbance and the part played by narcissism in human experience and development in general.

John Bowlby: attachment theory

John Bowlby (1907–1990), a child psychiatrist and psychoanalyst, was influenced by his experiences with delinquent youngsters and by reading the work of the ethologist Konrad Lorenz (Lorenz, 1952). Bowlby used

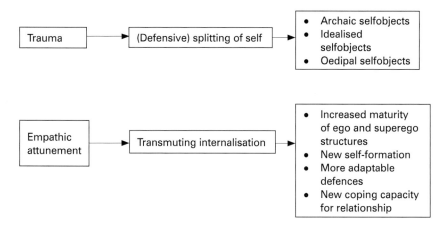

Fig. 3.1 Comparison of the effects of trauma and empathic attunement

the newly emerging science of ethology to link psychoanalysis again to its 'biological' origins through his attachment theory (Holmes, 1993*a*, *b*).

The biological origins of psychodynamic theory can be lost in the wide social application of psychoanalytic ideas that has taken place since Freud founded psychoanalysis. An antithesis between 'biology' and 'psychodynamics' may seem most marked with object relations theories that emphasise the personal social environment of the developing child within the family more than they emphasise the child's internal biological needs. However, if the child is viewed as meeting its biological needs by making dependent relationships, the dichotomy fades away.

Freud, being a neurologist, originally formulated psychoanalysis as a bridge between physical biological bodily states and mental experience. Instincts are linked to bodily functions and needs. Body-related instinctual drives within the mind make the bridge when they become psychological experiences as motives, emotions and thoughts. Attachment theory adds a further dimension to the understanding of the biological basis of motivation and behaviour. Studies of birds and primates suggest that feeding is not necessarily the main intermediary in the infant–mother relationship.

Attachment is the name given to the observable state and quality of an individual's attachments as well as that individual's experience of them. Attachments may be secure or insecure. The nature of the human attachment relationship alters when the infant is about 7-months-old to become what Bowlby regarded as attachment proper and called the primary attachment relationship. Before this age foster children may move family without extreme outward reactions, but typically after about 7-months-of-age stranger anxiety usually appears. Separation from the attachment figure in young children, and illness, fatigue or fear in adults, evokes proximity seeking. Separation from an attachment figure results in separation protest with angry striving for reunion.

The secure base phenomenon results when a person feels securely attached; young children who feel safe in this way feel able to engage in exploratory behaviour. The more attachment behaviour there is (i.e. seeking and clinging to an attachment figure) the less exploratory behaviour is possible and vice versa. Loss (lasting separation) injures the means of feeling secure and curtails exploration and general interest in the environment.

The influence of attachment continues throughout life and healthy development aims not so much for complete separateness and total independence as moving from dependence to mature dependence. The internal working model is a map that each person has of likely patterns of interaction between themselves and their attachment figures.

A significant amount of empirical research, particularly carried out in North America, has used measures devised specifically to investigate attachment patterns in Bowlby's theory. The Strange Situation Test (Ainsworth *et al*, 1978) and the Adult Attachment Interview (George *et al*, 1984) were devised and used by Mary Ainsworth and Mary Main. From this research they have outlined several different forms of attachment:

- anxious–avoidant
- secure
- ambivalent/anxious (or resistant)
- disorganised
- reverse attachment.

Reverse attachment is a newly added subcategory of anxious–avoidant attachment in which the child clings to acts of parenting the parent. These common patterns of attachment behaviour are remarkably consistent and durable for each individual person. They also appear as relationship patterns that psychoanalytic therapists observe and hear about in therapy sessions.

Bereavement, grief and mourning

Bereavement, grief and mourning are crises within the life cycle of an individual or group, but are also an integral aspect of normal living.

Freud formulated successful mourning as the way in which a bereaved person comes to accept that they will not be outwardly reunited with their lost loved one but instead internalises the lost person in the form of an internal object. Bowlby and Colin Murray Parkes (Bowlby, 1980; Parkes, 1972) studied reactions to separation and loss, especially in grief and mourning, and described the attachment behaviour that mediates this process in a series of steps:

- numbing
- distress and anger
- yearning and searching

- disorganisation and despair
- reorganisation.

Bowlby showed that children mourn in essentially the same way as adults, and that the sequence of events after a profound loss is similar to the sequence of the young child who has lost an attachment figure:

- protest
- despair
- detachment.

Bowlby's theory of normal attachment behaviour and psychoanalytic theories of regression and pathology

Bowlby felt that the potential for attachment behaviour is active throughout life. Therefore it is an error that attachment behaviour in an adult is indicative of pathology or of regression to immature behaviour. He rejected other psychoanalytic theories of regression that are based on orality and dependency as being out of keeping with the evidence. Psychopathology for Bowlby occurs because development has followed a deviant pathway, not because of fixation and regression to an earlier stage. In Bowlby's attachment theory common developmental diversions result in:

- anxious attachment; when attachment behaviour is elicited too easily
- partial or complete deactivation of attachment behaviour.

The pathway along which an individual's attachment behaviour develops and the ways that it becomes organised are a result of the experiences that the person has had with attachment figures while growing up through infancy, childhood and adolescence. Bowlby held the view that the way that a person's attachment behaviour organises in their personality determines the pattern of affectional bonds that person makes during the whole of life.

The place of Bowlby's theory in psychodynamic practice

There is no specific Bowlby school of psychotherapy and his greatest influence has been on child care practice. Nevertheless, attachment theory can be applied in clinical practice if the psychotherapy setting is regarded as a secure base, and the transference relationship as an interplay of attachment bonds.

In Bowlby's opinion, the attachment bond and the motive to form it represent an underlying instinctual impulse different from, but of the same order as, feeding, sexual and aggressive instincts. Attachment bonds continue to operate while, on the surface, different stages of attachment behaviour are activated or terminated by different situations. For example, attachment behaviour may be activated by strangeness, fatigue, anything frightening, or the unavailability or unresponsiveness of an attachment figure such as the parent for the child. In the transference, the therapist may fall into these roles for the patient. The resultant attachment behaviour may be terminated or altered by circumstances such as finding a familiar environment, or the ready availability and responsiveness of an attachment figure. When strongly aroused, attachment behaviour may not be brought to a halt without touching or clinging or an equivalent actively reassuring behaviour from the attachment figure (Bowlby, 1980).

In therapy this means that the therapist may respond to anxiety in the transference and threats to the therapeutic alliance between patient and therapist, by reassuring rather than interpreting (Holmes, 1996). Many psychoanalysts have felt that Bowlby's aim in this was quite different from the psychoanalytic aim of uncovering hidden meanings, and that psychotherapy based on attachment theory is different in principle from psychoanalysis. Others feel that some degree of enactment of mutual attachment is an inevitable part of any psychoanalytical encounter with a patient, and that therefore the distinction is more one of emphasis than absolute.

Psychodynamic psychiatrists, psychotherapists and psychoanalysts continue to be divided over attachment theory. By combining empirical research with psychoanalytic insight into the significance of early relationships, attachment theory provides an approach to the basic question for all psychodynamic theories of how externally observable behaviour and internal mental experience are to be linked together. In summary, attachment theory continues to be widely influential but is not universally accepted.

Mentalisation, attachment and borderline personality disorder

Peter Fonagy, a British contemporary Freudian psychoanalyst with active research interests in developmental psychology and attachment theory, has elaborated a theory of the development of self, based on both attachment within the social environment of the young child and on the capacity of the healthy young child to observe and internalise responsive states of mind in another human being. He called this capacity mentalisation. While this is necessary for healthy self-development, failure of mentalisation may occur through the interaction of the genetic vulnerability of the child and failure of the social caring (attachment) environment surrounding the child, leading in severe failure to borderline personality disorder. Mentalisation is the capacity to recognise both the mind of another person and one's own mind, not simply as a mirroring reflection of one another but as an agent of mutual interpretation and response. Beginning in the infant, who is in an emotionally significant relationship, mentalisation is the capacity to observe the ability of the other to interpret both their own and the infant's own states of mind, and through this to think of mutual human interaction in mental state terms.

Within a secure attachment environment, mentalisation leads to mutual emotional responsiveness. Frequently, vulnerable children who have grown up in abusive circumstances seem to close their minds to the minds of others as if the idea that their attachment figures harbour malevolent intent towards them is too painful to conceive. Instead they may develop the characteristic paradoxical combination of seeking physical proximity and clinging, but at the same time seeking mental distance. When the resulting mental state is closed to mutual intersubjectivity and therefore closed to mentalisation, the outcome may be borderline personality disorder.

Based on this theory of mentalisation, Bateman and Fonagy have manualised a treatment regime for borderline personality disorder they call mentalisation-based treatment combining group and individual psychoanalytic psychotherapy within a partial hospitalisation setting (Bateman & Fonagy, 2004).

Kleinian and post-Kleinian psychoanalysis

The term 'Kleinian' is commonly used for:
- Melanie Klein's personal approach
- later 'post-Kleinian' developments by other Kleinians, especially Wilfred Bion.

The existence of a distinct post-Kleinian group depends on a view that Bion and some of his Kleinian colleagues significantly surpassed Klein's own work. This idea has been advanced by Bion's supporters, notably Donald Meltzer.

Donald Meltzer

Meltzer (1922–2004) was an American child psychiatrist with a special interest in children with psychotic disorders and autism. He settled in the UK after training in psychoanalysis with Klein in London. While he retained a special interest in work with children, he was also at the forefront of those post-Kleinians who observed how borderline personality can represent a perverse personality structure organised around destructive aggression. His detailed studies of the analytic process during sessions has been widely influential, as was his account of the work of Freud, Klein and Bion (Hinshelwood, 1989). In particular in his later work he cultivated and promoted Bion's theory of thinking and experiencing.

Wilfred Bion

Wilfred Bion (1897–1979) is widely known in psychiatry for his pioneering approach to groups (see Chapter 9, Group psychotherapy). In fact group work only occupied him for a relatively short period during and shortly after the Second World War. From the 1950s onwards he concentrated on psychoanalysis with individuals. The range and originality of his work was perhaps second only to Klein herself within the Kleinian group (Hinshelwood, 1989). Bion, who had been born in India, had settled for most of his life in Britain, also travelled widely promoting a Kleinian approach in South America, and settled for a time in the 1970s in California before returning to Britain shortly before his death.

Klein based her theories of infant development on the analysis of children from about 2.5 years upwards in age. Bion, with a group of Kleinian psychoanalysts, concentrated instead on the treatment of adults with psychotic disorders. Their work assumed that the apparently senseless thinking of these individuals can be understood.

Klein's paranoid–schizoid position, with its distinctive quality of anxiety and defence, was used to formulate the kind of disturbed object relations with early infantile qualities that patients with schizophrenia bring into the transference. This led to detailed studies of the process of thinking used by these patients. These observations were then related also to narcissism, borderline states, confusional states and theories that link some forms of homosexual expression, and fear of homosexuality, with paranoia.

Psychotic and non-psychotic parts of the mind

Freud had distinguished neurosis from psychosis in terms of the reality principle. The ego seeks to know reality through the internal and external senses, by thinking and through consciousness. In neurosis, when instinctual needs are in conflict with the reality that the ego senses, instinctual needs (part of the id) are repressed in the service of the reality principle. In psychosis, conflict of this kind is resolved by abandoning the reality principle and finding some substitute, such as a delusion or hallucination. Freud introduced the idea that we all have some capacity for psychotic thought defined in this way – as a tendency to withdraw from external reality.

Klein saw anxiety as the key to understanding psychosis. She suggested that the earliest anxieties in normal infancy are psychotic in nature and ordinarily are 'bound, worked through and modified' in the course of development. Binding and working through are both concepts first introduced by Freud to explain symptom formation and resolution. Binding refers to the way that anxiety can be stabilised in the mind, for example attached to a symptom or to a positive developmental step, instead of being freely expressed as conscious anxiety. Working through is the psychic work involved in removing both repression and the compulsion to repeat. When infant development is disordered, instead of binding, working through and modifying, insufficiently modified primitive anxieties and terrifying figures can dominate the mind of the infant, and similarly the mind of the adult with psychotic disorder. The ego typically then uses excessive defensive splitting and projective identification to survive this internal situation.

Rosenfeld noticed how the psychotic patient quickly forms what he called a transference psychosis in which instantly formed projective identification with the therapist takes the place of more easily comprehensible forms of communication (Rosenfeld, 1954).

Bion described psychotic parts and non-psychotic parts of the mind (Bion, 1957). The psychotic personality or psychotic part of the personality arises from avoidance of having consciousness, instead of tolerating it: a state of mind rather than a psychiatric diagnosis. Consciousness in this context is as Freud defined 'a sense organ for the perception of psychical qualities' (Grinberg *et al*, 1975). As an internal state of mind, Bion regarded the psychotic part of the personality as always coexisting with a non-psychotic part of the personality. A psychotic state in part of the mind may or may not give rise to outward behaviour that leads to a psychiatric diagnosis of psychosis, depending on the balance of psychotic and non-psychotic parts.

In the psychotic personality, destructive impulses and deep intolerance of frustration result in violent hatred of internal and external reality. Love is turned into sadism, and the struggle between life and death instincts continues without end or resolution. Fear of annihilation predisposes in the transference, and elsewhere, to the hasty establishment of precarious and fragile relationships that are nevertheless tenaciously grasped. Aggressive attack directed towards the self mutilates the perceptual senses, damaging the link in the mind with both loved and hated objects, destroying mental activities such as thinking, and transforming them in unconscious fantasy into what Bion called emotionally charged 'particles' that are violently expelled through pathological projective identification. Once 'evacuated' these particles are fantasised as being independent and therefore beyond control. Having previously threatened from within, they are now experienced as dangerous threats from outside.

The non-psychotic part of the personality characteristically strives to maintain contact with reality. For example, whatever psychotic parts also exist, a patient usually attends psychotherapy sessions because a non-psychotic part of the personality recognises a need and recognises that something needs to be done about it.

'Pathological' and 'normal' projective identification

Bion clarified how projective identification can be recognised in 'normal' as well as 'pathological' forms:

- pathological projective identification occurs as a violent primitive defence of the kind observed in the psychotic part of a personality functioning mainly in the paranoid–schizoid position
- normal projective identification is the attribution of parts of the self (internal objects) to others (external objects) in the form of empathy operating largely within the depressive position.

Projective identification and the concept of container and contained

Bion applied the relationship container/contained:

container ◄─────► contained

to the form of projective identification in which an infant projects those parts of the mind having uncontrollable emotions into the good breast container (mother).

In Bion's theory of container/contained, when the infant projects parts of the mind that contain uncontrollable emotions into the good breast container, these parts of the mind and their associated feelings are emotionally detoxified by the container (in reality by the active participation of a more mature thinking and feeling mind, typically that of mother) and then are received back by the infant in a more tolerable form. This can be part of the normal empathic relationship that promotes healthy development, or when suffused with excessive envy, container and contained may be pathologically stripped of personal meaning and the capacity for developmental growth. In this sense container and contained refers to the relevant part of mother (container) and the relevant part of the infant (contained) in relation one to another.

By extension, the active process in a psychotherapist's mind (container) of thinking and feeling about the patient (contained) is an essential component of therapy. Therefore psychoanalytic psychotherapy takes place within a reciprocal (although asymmetrical) relationship that always includes consideration of what is going on in:

- the patient's mind
- the analyst's mind
- the transference
- the progress of treatment as a whole.

Joseph Sandler: projective identification, communication and actualisation

The contemporary Freudian psychoanalyst Joseph Sandler (1927–1998) critically appraised the theory of projective identification and connected it as a central post-Kleinian concept with contemporary Freudian practice. He did this by adopting the term actualisation for the way that one person in a particular emotional state through their behaviour induces the same feelings in another person's actual experience (Sandler, 1987).

Projective identification in post-Kleinian theory is both a means of communication between individuals through exchanges of emotion and unconscious fantasy, and refers to an individual's fantasy (as a solely internal activity). Bion used projective identification in both ways, without separate terms for the fantasy and for the actual behaviour that evokes a feeling in the other person. This dual use is confusing and has invited criticism.

From Sandler's point of view actualised projective identification is a wish fulfilment within an object relations framework. Sandler uses the example of a child who has a wish to cling, and as part of this wish has a mental representation of clinging to someone else, but also has a representation of that object responding to his clinging. When these role relationships appear in the transference and are actualised they represent a wishful aspect of unconscious fantasy life to which the receptive analyst or therapist responds in actual countertransference emotional experience.

Schizophrenia, splitting, projective identification: Rosenfeld and Segal

Kleinian accounts of pioneering psychoanalytic treatment with adult patients with schizophrenia were published by Rosenfeld in 1947 and Segal in 1950. Herbert Rosenfeld (1909–1986) was a refugee from pre-war Germany who moved into psychoanalysis while working in British general psychiatry with patients with schizophrenia. Hanna Segal came from Poland, trained in medicine and psychoanalysis in Britain, and settled in London. They demonstrated the importance of two mental mechanisms in schizophrenia:

- splitting
- projective identification.

Splitting and projective identification are often in this context also referred to as primitive or psychotic defences. In schizophrenia they contribute to instablity of the ego and instability of its identity, loss of affect, cognitive defects and impairment of symbol formation (Hinshelwood, 1989).

Rosenfeld's first patient with schizophrenia used splitting so that the patient felt not only divided in herself but that her thoughts and her actions were fragmented many times over. When this was associated with omnipotent fantasy of concretely getting inside the analyst, the patient experienced herself as omnipotently located in pieces within the analyst and confused with the analyst. In other words this individual experienced confusion through fragmentary splitting and projective identification with the analyst.

Segal discovered that when her patients with schizophrenia began to experience depression, this part of the patient's ego, finding the experience intolerable, would be split off and projected into the analyst. This gave the individual a superficial appearance of lack of affect and therefore an appearance also of failing to form transference (a feature that Freud had thought to be characteristic of psychosis). It is worth noting that this kind of projected depression, when experienced by the doctor or therapist of an individual with schizophrena, may contribute to undue pessimism about the possibility of successful treatment over and above their realistic judgement about the severity of the individual's impairment (which may also, of course, lead to a pessimistic outlook). Many psychoanalysts have in fact followed Freud's lead in feeling little psychotherapeutic optimism with individuals with schizophrenia.

Symbolic equation and symbol formation proper

Segal (1957) distinguished symbolic equation and symbol formation proper:

- symbolic equation is in the paranoid–schizoid position; the subject confuses the object with the symbol; the symbol is the product, in Bion's terms, of pathological projective identification. Segal's example is of the man who cannot play the violin because he believes he is masturbating in public (he cannot distinguish the fantasy from the concrete reality).

- symbol formation proper occurs in the depressive position when the symbol represents the object, but is not believed actually to be the object. Any violin player may know that violin playing can represent an erotic act while being clear that it is not the sexual act itself. This is a more mature developmental state of mind.

Bion's theory of thinking and knowledge

Bion was interested in philosophies of science often regarded as opposed to psychoanalysis, particularly empiricism and positivism. His theory of the origins of thinking bridges between psychodynamic theory and cognitive science, and with Emmanuel Kant's widely influential philosophical theory of knowledge. Bion's theory of thinking is based on the Kleinian approach to projective identification and symbolism.

Bion investigated three ways in which the mental activity of thinking occurs:

1. Pre-conception and conception. Pre-conception of 'something', for example a breast, meets a positive realisation of that 'thing' (in the example, an actual breast) giving rise to a conception. For Bion the pre-conception is an innate capacity, a form of predesigning as it would be called in developmental psychology (Stern, 1985), similar to Klein's idea that the infant has an inherent notion in unconscious fantasy of the mother and the breast.

2. Transformation of negative realisation. If a pre-conception meets a negative realisation (no satisfying breast is there) then the infant's capacity to endure frustration is tested. A frustrating object is felt to be a bad object. Bion suggested that if the infant has sufficient capacity to withstand the frustration then the 'no breast experience' is transformed into a thought. This is the first step towards being able to link frustration to the idea that there is, nevertheless, a good object that is absent at least for the moment.

   Alternatively, if the infant's capacity for tolerating frustration is low, the absence is likely to be experienced not as the existence of a good breast that is absent, but as a bad breast that is present. Because of its dangerous persecutory presence it may be omnipotently disposed of by projection. If excessive this prevents both symbols and thinking from developing.

3. Container and contained. The infant's experience of container and contained as already described provides the third model of thinking. The infant evacuates bad feeling and behaves in ways that evoke the same kind of feeling in mother. What happens next depends on the mother's capacity for reverie. Reverie is the mother's capacity to accept feelings actively, to process and 'metabolise' feelings into more tolerable forms, and thereby avoid impulsively returning bad feeling like an infant

herself. Bion called this kind of transformation alpha (α) function. If it goes well, the infant re-introjects (takes back in) feelings that can now be experienced as tolerable. Also in time the child takes in the alpha function itself for future use.

This is how growth can begin in the infant's ability to tolerate frustration and use symbols and thought. This is required for the emotional process of learning from experience. If instead the infant identifies with a parent who wilfully misunderstands and rejects such feeling, or if the infant cannot tolerate the mother's capacity for reverie because of excessive envy, then the infant develops internal objects that reject reality testing, reject symbolisation proper and rational thought, and therefore predispose towards psychosis.

In essence, Bion's theory of knowledge states that a subject makes a link with an object in order to know it. Knowledge therefore implies the existence of an object relationship. The links involved in knowledge are part of the emotional experience when two people, or two parts of a person, are in relationship one to the other. According to Bion there are three emotions that are intrinsic to this kind of link between two objects:

- love
- hate
- knowledge.

Bion's use of mathematical symbols

Bion's method of writing included mathematical symbols so that each idea can be thought about without premature conception of the underlying, unknown mental operations. The example given in the previous section is of Bion calling the most rudimentary form of thinking α function. This operates on sensory impressions and emotions to form α elements. They are the prerequisites of symbolisation and language in dreams and conscious thought.

Bion arranged the mathematical symbols into a grid of mental functions and elements. Detailed description of the grid is beyond the scope of this book. In the main, it is only used by those with a specialised interest in Bion. In reading Bion, whose style is dense, it is helpful to notice that at the same time as describing a particular function he requires the reader to use that method of thinking. To think about his concept of α function it is necessary to use one's own alpha function and α elements stimulated by the use of the abstract mathematical sign 'α'.

Thinking, Oedipal situations and attacks on linking

Bion also introduced a further function or process, the dynamic interaction between paranoid–schizoid position (Ps) and depressive position (D):

Ps ◄───► D

The paranoid–schizoid position (Ps) involves omnipotent strategies for avoiding the experience of pain, thereby bypassing creative adaptation. In the depressive position (D) knowledge can be used to modify psychological pain, with potential for creative adaptation as a result. Any individual is at all times somewhere between these two positions, moving dynamically between them.

There is a cross-reference to note here with the Oedipus complex in Freudian theory. The Oedipus myth from classical Greek mythology was used by Freud to illustrate a phase of development. Clinical reappraisal has highlighted how each child generates a private myth if he or she is to understand and know, or link, a relationship with the parental couple. Bion observed that this private myth, which he regarded as the link that forms the basis of all knowledge, can suffer destructive attacks from excessive envy, greed and sadism. In the clinical situation, understanding and creatively surviving these attacks on linking is a central task for the psychotherapist.

In essence, within the transference/countertransference relationship, in what Sandler would describe as the actualised form of projective identification, attacks on linking are experienced by the analyst as an inability within oneself to think and to know what is happening between oneself and the patient. The psychotherapist's experience of this may be as though one's own apparatus for learning from experience has been fragmented and scattered.

Emotion and cognition

Bion lessened the divide between emotion and cognition through the concept of 'normal' or empathic as well as 'pathological' projective identification as a method of communicating, and through the concept of container/contained. The centrality of object relations was retained because it is through mental understanding of another person that an individual is able to develop their own mental understanding, to create a mind of their own, and to acquire awareness that others also have independently thinking minds.

Dispersal and disintegration, and integration

Bion also reformulated his concept of the development of thinking during fluctuation between paranoid–schizoid and depressive positions in terms of dispersal and disintegration versus integration:

Paranoid–schizoid position ◄─────► Depressive position

Dispersal and disintegration ◄─────► Integration

This can be criticised as an oversimplification, especially because narcissistic states of mind can intervene between the paranoid–schizoid and depressive positions. Nevertheless Bion's idea, although a simplification, is useful in clarifying a possible relationship between:

- thinking
- the achievement of a depressive position
- the integration of object relations within the framework of the Oedipal situation.

Recent post-Kleinian developments

Bion and the post-Kleinians who took up his ideas have raised the profile of thinking (cognition), within psychodynamic theory, which had previously been dominated by theories of emotion (affect), unconscious motivation (conation), and unconscious aspects of relatedness. That these core concepts should be joined by thinking as a basic mental function that transforms and alters perceptions and thoughts has especially been taken forward and developed in Britain by Edna O'Shaughnessy, Ronald Britton, and John Steiner.

Britton (1989) and O'Shaughnessy (1989) described how failure to integrate observation and experience represents failure to internalise any recognisable Oedipal triangle. The child's failure to realise the existence of the Oedipal situation is a failure to recognise the parents' relationship, a failure that characteristically arises from a previous failure of maternal containment. This occurs if pathological projective identification takes over as a way of coping with object relationships. Then the realisation of a third side to form a triangle of relationships is intolerably painful. This is because the third side is a link between the original object (mother or part of mother) and another object (father or part of father). Therefore, if recognised for what it is, it must be equated with no longer having exclusive omnipotent possession of the object (mother), and at the same time equated with a requirement to move from the paranoid–schizoid to depressive position.

The denial of the existence of an Oedipal triangle and failure to internalise the original object and her relation to a third person is characteristically an aggressive rejection of depressive pain and depressive realisation. This kind of denial is typically evident in borderline and narcissistic personality.

Such forms of defensive retreat have been variously described. Britton talks of Oedipal illusions. A number of post-Kleinian analysts including Betty Joseph, Donald Meltzer and Herbert Rosenfeld have described patients who seemed to achieve an uneasy stability somewhere between the paranoid–schizoid position and the depressive position, but gripped by a perverse relationship between destructive parts and dependent parts of the personality. This is a sexually exciting but essentially destructive, narcissistic process that blocks progress in treatment and prevents creative contact between patient and therapist. Steiner has argued for the use of the term pathological organisation to describe the outcome of this process. The pathological organisation is a state of mind that:

- achieves an equilibrium and developmental stasis
- avoids depressive anxiety and pain

- varies from individual to individual in the degree to which there is a malevolent and destructive influence on realistic thinking, on realistic perception and on emotional responsiveness within relationships (Steiner, 1987, 1993).

Perversions, narcissistic states and pathological organisations

There is no single universal definition of perversion that applies to all psychodynamic theories and all therapeutic situations. This mirrors the difficulty inherent in defining the boundaries of 'normal' sexuality. Perversions are sometimes defined as any sexual behaviour in which gratification through heterosexual intercourse is not the aim, but this definition is criticised for being over inclusive and judgemental. Alternatively perversion can be characterised as aggression that is masked by apparently erotic aims. The term perversion is also used within psychoanalytic theory to refer to normal aspects of infantile development in which a child expresses sexuality through bodily experience other than genital sexual intercourse.

Freud regarded infantile sexuality as being multiply perverse, including sadistic, masochistic, voyeuristic and homosexual elements (Hinshelwood, 1989). He also noted that perversion has a relationship with neurosis, in that the perverse individual enacts sexual impulses that the neurotic represses. In this view, a perverse relationship always implies some form of aggression and violence, in that there is a potential heterosexual relationship and Oedipal resolution that in unconscious fantasy is being destroyed or seriously distorted through the perversion.

Sadomasochistic violence aims to keep an object going so that the object can be made to suffer, distinct from self-preservative violence, which aims to remove danger and to neutralise a threatening object (Glasser, 1998).

Perverse mental mechanisms can be either:

- a system of defences (for example, defending against psychotic disintegration, confusion or helplessness), or
- a primary addiction aimed at erotic gratification.

Both forms of perverse organisation may exist simultaneously.

Sadism and sadistic cruelty occupied a central position in Klein's thinking about sexuality and aggression during childhood development, rather than forming part of a specific theory of perversions as such. However, the post-Kleinians Rosenfeld and Steiner both observed that perversion as an internal state of mind involves perverse relationships between different parts of the self that lead to narcissistic states and pathological organisations (Rosenfeld, 1971; Steiner, 1982, 1993).

Bion's theory as a bridge to object relations theory and self psychology

Through theories of thinking, particularly the concept of container and contained, Bion provided a bridge not only between Kleinian theory and those who developed object relations theory (such as Suttie, Fairbairn, Winnicott, Balint and Bowlby), but also with Kohut's self psychology. Object relations theory emphasises a personal environment and how a parent behaves with an infant, alongside the influence of the infant's internal fantasy of what is going on. Fairbairn, studying severe schizoid states, and Kohut, studying narcissistic states, both saw an apparent lack of Oedipal material in the treatment of these individuals. They argued that Freud and Klein were wrong in their opinion that the Oedipus complex or situation is a ubiquitous issue in all mental life (Klein's broad position), or at least central from a fairly early age in childhood onwards (Freud's broad position).

Post-Kleinians, following on from Bion, have refuted Fairbairn and Kohut on this issue. They see an apparent lack of Oedipal situations and the depressive position in the treatment of these individuals as being because these, on the contrary, are central, but psychic pain generated by these mental states leads to their rejection and the individual to retreat from them.

This is another aspect, alongside the contribution of perversion described in the last section, of how narcissistic states and pathological organisation arise in the development of personality and character disorders, notwithstanding the range of opinions that exist regarding the role of Oedipal situations in the implied splitting of the self and its object relations.

The British independent group

Fierce debate between the Freudians led by Anna Freud, and the Kleinians led by Melanie Klein crystallised in the British Psycho-analytic Society in the 1940s in what became known as the 'controversial discussions' (King & Steiner, 1991). The independents, formerly known as the 'middle' group, generally wished to agree wholeheartedly with neither the Freudians nor the Kleinians. Some trace their origins to the early years of the British Psycho-analytic Society before the arrival in London of Melanie Klein and Sigmund and Anna Freud. In practice, the British independents are a diverse group of psychoanalysts loosely united by an object relations approach, while also drawing on many classical Freudian and Kleinian ideas.

Object relations theory is a broad term for their theories that give a central place to object relationship and regard Freudian instinctual drives alone as insufficient to explain human relationships. The main strands of object relations theory as evolved by the independents are (Rayner, 1991):

- emotions (also referred to as 'affects' and as 'feelings') are the states of mind that allow intuitive evaluation of the current state of self and object relationship
- symbols and artistic creativity arise in emotional states between object and subject, in the beginning between infant and mother
- object and subject move rhythmically in and out of states of differentiation and combination.

Fairbairn, Winnicott, Balint and Bowlby are independents already considered in Chapter 2 (Psychodynamic theories I) and earlier in this chapter. The work of Paula Heimann (1899–1982) and of Masud Khan (1924–1989), to be described next, link those earlier independent theories to the work of contemporary independents from where the works of Christopher Bollas, Harold Stewart and Patrick Casement are selected as broadly representative.

De-differentiation: self and object combined or merged

It seems a paradox that human beings experience states of combination (merging) with objects, yet in order to experience a relationship in the first place there must be some differentiation between subject (self) and object (for example, mother). Rhythmic movement back and forth between differentiation and combination solves this apparent contradiction. States of combination, merging or de-differentiation between self and object have been described by many psychoanalytic writers of all persuasions.

The independents include:

- Marion Milner (illusion of unity)
- Margaret Little (basic unity)
- Michael Balint (primary love; object as primary substance)
- Donald Winnicott (merging; transitional phenomena; good enough environment; ordinary devoted mother; medium; primary maternal preoccupation; holding function of mother; facilitating environment)
- Masud Khan (protective shield)

Those from other schools who have also described these states include:

- Anna Freud (need-satisfying object)
- Heinz Hartmann (average expectable environment)
- René Spitz (mediator of the environment)
- Margaret Mahler (extra-uterine matrix).

Paula Heimann

Paula Heimann (1899–1982) in earlier years was a leading member of Klein's group in London. She clarified the distinction between aggression serving various forms of creative self-assertion upon the environment; and aggression in the service of cruelty in which natural aggressiveness is perverted into sadistic and masochistic impulses (Heimann, 1969).

This basic distinction led her in 1955 to break away with a group of former Kleinian psychoanalysts to join the independents. They disagreed with Klein's argument that envy always means aggressive death instinct and therefore is always destructive and sadistic (Klein, 1957). Among Heimann's group were analysts who recognised forms of envy that lead to creative emulation of the object and of good qualities possessed by the object.

Heimann also described as normal a capacity for temporary narcissistic withdrawal. This narcissism is part of the mastery of anal function, which she linked with the achievement of healthy independence in a young child's development and also with the capacity thereafter for creativity throughout life. Heimann observed that some narcissistic withdrawal is necessary for the individual to attend to bodily functions, particularly defaecation. Narcissistic withdrawal is also needed to support activities such as writing or other artistic endeavours. These activities generally involve the writer or artist in maintaining a state of relative social withdrawal and self-preoccupation in order to create an environment and frame of mind in which creative production can occur (Heimann, 1962). Heimann's observations on the link between anal characteristics and narcissism in healthy development can be contrasted with the description by Donald Meltzer of anality and narcissism in states of 'pseudomaturity', and by the American psychoanalyst Leonard Shengold who elaborated the relationship of body ego, anal defensiveness and narcissism in severe character pathology and perversion (Meltzer, 1966; Shengold, 1992).

The use of countertransference

Heimann's classic 1950 paper 'On counter-transference' was bold and concise:

- countertransference is a concept that covers all the analyst's emotional response experienced towards the patient
- it is the patient's creation
- it is an instrument for research into the patient's unconscious.

Heimann captured the mood of a new era in psychoanalysis, challenging the classical view of countertransference resistance, even though before this Ella Sharpe (1875–1947), in London, had already been teaching that the analytic relationship is an unfolding, serious dramatic play, in which the analyst is in a dialogue with his or her own feelings, and has those feelings available for use (Rayner, 1991).

In contrast to the simplicity of these earlier published views, Heimann later said that the psychoanalytic situation viewed as a relationship between two people implies two transferences, two resistances, two unconsciouses; and that the transference of the analyst on to the patient should be acknowledged and distinguished from what she meant as countertransference (Kohon, 1992). Pearl King has advocated a return to the original meaning of the term transference, namely the arousal in the analyst of a transference response to the patient related to the analyst's own unconscious needs that may be inappropriate and alien to an understanding of the patient at that moment. King prefers to refer to the totality of emotions that an analyst has towards a patient as the analyst's affective response (King, 1992).

Heimann's study of countertransference was a major turning point and prepared the way for a development that has spread throughout Kleinian, contemporary Freudian and independent practice. Psychoanalysts and therapists today make greater use of their countertransference experiences (i.e. what it feels like to be with the patient) as an additional source of information about the patient, reflecting what the patient may be experiencing, or what the patient may be projecting into the analyst to avoid experiencing themselves. Heimann was very critical of those who regarded her work on countertransference as a carte blanche to justify any interpretation on the sole evidence of the analyst's own feelings without checking that the patient's communications provide evidence in themselves. However, countertransference observations are particularly useful to direct an analyst's attention to emotionally charged issues that might otherwise be overlooked.

Masud Khan

Masud Khan (1924–1989) was described by his obituarist Adam Limentani as 'gifted and disturbed'; 'full of contradictions' and 'leaving behind a remarkable degree of hostility and criticism'. The final years of his life were marked by eccentric and abrasive behaviour, mutilating surgery for cancer, and personal alienation. Transgressions beyond acceptable limits of professional behaviour by socialising with patients and trainees and exploiting his position, led to his removal from the status of training analyst. Khan's fall should stand as a firm reminder that ethical behaviour of the highest order is required for psychotherapy of any kind in keeping with the personal trust involved between patient and analyst. He was expelled altogether from the British Psycho-analytical Society after publishing his last book *When Spring Comes*, about which 'not even Khan's best friends have been able to find anything good to say' (Limentani, 1992).

To leave out Khan altogether as too controversial and inconsistent would be to ignore the influence and quality of his prolific earlier writing. Khan ranged widely, connecting Balint, Fairbairn and Winnicott with Kleinian and more recent independent perspectives. Over many years there had been a trend in psychodynamic theory towards emphasising traumatising influences that occur very early in infancy. This was the focus for Fairbairn, Balint, Winnicott and Bowlby. Khan redirected attention back to the effects of trauma occurring later in life than infancy in keeping with the classical Freudian tradition. Khan also added the new concept of cumulative trauma (Khan, 1974). This is the idea that trauma can operate silently and repeatedly with effects remaining hidden until they surface later in adolescence.

Khan on character and perversion

Fairbairn and Winnicott analysed character impairments; Fairbairn did this through his theory on schizoid character as the interaction of sub-selves within split internal mental structure; and Winnicott did it through his theory of false self, in which false self as pathological defence disinherits true self, because true self requires transitional activity (rather than defensive activity) to flourish. Both Fairbairn and Winnicott had been influenced by Klein, but also then departed from her theories. Winnicott also felt his theories to be at odds with Fairbairn's position.

Khan integrated the ideas of Fairbairn and Winnicott in a theory of schizoid character and perversion. His theory also extended Klein's concept of reparation, i.e. repair of an object that has in fantasy been damaged. Khan's theory was that a perversion is an attempt at repairing damaged narcissistic feeling about the self (Khan, 1979).

In Khan's view narcissistic damage in perversions, in both women and men, is the result of developmental failure of self (sometimes also referred to as ego) integration in the face of deficiencies in the mother and child relationship. Emotional need, existential fear of the self's own nothingness, and aggression, are all hidden in specific perverse activities. These perverse activities are sexual forms of manic defence, and seek to involve another person in a kind of transitional state in which temporary loss of separate identities is a manipulative substitute for authentic intimacy. The French analysts Joyce McDougall and Janine Chassaguet-Smirgel, known in the English-speaking world for their writings on psychosomatic illness and gender disorders, have followed a similar line, particularly in McDougall's 'neo-sexualities' (Chassaguet-Smirgel, 1984; McDougall, 1986).

Christopher Bollas

Christopher Bollas is an American settled in the UK and a member of the British independent group of psychoanalysts, whose first academic career was in English literature. He was especially influenced by Winnicott's concept of transitional activity in the development of a capacity to symbolise. Transitional activity is critical for healthy character growth. Character defects arise from damage or distortion to the transitional ability to symbolise emotions (Rayner, 1991).

Bollas conceives character as a quality of being separate in identity as an individual, yet emotionally open to others, and that this is a state of mind achieved through individual creativity. Drawing on Freud's classical vision of the dream as a model for all unconscious mental experience and individual creativity, he suggests that emotionally significant experiences in everyday life in healthy individuals are constantly broken down in the mind and recombined.

Thus, a classical emphasis on reconstructing the past to give meaning to an individual's personal history in ordinary health or during psychotherapy takes on a new significance in the present. The present moment in time for any person is always made up by breaking down and recombining emotional experiences from the past in ways that inform current experience. This reconstructed history makes up both consciously known identity and unconscious experience of self. It can be open to new interpretation and creative understanding of experience, or it can be closed and a stultifying experience of clinging defensively to rigidified representations of the past (Bollas, 1992, 1995).

91

Harold Stewart: control, collusion, aggression and regression

The British independent psychoanalyst Harold Stewart (1925–2005) began his career as a general practitioner studying hypnotherapy before shifting his attention to psychoanalysis, searching for 'a more sensitive, productive and far-reaching method of exploring patients' problems' (Stewart, 1992). He explored control and collusion between patient and therapist in the Oedipal situation and in its equivalent in Greek mythology, through the idea that there was knowing collusion in their sexual crime between Jocasta and Oedipus. They represent mother and son, as well as therapist and patient in a transference relationship. Control and collusion play a role in hypnosis. Stewart noted that hypnosis is impossible once a patient is freed to contradict and hence be consciously aggressive to the hypnotist. Remaining close to clinical experience, he recognised aggression working in 'healthy' ways as well as working 'pathologically'. As illustrated by the patient who contradicts the hypnotist in an act of adaptive independence, freedom of aggressiveness within the limits necessary to counter the influence of excessive control is necessary for development and for the autonomous self to flourish.

Stewart follows a trend within the independent analysts group not necessarily to speculate theoretically about whether there is an innate basis for aggression as well as aggression secondary to frustration. This lends a different emphasis to destructive aggression compared with Kleinian theory, even though Stewart, like his teacher Balint and like Winnicott, was sympathetic to much of Klein's thinking. The concept of therapeutic regression is another area in which they depart from Kleinian theory.

Regression has held a central but controversial place in psychodynamic theory. The basic concept of regression is that of returning to some stage of early childhood experience by returning to an earlier state of mind, and to an earlier mode of functioning.

Freudian theory emphasises defensive regression in which the subject avoids anxiety by returning to earlier developmental stages (of libido and ego) called fixation-points. While a significant body of opinion regards any regression as therapeutically unhelpful, Fairbairn, Balint, Winnicott and Khan are prominent among those who have described therapeutic regression as a factor for potential psychological growth and change. Harold Stewart drawing particularly on the work of Michael Balint, elaborates this theory.

Beneficial change during regression is referred to as benign regression. Adverse change during regression is referred to as malignant regression.

Regression is also an example of a therapeutic factor that is not a classical Freudian transference interpretation. It is part of a broader independent view that transference interpretation is not the only factor that can bring about therapeutic change in a patient. Stewart (1992, p. 118) strikes a particularly clear balance. This is not to 'deny or denigrate the vital importance of interpretative work; it is to dispute its exclusive role as a therapeutic agent in analysis'.

The explicit concept of therapeutic regression is virtually absent from the current literature of both contemporary Freudians and Kleinians. Yet a wide range of psychodynamic ideas touch implicitly on the topic of regression and some post-Kleinian concepts are particularly useful in understanding and dealing creatively with regression. These include Bion's containment and contemporary reappraisals of the Oedipal situation which bridge with the concept of pathological organisations.

The post-Kleinian formulation of pathological organisations links to unresolved Oedipal issues, but this is not an explicit connection made in Stewart's writing. The distinction between benign and malignant regression also overlaps with Fairbairn's formulation of dependence, and bridges to self psychology and to Kernberg's work with borderline states (Bacal & Newman, 1990). Here then is a prime example of apparently divergent psychodynamic theories converging around a common theme.

Patrick Casement: internal supervision and trial identification

Casement's book *On Learning From the Patient* (Casement, 1985) quickly established itself as a standard reference for psychotherapists working in all settings. Subsequently he expanded on his earlier work in a sequel *Further Learning From the Patient* (Casement, 1990). In the independent group tradition orthodox Freudian emphasis on transference interpretation is combined with post-Kleinian developments. He suggests factors other than interpretation of the transference can be effective in bringing about change in a patient.

Casement uses the concepts of internal supervision by the analyst directed at his or her own responses, and trial identification with the patient, so that the analyst maintains touch with the patient's point of view and experience.

Criticism can be levelled against Casement that he does not take sufficient account of the devious, malicious nature of psychopathology that surfaces across the range of therapeutic settings, including depth psychoanalysis, less intense psychotherapy, or routine psychiatric consultations. Thus malign psychopathology can be observed arising from both the intrinsic nature of a patient's pre-existing psychopathology and malignant regression within the analytic session.

Both require emphasis in any balanced view. Casement's aim in this is not to discard 'tough-mindedness' on the part of the analyst but to examine additional factors that promote successful psychoanalytic therapy.

Therapeutic factors in psychodynamic psychotherapy

Those positive elements that make a difference to the mental state of a patient are sometimes called 'therapeutic factors'. The theme of these chapters is that there are differences of opinion about which factors are most important and valid, but there are also wide areas of overlap between the main psychoanalytic groups on this specific question of what kind of patient and therapist 'activities' contribute to a satisfactory outcome.

Stewart (1992) and Casement (1985, 1990) provide examples of this kind of inclusive approach to the application of theory to clinical practice. In this final section we draw together their accounts and offer a summary of the principal therapeutic factors, some or all of which may determine outcome in any particular psychodynamic psychotherapeutic encounter.

Therapeutic factors can be grouped under the following headings:

- attitude, or general stance of the therapist towards their patient
- qualities that emerge in the relationship between analyst and patient
- the aims of psychotherapy in terms of internal psychic structures
- the aims in terms of more external clinically observable change
- specific therapist activities in psychotherapy that promote change
- the social environment within a session.

The attitude, or general stance of an analyst towards the patient may include:

- every effort being made to examine everything the patient says for what it tells about the transference
- therapist in a spirit of 'open mindedness' assuming that not everything the patient says is only about the transference; for example, what a patient says about the analyst may be true, not 'just' fantasy
- a state of mind of 'not knowing' being valued as well as that of 'knowing'
- recognition and valuing of the mutual nature of the positions of patient and analyst, as well as valuing contrasts between them
- the therapist following the patient and resisting dogmatic certainty about the meaning of what is happening in each session
- interpretation aimed at gaining fresh insight (as opposed to, for example, repeating cliché-ridden interpretations to the patient in a way that promotes intellectuality at the expense of emotional immediacy or authentic insight)
- the patient discovering as much as possible for themselves, but the therapist also being prepared to lead the way
- the therapist being prepared to be subjective but on the other hand recognising that his/her countertransference will be of no use to a patient unless it relates to where the patient's experience already is
- trauma may be felt to be repeated in psychotherapy, but this experience of repeating can be of therapeutic use only if what occurs in psychotherapy is clearly different from the original disaster
- the therapist assuming that a patient is aware of some hope, at least unconsciously, for the possibility of 'growth' and has some awareness of the needs that will sustain that growth.

Creative qualities in a relationship between therapist and patient may emerge as:

- space to play with feelings and ideas together
- the human warmth of empathy
- consistency and fairness
- the availability of therapist to be used by patient as a kind of self-extension
- that therapist can be trusted by patient to accept different feelings.

What is meant by psychic change is a complex issue that varies according to the theoretical stance from which the question is asked. In clinical practice, therapeutic psychic change will usually be related to the following three basic aims for internal structure:

- the aim of modifying the relationship between the id, ego, and superego by augmenting the influence of the ego and moderating the strength of both the superego and the id
- the aim of recovery of previously split off parts of the self and their re-integration
- the aim of altering the relationship between internal and external objects in terms of the paranoid–schizoid and depressive positions (taking account also of any idiosyncratic pathological organisations that may be interposed by the patient between these positions).

Some broad criteria for more external, clinically observable psychic change include:

- changes in the nature of the impulses, affects, and attitudes towards objects, both internal and external
- changes in the tolerance of impulses and affects, particularly anxiety, shame and guilt
- changes in the main modes of mental functioning, such as the modes of thinking and dreaming
- changes in dreams and dreaming in terms both of the dream content and the ways of experiencing dreams
- changes in the experiencing of self in terms of realness, fullness and wholeness
- changes in the presenting symptoms, although this in itself does not necessarily indicate permanent improvement.

Specific therapist activities that are agents for psychic change in psychoanalytic psychotherapy are as follows (Stewart, 1992):

- transference interpretations
- interpretations outside the transference, sometimes called 'extra-transference' interpretations
- reconstructions
- therapeutic regression
- techniques, other than interpretation, to overcome analytic impasse
- the therapist remaining silent, especially when the patient, filled with intense emotion, is recovering contact with a lost original object.

(Different types of therapist activity are further elaborated in Chapter 4.)

Different types of transference interpretation described from an object relations point of view can be summarised as follows (modified from Stewart, 1992):

- interpretations aimed at understanding drive–anxiety–defence conflicts between patient and analyst in a dependent type of relationship
- interpretations aimed at understanding the experiences and vulnerability of patient with the analyst in a narcissistic type of relationship
- an extension of the latter to include the interpretation of failure to achieve mutual understanding in the face of a narcissistic relationship
- interpretations aimed at understanding and clarifying the atmosphere or mood (identifying the affect) between patient and analyst, which might be in either type of object relationship, dependent or narcissistic
- interpretations aimed at understanding the patient's idiosyncratic unconscious response to the analyst's interpretations, which is especially relevant with a patient who is in a regressed phase of therapy.

Not included here under the heading of 'transference interpretation' are variations on the kind of vague reference by a therapist of all the material presented by the patient to the transference that lead to statements of the 'you-mean-me' kind, such as 'you feel this about me now', or 'you are putting your anger into me', or 'you are doing this to me', or 'you are making me experience your confusion'. Unless such observations as these are supported clinically by the patient's reported experience and associations, then they sound to a patient like magical thinking by the therapist, or a sign of the therapist's lack of understanding.

The social environment, as well as internal forces, influence the maturing self. Fairbairn, Balint, Bowlby and Winnicott all described the infant as primarily oriented towards finding affection within intimate relationships with other people, not merely oriented to oral libidinal satisfaction. The innate potential of an infant, or regressed child patient, or regressed adult patient, interacts with an environment. That interactive environment may be helpful and sympathetic, may be harsh and traumatic, or may be somewhere between these extremes. Psychopathology arises at this interface between innate potential and the interactive environment. It is also at this interface that psychodynamic psychotherapy and psychoanalysis operate effectively.

It follows that a psychodynamic therapist or analyst can think of themselves as a social environment for their patient in psychotherapy and find their own personal style and personal theoretical base from among the basic principles of psychoanalysis. A therapist can be not only a knowledge base but also a personal environment with whom patients engage.

The emphasis of interpretion alters according to whether the patient is:

- re-experiencing remembered earlier or recent traumatic events
- re-enacting distressing patterns of unconscious fantasy
- expressing aggression destructively towards self, therapist or the therapeutic situation as a whole.

At the same time as interpreting in words, the therapist may psychologically move to and fro in empathic closeness to, or observing distance from, the patient. This will be experienced by the patient as emotionally synergic with, or at the other extreme as confronting of, the patient's destructive and defensive strategies, i.e. the therapist moves between:

empathic closeness to patient ◄──► observing distance from patient

while the patient's experience potentially moves between:

emotional synergy with defences ◄──► confronting defences.

Conclusion

The independents emphasise an affectionate responsive human environment for healthy development in childhood and for creative change during therapy. In the classical Freudian tradition, innate instinct (libido and aggressive drives) underpin development and personality change. Kleinian and post-Kleinian approaches also emphasise innate characteristics rather than environmental factors, and therefore advocate that the *only* route to empathic emotional synergy is through interpretation of the patient's defensive and aggressive activities, because these defensive and aggressive activities are ubiquitous and universal (Kleinian and a strand of later Freudian theory). Others say defences and aggression are relative to experience in the human environment of relationships (British independent, and other Freudian lines, ego psychology and Kohut's self psychology). The view that the only agent for change in depth in analytic work is interpretation of the transference (especially if the emotional containment provided by interpretation of the transference is included under this heading) is more characteristic of the position adopted by many Kleinians and post-Kleinians. Most contemporary Freudians and most independents do not regard interpretation of the transference as the only important therapeutic factor. Nevertheless, understanding the transference and when to interpret it is a central shared feature of the approach taken by all psychoanalytically oriented psychotherapists.

References

Ainsworth, M. D. S., Blehar, M. C., Waters, E., *et al* (1978) *Patterns of Attachment: A Psychological Study of the Strange Situation*. Hillsdale, NJ: Erlbaum.

Bacal, H. A. & Newman, K. M. (1990) *Theories of Object Relations: Bridges to Self Psychology*. New York: Columbia University Press.

Bateman, A. & Fonagy, P. (2004) *Psychotherapy for Borderline Personality Disorder: Mentalization-based Treatment*. Oxford: Oxford University Press.

Bion, W. R. (1957) Differentiation of the psychotic from the non-psychotic personalities. *International Journal of Psychoanalysis*, **38**, 266.

Bollas, C. (1992) *Being a Character*. London: Routledge.

Bollas, C. (1995) *Cracking Up*. London: Routledge.

Bowlby, J. (1980) *Attachment and Loss, vol. 3. Loss. Sadness and Depression*. London: Hogarth.

Britton, R. (1989) The missing link: parental sexuality in the Oedipus complex. In *The Oedipus Complex Today: Clinical Implications* (ed. J. Steiner), pp. 83–101. London: Karnac.

Casement, P. (1985) *On Learning From the Patient*. London: Tavistock.

Casement, P. (1990) *Further Learning From the Patient*. London: Tavistock/Routledge.

Chassaguet-Smirgel, J. (1984) *Creativity and Perversion*. London: Free Association Press.

Erikson, E. H. (1968) *Identity: Youth and Crisis*. London: Faber and Faber.

George, C., Kaplan, N. & Main, M. (1984) *Attachment Interview for Adults*. Berkeley, CA: University of California.

Glasser, M. (1998) On violence. A preliminary communication. *International Journal of Psychoanalysis*, **79**, 887–902.

Greenberg, J. R. & Mitchell, S. A. (1983) *Object Relations in Psychoanalytic Theory*. Cambridge MA: Harvard University Press.

Grinberg, L., Sor, D., Tabak de Bianchedi, E. (1975) *Introduction to the Work of Bion*. The Roland Harris Educational Trust. Reprinted (1985) in London by Karnac.

Heimann, P. (1950) On Counter-transference. Reprinted (1989) in *About Children and Children No-Longer: Collected papers 1942–1980 of P. Heimann* (ed. M. Tonnesman), pp. 73–79. London: Routledge.

Heimann, P. (1969) Evolutionary leaps and the origin of cruelty. Reprinted (1989) in *About Children and Children-No-Longer: Collected Papers 1942–1980 of P. Heimann* (ed. M. Tonnesman), pp. 206–217. London: Routledge.

Heimann, P. (1962) Notes on the anal stage. Reprinted (1989) in *About Children and Children-no-longer: Collected Papers 1942–1980 of P. Heimann* (ed. M. Tonnesman), pp. 169–184. London: Routledge.

Hinshelwood, R. D. (1989) *A Dictionary of Kleinian Thought*. London: Free Association Books.

Holmes, J. (1993a) Attachment theory: a biological basis for psychotherapy? *British Journal of Psychiatry*, **163**, 430–438.

Holmes, J. (1993b) *John Bowlby and Attachment Theory*. London: Routledge.

Holmes, J. (1996) *Attachment, Intimacy, Autonomy: Using Attachment Theory in Adult Psychotherapy*. London: Jason Aronson.

Kahn, M. M. R. (1974) *The Privacy of the Self*. London: Hogarth.

Kahn, M. M. R. (1979) *Alienation in Perversions*. London: Hogarth.

King, P. (1992) Foreword. In *Psychic Experience and Problems of Technique* (by H. Stewart). London: Routledge.

King, P. & Steiner, R. (1991) *The Freud–Klein Controversies 1941–1945*. London: Routledge.

Klein, M. (1957) Envy and Gratitude. Reprinted (1975) in *The Writings of Melanie Klein. Envy and Gratitude and Other Works 1946–1963*, pp.176–235. London: Hogarth.

Kohut, H. (1959) Introspection, empathy, and psychoanalysis: an examination of the relation between mode of observation and theory. Reprinted (1978) in *The Search for the Self: Selected Writings of Heinz Kohut: 1950–1978, Vol. 1* (ed. P. H. Ornstein), pp. 205–232. New York: International Universities Press.

Kohon, G. (1992) Review of Paula Heimann's collected papers. *International Journal of Psychoanalysis*, **73**, 164–165.

Limentani, A. (1992) Obituary for M. Masud R. Khan. *International Journal of Psychoanalysis*, **73**, 155–159.

Lorenz, K. (1952) *King Solomon's Ring*. London: Methuen.

McDougall, J. (1986) *Theatres of the Mind*. London: Free Association Press.

Meltzer, D. (1966) The relation of anal masturbation to projective identification. Reprinted (1988) in *Melanie Klein Today: Developments in Theory and Practice, Vol. 1. Mainly Theory* (ed. E. Bott Spillius), pp. 102–116. London: Routledge.

O'Shaughnessy, E. (1989) The invisible Oedipus complex. In *The Oedipus Complex Today* (ed. J. Steiner), pp. 129–150. London: Karnac.

Ogden. T. H. (1989) *The Primitive Edge of Experience*. Northvale, NJ: Jason Aronson.

Ornstein, P. H. (1978) The evolution of Heinz Kohut's psychoanalytic psychology of the self. In *The Search for the Self: Selected Writings of Heinz Kohut: 1950–1978, Vol. 1.*(ed. P. H. Ornstein), pp. 427–460. New York: International Universities Press.

Parkes, C. M. (1972) *Bereavement. Studies of Grief in Adult Life*. London: Tavistock.

Rayner, E. (1991) *The Independent Mind in British Psychoanalysis*. London: Free Association Books.

Rosenfeld, H. A. (1954) Considerations regarding the psycho-analytic approach to acute and chronic schizophrenia. Reprinted (1965) in *Psychotic States: A Psycho-analytical Approach* (ed. H. A. Rosenfeld), pp. 117–127. London: Hogarth.

Rosenfeld, H. A. (1971) A clinical approach to the psychoanalytic theory of the life and death instincts: an investigation into the aggressive aspects of narcissism. *International Journal of Psychoanalysis*, **52**, 169–178.

Ryle, A. (1995) *Cognitive Analytic Therapy*. Chichester: Wiley.

Sandler, J. (1987) The concept of projective identification. In *Projection, Identification, Projective Identification* (ed. J. Sandler), pp. 13–26. Madison, CT: International Universities Press. Reprinted (1988) in London by Karnac.

Segal, H. (1957) Notes on symbol formation. *International Journal of Psychoanalysis*, **38**, 391–397. Reprinted (1981) in *The Work of Hanna Segal*, p. 76. New York: Jason Aronson.

Shengold, L. (1992) *Halo in the Sky: Observations on Anality and Defense*. New Haven, CT: Yale University Press.

Steiner, J. (1982) Perverse relationships between parts of the self: a clinical illustration. *International Journal of Psychoanalysis*, **63**, 241–251.

Steiner, J. (1987) The interplay between pathological organisations and the paranoid–schizoid and depressive positions. *International Journal of Psychoanalysis*, **68**, 69–80. Also in (1988) *Melanie Klein Today, Vol. I. Mainly Theory*, (ed. E. Bott Spillius), pp. 324–342. London: Routledge.

Steiner, J. (1993) *Psychic Retreats: Pathological Organizations in Psychotic, Neurotic and Borderline Patients*. London: Routledge.

Stern, D. N. (1985) *The Interpersonal World of the Infant*. New York: Basic Books.

Stewart, H. (1992) *Psychic Experience and Problems of Technique*. London: Routledge.

Sutherland, J. D. (1980) The autonomous self. In *The Autonomous Self: The Work of John D. Sutherland* (ed. J. S. Scharff), pp. 61–65. Northvale, NJ and London: Jason Aronson.

Sutherland, J. D. (1989) *Fairbairn's Journey Into the Interior*. London: Free Association Books.

CHAPTER 4

Psychodynamic therapy with individuals

Sandra Grant

For the beginning therapist, the wealth of intellectual knowledge and debate summarised in the last two chapters can be fascinating but daunting. It may seem far removed from the stress of the consulting room, where one has to think of what to say next (or what to stop oneself saying). Psychoanalytic theory is developed from years of painstaking clinical observation, not in a vacuum: most psychoanalysts see each patient 4 or 5 times a week for several years. Such in-depth knowledge of the theoretical background may not be necessary except for the specialist, but it is important to realise that there is a solid body of clinical work that lies behind the common constructs used in psychotherapy. When something arises in therapy that suddenly brings a theoretical premise into mind that makes sense of a complex situation, it reminds us that the theory has arisen largely from painstaking observation working directly with patients.

The difficulty translating this theory into practice can lead to a sense of inadequacy or to an intellectualisation of the process. Some people reject psychodynamic approaches in favour of more simple paradigms and feel uncomfortable being compelled to undertake such work as part of training. Many people, however, come back to a psychodynamic approach later in their professional careers, driven by a need to acknowledge and recognise the complexity of human relations, the uniqueness of individuals and the importance of the therapeutic relationship as well as technical skills. From such a vantage point, the capacity to tolerate not knowing and to avoid easy answers becomes an important therapeutic skill.

The therapeutic challenge is to utilise psychoanalytic understandings when appropriate to inform briefer, or longer but less frequent, work. Less intensive therapies are not to be seen as 'second best' to psychoanalysis.

While this book as a whole is targeted at a wide audience from beginners to specialists, this chapter is written primarily for psychiatrists working within the National Health Service who are not specialist psychotherapists, but who are either undertaking psychotherapeutic training as part of general training, or who wish to develop such skills within other branches of psychiatry. The aim is to provide practical examples reflecting some of the important themes discussed in the earlier chapters, by telling the stories of moments in time during therapy.

To simplify terminology, the general term 'therapist' will be used to signify a psychiatrist carrying out psychotherapy with an individual patient (although the chapter will also be relevant to non-medical therapists). The traditional term patient has been retained rather than service user or client because of the NHS setting where the work described was undertaken.

Only individual therapy is described, the other modalities are covered in other chapters.

Beginning therapy

The assessment process has been covered in detail in Chapter 1. Most patients entering a psychotherapeutic relationship have minimal knowledge of what is expected of them. Some basic information about what can be expected will have been discussed before beginning. The injunction to say whatever comes to mind, free association (rather than pursuing a logical train of thought) may feel alien to many people, who understandably want to tackle the perceived problems head on. The timescale (brief or long-term) will have been agreed and an understanding reached about the reasons for the choice. Brief therapy will be focused around a particular issue, for example, bereavement or childhood sexual abuse.

Often there is an idealised expectation of what psychotherapy can achieve in a magical way, providing new parents, undoing all past trauma, removing symptoms and leading to happiness. Conversely, there may be a negative view that talking can do nothing. The patient may have a need to do well, to please the therapist, to remain in control etc. In other words the way the person approaches therapy is itself information about inner conflicts and anxieties and about a style of relating.

At the assessment stage a brief discussion of such themes, combined with experience of one or two trial interpretations will enable the individual to make an appropriate choice about whether to enter this form of therapy, and will prepare him for what is to come. Too often the emphasis is on one side only; the therapist's decision whether or not to offer therapy, yet it is a joint process. Basically, for the patient, the issue is one of trust rather than objective criteria or evidence. Will he trust the professional's knowledge and skills? Given our human propensity to seek good parental objects the benefit of the doubt is usually given to the putative therapist unless there are major difficulties in establishing basic trust. The therapist therefore has to take responsibility for enabling the individual to make as informed a choice as possible, while recognising that this choice will be as much subjectively as objectively determined.

Evidence-based medicine shows psychotherapy is effective in many situations, but cannot predict whether one particular therapist will effectively help one particular patient. The paradox is that it is those who have had earlier damaging relationships who will be least able to trust, yet need help the most. A good therapist will recognise the element of doubt and cynicism about therapy and acknowledge it where possible. He will provide hope but not guarantees and will agree that it is a major step and difficult choice to enter a therapy that may be emotionally painful.

The preparation for starting therapy consists only partially in informing the patient what is expected. It requires the therapist to reflect and judge himself. Can I get in touch with this person's pain? Can I bear it? Can he/she bear it? Will I be available as long as necessary? Have I got adequate support/supervisory arrangements? This applies at all stages of training or seniority. The therapist may have worked with several hundred people, but for each specific patient this is likely to be the one chance to work things out. Honesty, humility and humanity are basic requisites the psychotherapist must have to back his theoretical knowledge.

Practical issues

Consistency

If a person is to be open about hopes, fears, inadequacies and a personal life history, it will be easier to receive therapy in a secure, reliable, familiar setting to supplement the holding environment of the therapist's mind. Therapy should take place at the same time(s) each week, in the same place, with the same person. The length of each session will be the same (usually 50 minutes). The phrase for announcing the session has ended will usually be the same. Cancellations by the therapist will be rare and announced well in advance where possible (for example for holidays). The impact of such changes must be explored if it seems to be an issue.

Case vignette

Donald had stated that he did not mind that a session had been cancelled at short notice, but at the next meeting he talked of being in two minds about coming, and later mentioned his exasperation with several people who had not stuck to agreed plans. The therapist suggested that this theme was also important between the two of them. After initial denial, he agreed and talked of his disappointment about the cancelled session. This led to him recalling incidents in childhood when he had been severely let down and the realisation that his sensitivity about such issues was now sometimes excessive. Although he had thought he had hid it from his friends, his prickliness and apparent neediness was driving people away.

Comfort

The physical environment for the therapy session should be welcoming, relaxing and quiet, domestic rather than clinical. The therapist has to guard against interruptions from pagers or telephone. Both people need comfortable chairs at the same height, set at an angle to each other and without a desk in between. A clock visible to patient and therapist will allow mutual adherence to time boundaries without surreptitious glancing at watches (seen as signifying anxiety or boredom by both parties).

Constraints

In order to provide the consistent boundaries that are necessary to enable the development of the transference neurosis in longer-term work, the therapist has to endure a state of relative anonymity and neutrality, which may be experienced on both sides as a deprivation. The clearest constraints are against a sexual relationship (as in all therapeutic contexts) or other physical contact. There is also a barrier about the therapist revealing too much personal information. The patient may describe events, beliefs or interests highly pertinent to the therapist in his or her personal life, but it is rarely correct to reveal this. The delicate task is to be hidden but human, and not defensive or overly guarded.

Case vignette

Mary had close connections to the lead singer of a pop group and would describe private meetings on the assumption that her psychiatrist shared the same musical tastes. The important issue therapeutically was for the psychiatrist to resist the temptation to enter musical debate or to become fascinated with secrets being shared. Instead they needed to understand together Mary's low self-esteem and her attempt to gain vicarious status.

This is another example demonstrating how the patient's way of relating to the therapist can give significant information about internalised object relations.

Confidentiality

Particular attention needs to be paid to the issue of confidentiality. The therapist needs to keep notes for a variety of purposes, recording activity, communicating with colleagues who may also be seeing the patient, keeping a record for supervision, legal reports etc. Notes should not be taken during the session, but at its conclusion when the patient has left. The therapist should not generally make detailed process notes in the general psychiatric casenote. Often the therapist will be inexperienced and in training and require to make process notes for their own use in supervision. Each therapist should be responsible for recording their own work with their patients and be clear about the procedures and protocols within their own particular service for doing this.

At times the patient's need for confidentiality may have to be challenged (see case vignette below). To break confidentiality is a serious matter but, if there are real concerns about the patient (for example serious abuse or violence to another person or child) this may have to be done. As a rule, this should not happen without consultation with senior colleagues.

Case vignette

Caroline was referred for psychotherapy when she 'fell to pieces' after accusations of non-accidental injury to her disabled daughter. After 20 sessions she admitted that she had in fact tried to kill her. The therapist had a paramount responsibility to protect the child and told the patient this, although in discussion she suggested the patient had disclosed the information because she was scared of what she had done and might do and wanted the therapist to help set some boundaries to protect her daughter.

Disclosure to the therapist enabled Caroline to immediately inform the social workers and police herself and the child was taken into care.

Consultation/supervision

Given that the therapeutic relationship is the cornerstone of dynamic psychotherapy it is necessary that staff at all levels have the opportunity to discuss this relationship with an uninvolved, experienced other person. This will mean a supervisory relationship, peer review or consultancy on a frequent basis. Ensuring this and preserving the time in the face of other demands, is the essential bedrock of good practice.

Starting therapy is difficult for all concerned, the therapist, the patient and often the patient's partner and family. The therapist has to tolerate his own anxiety about not knowing the patient, accepting that it will take time to become attuned to the patient's personal style of communication. The task is to establish the basic ground rules and framework for the therapeutic relationship while ensuring that the patient has the opportunity to be listened to and heard, then understood.

From the start a model of cooperative working should be developed that allows the patient space to be talkative or silent in the presence of someone who is alert and attentive. The therapist may occasionally make a comment to clarify, elucidate, acknowledge or make links between previously unlinked phenomena. The novice therapist has to learn to negotiate a place in the spectrum of activity between being over-talkative and completely silent. The temptation to make premature interpretations should be resisted. Such issues will be discussed in the supervisory setting.

Case vignette

Philip, a trainee therapist, was very keen on psychotherapy and wanted to show how much he had learnt. On the second session with a patient he interpreted the patient's distress about his father's suicide as being due to his guilt about having unconsciously wished him dead.

At such an early stage in therapy the main anxiety will usually be about trust and hope in establishing a relationship with the therapist that will help a person 'get better'. There was no evidence for the interpretation given above and such a comment would have been experienced as confirmation that the death was indeed his fault. The timing was wrong and the remark could not help the development of a therapeutic alliance.

Getting the balance right might seem difficult. While premature wild interpretations should not be made, caricaturing the legendary blank screen is another common problem for beginners.

Case vignette

Joan, a trainee therapist, was so terrified of making a mistake she only remembered negative injunctions about not asking questions and not making premature interpretations. The patient asked to see the assessing consultant with the complaint that the doctor said nothing and avoided eye contact. 'How would that help?' The patient said she 'needed to know that the therapist was alive'.

The supervisor has to balance an understanding of the subjective and objective realities of such experiences. There is obvious legitimacy in the patient's complaint that the 'expert' she came to for help appeared to be doing nothing. Knowing her history it would have been legitimate to suggest that this may possibly also reflect the patient's anxiety about her ill mother when she was a child. This would have been premature in a first session (unless with an experienced therapist) and would appear to dismiss the reality of what the patient felt in the present. The trainee would perhaps have been best to acknowledge the patient's feelings and her need to have a response, then discuss the difficulty with her supervisor. It would also be important for the trainee privately to consider whether there was something about the patient and her history that resonated with herself and made her shut off from the patient.

In 5-times-a-week work, long silences on both sides may be tolerable. For a patient starting once-weekly sessions such isolation is usually too much, and the time too precious. Remarks reflecting or mirroring the patient's statements, or remarks clarifying links that are being suggested, are not interpretations per se but are vital interventions to provide an infrastructure to enable exploratory work to begin.

For the patient, beginning therapy is a unique experience, coloured however by all his or her past experience of relationships. To the extent that the person's life experience has been good, the expectation that this new relationship will be fruitful will be enhanced. Those with negative experiences will anticipate the worst, although such trepidation may be scarcely conscious. Sometimes what is expressed is the opposite: unreal idealised expectations of an omnipotent healing.

Case vignette

Helen came to therapy desperate for help from a 'good' therapist as opposed to her previous 'bad' therapist who had 'abandoned' her, just as she felt rejected and unloved by her family. This was a warning of a potential negative therapeutic reaction and the need to be alert to transference issues. The therapist had to guard against identifying with the 'good' image, failing to appreciate the challenge to prove (disprove?) her therapist was a good clinician/mother. This countertransference awareness was essential in the ongoing therapy.

A therapist should be aware of the possibility of differing responses based on transference. The nature of the power-imbalance in therapeutic relationships, and the tenacity of early internalised relationships, means that doctors will tend to be viewed as similar to the parental figures of childhood. This can be especially disconcerting for a young trainee who is reciprocally struggling with the perception of an older patient as a parental figure. The consistent approach and self scrutiny of the therapist ensures that the picture that emerges is coloured in the main by the patient's inner template not the 'reality' of the therapist, nor the therapist's countertransference.

Case vignette

A therapist spent the morning with 3 patients. Although he thought he related to each with a similar level of warmth, interest and activity, the 3 people had different views of him. The first said in an exasperated way that he was a 'cold automaton robot'. The second said how she felt really understood and helped by him. The third teased him in a flirtatious way.

In each case the doctor had to review his own countertransference and behaviour, lest he had influenced the different perceptions. Satisfied that he had not done so to any significant degree he was able to build on his knowledge of each person's history to make sense of the different views about him.

The first patient had experienced his father as cold and remote. The therapist commented that the patient seemed to fear he was going to repeat the unhappy relationship with his father. This received the response that the doctor was not going to wriggle off the hook: he was cold and distant. The therapist replied that it seemed that hooking him or pinning him down was important. The patient's emotional tone changed as he went on to talk about his athletic skills as an adolescent and his desperation that father was always too busy to come and watch him run.

The second patient had spent her childhood trying to please her mother and the therapist felt she was saying what he wanted to hear (he himself had not felt any real contact or understanding with her). He said that maybe it was easier giving good feedback to him than letting him know her disappointments. She said there were no disappointments (silence for several minutes). She then apparently changed the subject to mention that her friend had 'failed to phone her as arranged, which was typical'. She was the one who always had to keep contacts going; nobody else seemed to treat friendship seriously. For the therapist this was confirmation of his intuitive sense that something more negative lay behind the congratulatory statements. He decided it would be premature to comment further at this stage.

With the third, flirtatious patient, he was aware that she had been sexually abused and that she was relating to him in a way that reflected this. He decided that it was too early to comment, lest it appear he was saying the abuse was her fault. He was alerted to the need to listen for indications of her feelings about him in future and to pay attention to boundary issues in the therapy (such as prolonging sessions).

The above examples relate to single session experiences, but as therapy continues a more fixed and consistent relation to the therapist will emerge, the transference neurosis. As therapy progresses further and the patient understands the origin of this attitude, he will perceive the therapist in a more realistic and flexible manner, a sign of change in his inner world.

At the beginning of therapy it is tempting to presume one knows what the dynamics are and how therapy will proceed, given the personal and family history and the presenting complaint. It is important to record such formulations in order to reflect back afterwards and refine one's assessment skills in the light of experience. Of course there is the potential for turning the original formulation into a self-fulfilling prophecy, one of the reasons for the therapist being relatively silent and non-intrusive. The debate about 'false memory syndrome' about sexual abuse is a good example of this. It is important for the therapist to be able to tolerate uncertainty and to keep an open mind.

The process of therapy

If the core theoretical premises of psychoanalysis are a dynamic unconscious and the transference and transference/countertransference relationship, how are these manifest in the broad range of applied psychodynamic therapies? A therapy has a psychodynamic component if an understanding of underlying themes based on psychoanalytic awareness is used to inform or guide a treatment plan or specific intervention.

Psychodynamic therapies are often designated as insight-oriented (a remarkably neutral term for the awareness of so much pain and conflict). The aim is to 'make the unconscious conscious', although insight is not merely cognitive and requires 'working through'. For the patient it has an essential emotional component or 'gut-reaction' combined with an intellectual understanding. The therapist puts into words what is implicit in what the patient is saying and the patient takes it further so that jointly a new understanding is reached. This requires an intimate analytic relationship between therapist and patient that has clear boundaries and constraints and is underpinned by a clear theoretical model.

The relationship the patient develops with the therapist is based on a number of factors, including past history of relationships and unconscious fantasy as well as how the therapist actually behaves. The extent to which this transference relationship is interpreted depends on the main theoretical focus and usually on the length of therapy.

One differentiating factor of psychodynamic therapies is that the therapist is a participant observer, while also maintaining clear boundaries. The therapist has to recognise and understand his or her own emotions, thoughts and behaviour in relation to the patient as far as possible. The information gained, or awareness of the countertransference in a broad sense, is used to guide the therapeutic process. This is not easy, especially when projective identification takes place and the therapist may be experiencing feelings that originate from the patient.

Case vignette

Anne was receiving brief intensive psychotherapy following the failure of behavioural treatment for a recently developed phobic condition that had prevented her performing on stage, her professional career. The driving forces and triggers were found to be her impending marriage in the context of an intense work culture that involved travelling away from home, when sexual relationships often developed and had taken place in her fantasy. The phobia was partly an unconscious defence against such temptations (or instincts) and was related to childhood experience of parental infidelity (which she witnessed) and marital breakdown.

The symptom was over-determined, with an important component being her current experience as a woman in a male-dominated competitive work context. The transference relationship started from an expectation of further failed therapy (inadequate desexualised homemaker/mother), then became an idealised view of a sexually secure, professionally successful mother. Insight was gained into her forgotten earlier experience of a supportive nurturing mother, now re-experienced in the relationship with her therapist.

The countertransference awareness, which influenced interpretations, was about the therapist feeling a great need to perform well. This had multiple components, including projective identification: the patient felt more relaxed about going on stage again, whereas the therapist now felt her need to 'perform' well. In addition the therapist had to recognise the internal pressure of needing to 'prove' psychotherapy could work when other treatments failed.

Another basic premise about psychodynamic work is the recognition of internal conflict and contradiction. A person may hold several opposing points of view. Some of those viewpoints may not be conscious and overt but will influence behaviour nevertheless. Opposites can coexist; this applies not only to drives and defences against them, but also to thoughts and feelings ('methinks he doth protest too much').

Case vignette

Sheila had been in an incestuous relationship in her teens and was upset when this ended, believing the relationship had been very positive. She developed bulimia and began, then discontinued, therapy. It was not until 5 years later that she realised she also hated her father: these feelings had been blocked off. In the second phase of therapy she repeated this pattern, idealising her therapist then becoming angrily disappointed. Gradually she came to realise this pattern also applied to her eating problem. Her therapist had to understand and manage her own ambivalent feelings about the patient in order to help the patient tolerate feeling such contradictory things at the same time rather than splitting them into extremes.

Psychodynamic psychotherapy makes us face both internal and external reality and responsibility and is no soft or easy option as is evident from the above example. Bion's assertion of the human being's paramount need for truth (Grindberg *et al*, 1975) is correct, but there are multiple truths and we can tolerate only so much at a time.

Adopting a psychodynamic stance means listening with a 'third ear' to latent communications, to what is not being said and what is revealed in speech, body language or behaviour. For example, being late once may be a mishap, but being late 3 times could be a communication, just as being obsessively punctual could reveal information. This is an example of psychic determinism. (For discussion of the issue of lateness as possible resistance, and how to deal with it, see Bateman & Holmes, 1995.)

What an unconscious communication such as this means cannot be determined in the abstract, but is relatively unique to the individual and needs to be explored by both patient and therapist. Whether or not this communication is translated or interpreted by the therapist to the patient (or indeed the patient to the therapist) depends on the extent to which the therapy is exploratory and intensive or focused on agreed themes, which is usually but not always reflected in the frequency and time-scale of therapy. The therapist may have a sense about the underlying meaning of some behaviour and holds this idea in his mind as a hypothesis, waiting for further evidence to confirm or refute the theory. When the idea seems near the patient's consciousness because of repeated discussion of similar and related topics, a tentative interpretation is made suggesting this hidden meaning.

Case vignette
Bob, a man in his 50s who worked in the arts field, had depression interfering with his work. He would refer to literary and dramatic work frequently in every session. Although understandable in terms of Bob's profession, the therapist had a sense of intrusion and blocking of the therapeutic process, being first intrigued with the patient's depth of knowledge, then getting bored and taking his mind off the therapeutic task. There was no evidence of emotions. Somehow the content of the stories (however intellectually fascinating) did not appear to represent or engage with the patient's own troubles.

Awareness of this countertransference response led the psychiatrist to be alert to the use of this mechanism as a defensive way of relating (or not relating) and gradually the complex background to this communication style was looked at together. It was suggested (interpreted) to Bob that his far-reaching cultural knowledge did not always aid communication, but enabled him to hide more emotional aspects of himself. Perhaps this way of relating with only part of himself could get in the way of therapy?

He responded by talking about his mother whom he found intrusive and demanding (and who had minimal cultural knowledge). Doing well at school had helped him separate from her and create a separate self-identity that bolstered his self-esteem and allowed him to express his contempt for her. He denied that this mechanism was relevant to therapy and was astonished at the thought that maybe he needed his mother or the therapist. He confessed that his view of psychoanalytically-oriented therapy was to exchange intellectual ideas with an equal, not to be made upset.

Resistance in therapy should not be seen as a person being difficult or refusing help (although of course this is sometimes the conscious position). It is an unconscious way of protecting against repetition of earlier traumas. And sometimes the defensive structures are culturally supported and vindicated.

Although psychotherapy may seem to be a predominately verbal exercise, this example demonstrates that it is not merely the words and content that give meaning, but the way the words are used within the therapeutic relationship. Sometimes, however, the words themselves are directly describing the underlying process.

Case vignette

Linda had been off work for over a year with a mixed anxiety state and depression. She took the injunction to say what came into her mind seriously and recounted details of her past life and current circumstances in some detail. Progress was taking place in terms of insight into her regimented childhood and her need to conform.

Then she decided she needed to buy new curtains. And then described what type of curtain, what colour, what size, what shop, what they cost and so forth over several sessions. Questions about what the curtains meant were met with an exasperated 'To keep people from seeing in of course and anyway you told me to say what was on my mind!' A suggestion (interpretation) that this might also apply to not letting the therapist see how she felt was met with puzzlement 'Curtains are only curtains after all'. The symbolism was not apparent to her.

Nevertheless in the next session she explained that she might after all have been holding back. (It was important that this conclusion was reached by her and not forced by the therapist.) The experience of 'conforming' to rules was being repeated in therapy and yet the actual experience of blocked free association showed that there was actually a subversive non-conformist (probably healthy) side to her. Acceptance of this was felt as liberating and she felt safe enough to describe some more unusual non-conformist practices.

By the middle phase of therapy the therapist will usually have learned about the key relationships and major life events the patient has experienced both now and in the past. There will be a shift away from focusing on symptoms to a more holistic examination of thoughts, feelings and relationships. The transference will be becoming evident as the patient's relationships in the past, which have been reflected in current adult ways of relating, become repeated also in the therapeutic relationship. Malan describes this as the 'triangle of persons' (Malan, 1979).

Similarly the therapist and patient will have begun to understand the patient's 'triangle of conflict'. This consists of hidden feelings, the defences or coping mechanisms for dealing with them, and the anxieties about what will happen if such conflict is not kept under control. Abstract theory becomes demystified into a concrete human story where such connections can be recognised and where examples are only too evident within the consulting room itself.

Case vignette

Carol had been abused by her mother who had a highly ambivalent, physically controlling relationship with her daughter, especially in the area of femininity.

She dreamt of her therapist, and the fact her therapist had 'entered her head' by appearing in a dream scared her as being an intrusive attack similar to her mother's sexual attacks, even although in the dream the therapist seemed to be protecting her (just as mother had justified her actions as being to protect her from men).

The connections between the above patient's current distress and the family history would be apparent using most theoretical models. What a dynamic approach does is to show how the patient may see her therapist in a light coloured by such experience and how this can bring the dynamics alive in the here-and-now of their relationship. Whether or not the transference relationship is interpreted depends on the theoretical orientation and skill of the therapist, the intensity of the therapy, and the impact of the transference phenomenon on the treatment process.

Psychodynamic theory provides guiding principles and background knowledge, but cannot define specific interactions and interpretations to give for specific disorders, guiding the therapist as to what to say to a particular individual. Some potentially serious disorders can have quick resolution when the basic ego-strength is secure and the family context is supportive.

Case vignette

Louise, aged 16, had anorexia nervosa. She was an expert athlete, destined for real success and strongly supported/pushed by her father. A few individual sessions enabled her to confront her father with the fact she wished to be 'normal' and this was accepted and agreed by the family as a whole. She gave up professional sport and her symptoms gradually resolved. It was not thought appropriate to explore underlying factors.

For many people, brief therapy will be appropriate and sufficient, but increasingly NHS psychotherapists are being asked to treat people with severe personality disorders. It is possible to be simplistic and categorise people along a spectrum of psychological health, ranging from those with relatively healthy object-related functioning to those with narcissistic and borderline personalities. The transference is considerably different in each group as is inevitably the countertransference response. The first group of people with more neurotic phenomena were traditionally the patient group for psychotherapy, but this focus has gradually extended to utilising psychodynamic insights in working with people who have a severe personality disorder or those with conditions not traditionally seen as amenable to dynamic approaches.

Case vignette
Moira rubbished any comment from her therapist and insisted that her negative and nihilistic view of the world was the only valid one. When the therapist would attempt to empathically respond by acknowledging the patient's anger and despair, Moira would simply attack again. There was little material or information given for the therapist to work with and he had a sense of working very hard to establish any sense of contact: each session would feel like starting again. After some time he commented on this process, linking it to the previous failed therapy, and suggesting that a powerful repetition was occurring. The patient spontaneously said 'It's like with my mother!' and there was a sense of contact and opening up that proved to be the fragile start of a therapeutic alliance.

It should be noted in the above example that if the doctor had interpreted early on that she was behaving as she did with her mother (fairly obvious from the history) it would have been ineffectual. The theme had to come up again and again, before the pattern could be pointed out and the patient herself made and owned the 'interpretation'. This made it possible for this theme to be 'worked through' during the rest of the therapy.

Ending therapy

Finishing therapy can be painful on both sides, but usually is also an opportunity for recognition of a shared endeavour, despite seeming unbalanced in power and emotions (although the therapist can also feel powerless and have strong feelings this is not usually overt). Optimally, ending comes about by mutual agreement and planning, recognising that enough has been done, that diminishing returns would accrue from continuing work, and that the process of separating and ending itself is an important part of the journey.

In practice, many therapies are time-limited in advance especially in the light of research evidence indicating the efficacy of brief work. Resource constraints are a relevant factor, whether privately or publicly funded. Most NHS services are required to limit the duration of long-term therapies and often 2 years is regarded as an appropriate timescale. Other factors that impinge are life-choices and career moves on both sides. Also early symptom relief may be genuine not merely a transient 'flight into health'. Brief work may well be adequate. Early termination can certainly be 'resistance', but this does not stop the possibility that the patient can do no more at this time with this therapist. All these topics need to be open for discussion.

The final stages of therapy focus on themes of ending, separation, loss and liberation, with disillusionment and regret usually balanced by gratitude and hope. For the person who has had a good experience the process and the relationship will have been internalised and remain available as a source of comfort and learning for many years.

Case vignette
Gill sought out her previous therapist, after a 10-year gap, to discuss the death of her father. She said it seemed important to let him know that she had managed

to cope, although very upset, and had some very special times with her father before he died. They had got on a lot better after her therapy. Sometimes she would imagine what her therapist would have said about things, especially about not looking to the therapist for answers but relying on herself. She had briefly experienced a recurrence of the neurotic disorder that originally brought her into therapy, but realised it was to do with not facing her upset about Dad. In some ways her therapist had been a bit like a Dad to her, which was daft because he was actually a lot younger. She did not want to start therapy again but had wanted to say hello and thank you and let him know how the work they had done had helped so much later.

Brief therapy

In long-term psychodynamic treatment the therapist can wait to get a sense of the underlying dynamic issues before commenting or interpreting. In brief therapy a decision has to be taken whether to explore this at all in the brief time available. One particular theme is selected as a focus, for example separation anxiety, bereavement or previous traumatic events. Such a theme will be agreed jointly, with a given time-scale and follow-up. The aim is to tackle one specific important issue that will give the patient a way of working to understand himself that can be generalised to other issues. There is no interpretation of transference unless it is directly relevant to the theme. The therapist is more active.

The length of brief therapy is linked partly to the research base indicating that 10 sessions may be the optimal length, with diminishing returns after. It ensures a concentrated focus and minimises the development of transference separation difficulties. People who have circumscribed problems, but are relatively healthy, do better than people with a personality disorder.

Case vignette

David had been unable to cope with the death of his child. He entered therapy carrying literature reviews and checklists about post-traumatic stress disorder; he was clearly used to being in control. The 10 sessions of therapy focused on the grieving process and with an overt subtext about his fear of not having been able to control his child's illness. After initial anxiety about not being set specific tasks he started to welcome the less directive way of working. He gained symptomatic relief and an understanding that his defensive way of 'coping' by endless research into the illness had compounded the stress for him and his wife.

At the end he wished further sessions to look at himself more generally. He wanted in particular to explore how he related at work. This was declined on the basis of not being the original contract, and possibly being a repetition of his desire to know something completely (in this case psychodynamic therapy).

What if the chosen time-scale and focus is wrong? This can happen in two forms. The patient may not appear to have gained anything. Alternatively, he may have rapidly been able to work in this way, opening up new areas and would clearly be able to benefit from ongoing work. Should either or both be offered more or alternative therapy? In both instances sessions should stop after the planned number of sessions to keep to agreed boundaries. This is where re-assessment is needed, initially with the supervisor or team and then with the patient.

Psychodynamic assessment of the need for more therapy will no doubt have to be complemented with the reality of resource constraints and other practical considerations. If the therapy has not gone well is it because of a poor assessment, or poor therapy? It is rather too easy to see problems as the patient's resistance. Once again there are no hard and fast rules (unless operating within rigid constraints) and such decisions need to be taken after careful discussion with the supervisor.

A frequently asked question is whether to phase out sessions and whether to arrange a follow-up. The most common practice is not to do this but it depends on the nature of the problem and the nature of the therapy. This is a question best discussed in the supervision setting.

Supportive therapy

Apart from the highly specialised services, the current trend is for psychotherapy and psychiatry to become more integrated, focused on the needs of patients, not on narrow schools of thought. The anticipated psychological outcome of less intense approaches may be less global than those described by Stewart (1992) for psychoanalysis but nevertheless can lead to significant improvement in the quality of life.

Psychodynamic psychotherapists have learnt much from systems-based approaches and from cognitive therapies, and psychodynamic thinking has been open to new ideas and has developed. One of the most significant shifts over the past decades has been the acceptance of the high incidence of child sexual abuse and its aftermath, influenced by clinical work and criticism of psychoanalysis (Masson, 1984) and by the development of other theoretical approaches, such as attachment theory. This has refreshed psychoanalytic thinking about trauma (for example Welldon, 1988; Garland, 1991; De Zulueta, 1993) and has enabled non-specialist psychotherapists to understand their patients better and learn how to help them.

Psychotherapeutic skills are as relevant to biological illnesses and treatments as to the psychological. Freud himself proposed a biological basis for much psychopathology. Irrespective of aetiology, different patients view their illnesses, medication, hospitalisation and the doctor–patient relationship in different ways. Psychodynamic theory is one of several approaches to help us understand these varying attitudes and really hear what people are trying to say rather than presume we know.

The aim of supportive therapies is primarily external; to set limits, manage crises, reality test, educate and provide environmental support. Over time there is the possibility of the therapeutic relationship(s) and environment enabling greater independent and mature functioning.

For too long supportive therapy did not receive recognition of its place as the mainstay of psychiatric treatment relationships, requiring training and supervision. In essence the term refers to supporting the person's ego strengths rather than opening up the supposed dark world of the unconscious. In practice there may not be a clear distinction. In supportive work the therapist retains a holistic perspective and discusses psychosocial issues raised by the patient. There is less emphasis on transference interpretation.

When psychiatrists are limited to 15-minute appointments there is often little opportunity for the patient to raise issues of concern; time can be filled with discussion of symptoms, side-effects and drugs. Yet it is important that such medical themes are understood in the social context and emotional life of the patient. Too often patients describe their worries being discounted, 'Everything I say is seen as paranoid or not valid – just because I hear voices does not mean I am totally barking mad.' Aided by Bion's concept of psychotic and non-psychotic parts of the personality (Bion, 1967), the psychodynamically informed psychiatrist can work with the less disturbed part of the person's thinking, while not ignoring or denying the immense problems the patient is having to contend with.

Case vignette

Margaret, who has a bipolar disorder, was adamant when becoming ill again that she would not go into hospital and would kill herself if she was 'sectioned'. Recognising that for her this would symbolically mean both 'becoming' her psychotic father, and also being dominated by her invasive and controlling mother, enabled staff to acknowledge her requests and treat her on an intensive out-patient basis. The patient's drive for independence was construed as a healthy part of her, not as lack of insight. Team discussion centred on whether the psychiatrist should re-enact the 'controlling mother' by insisting on admission, and how the team did initially wish the psychiatrist to play this role because of their worries about potential self-mutilation and suicide.

Taking the risk not to admit her was possible due to a long-standing therapeutic relationship where the psychiatrist knew enough about the patient to believe her and to recognise that the therapeutic alliance with members of the team was strong enough to provide appropriate support and limit-setting. Margaret accepted increased medication, attended most days, used internet chat-rooms at night to talk to people with the same mental health problems, and recovered without the need for hospital admission.

Such an emphasis on patients' strengths is not always easy. There is a tension between the goal of empowering the patient yet acknowledging the legitimate need at times for external decision-making and control, especially when compulsory treatment is required. The increasing development of independent patient advocacy is articulating the concerns of those who have often felt unheard and the service-user movement is pushing for the development of partnership working with professionals.

Despite Freud's early emphasis on biological factors, it is tempting for those working psychotherapeutically to 'blame' the environment, especially the early parenting environment. It is therefore salutary to balance one's theoretical bias with experience of working with those who have endured difficult circumstances yet become emotionally and psychologically mature. There is a constant interplay between biological and environmental factors.

Case vignette

Frances at 60-years-old had been married for 35 years and raised two children to adulthood while working in a caring profession. Her childhood had been marred by the illness of her mother with Huntington's Disease, which caused the family to break up. At the age of 9 Frances had been attacked by her mother with an axe. When she was 13 her mother finally managed to kill herself with an overdose. Yet Frances grew up able to support an extended family suffering from the genetic disorder or the threat of it, until she herself (surprisingly late on) succumbed to the illness and the family support became mutual.

The therapist had reservations about the value of psychotherapy in this case (probably/possibly because it was too painful for her (the therapist) to cope with), but still went ahead. Frances in the first session talked of the great relief about finding someone who seemed able to accept things as they were and not rush to pity her or make false reassurances. She went on to benefit considerably from supportive psychotherapy, looking at some of the pain she felt in dying from an illness she had horribly witnessed in her mother and had passed on to her children (two had been detected positive following pre-symptomatic testing.)

Supportive therapy can be even harder with those with a primary diagnosis of personality disorder (a term mostly seen by patients as far from supportive). Reality-testing and limit-setting, coupled with genuine support and honesty may sound easy, but in practice the psychiatrist is often sorely stretched and has to struggle with negative feelings. Such patients are often so vulnerable to life's misfortunes or perceived narcissistic slights that emergency crises are frequent. Self-mutilation and self-harm raise anxiety and threat of harm to others even more so. Hospital admission may not resolve the crisis, merely exacerbating regressive behaviour.

The psychotherapist/psychiatrist and team need to understand the full range of psychotherapeutic treatments to manage the situations that arise and support the individuals involved. From the psychodynamic perspective, Tom Main's classic work 'The Ailment' should be starter reading (Main, 1957). In many settings borderline workshops have been established for joint management of such people by general psychiatrists and psychotherapists.

Conclusion

Psychodynamic approaches to working with individuals can be used in different ways and in different settings, ranging from long-term intensive psychotherapy to informing mainstream psychiatric practice. The work is highly rewarding and sometimes challenging, both intellectually and emotionally. It involves one's own personal attributes, weaknesses and strengths more than any other form of treatment. The dilemmas faced by patients will inevitably reverberate with aspects of the therapist's own history, past and present, conscious and unconscious. This may lead to blind spots and mistakes. That of course is inevitable, but it is why it is important that people planning to enter this field should have the opportunity to undergo therapy themselves.

It is also why, from beginning therapists to experienced professionals, discussion of one's clinical work is crucial. Supervision is fundamental to learning psychotherapy and remains key to continuing professional development at all levels.

References

Bateman, A. & Holmes, J. (1995) *Introduction to Psychoanalysis*. London & New York: Routledge.

Bion, W. R. (1967) *Second Thoughts: Selected Papers in Psycho-analysis*. London: Maresfield Reprints.

De Zulueta, F. (1993) *From Pain to Violence: The Traumatic Roots of Destructiveness*. London: Whurr Publishers.

Garland, C. (1991) External disasters and the internal world: an approach to psychotherapeutic understanding of survivors. In *Textbook of Psychotherapy in Psychiatric Practice* (ed. J. Holmes), pp. 507–532. Edinburgh: Churchill Livingstone.

Grinberg, L., Sor, D. & Tabak de Bianchedi, E. (1975) *Introduction to the Work of Bion*. Scotland: Ronald Harris Education Trust.

Main, T. F. (1957) The Ailment. *British Journal of Medical Psychology*, **30**, 129–145.

Malan, D. H. (1979) *Individual Psychotherapy and the Science of Psychodynamics*. London: Butterworth.

Masson, J. M. (1984) *The Assault on Truth: Freud's Suppression of the Seduction Theory*. Harmondsworth: Penguin.

Stewart, H. (1992) *Psychic Experience and Problems of Technique*. London: Routledge.

Welldon, E. V. (1988) *Mother, Madonna, Whore: The Idealization and Denigration of Motherhood*. New York: Guilford Press.

CHAPTER 5

Cognitive analytic therapy

Tom Murphy & Susan Llewelyn

Cognitive analytic therapy (CAT) developed from Dr Anthony Ryle's work on brief psychotherapy in the late 1970s. Originally a general practitioner, Ryle moved first to a university health service and then 15 years later to a National Health Service post as a consultant psychotherapist. His career has therefore allowed him to see (and research) both the very large population of those suffering from psychological problems, and also the woefully inadequate level of service provision, specialist and general, for this population. Understandably he looked to forms of brief psychotherapy as a way of providing a service.

During this time he was also interested in ways of integrating different psychotherapeutic approaches. In researching psychological problems he made use of Kelly's repertory grids from construct theory (a method that elicits people's understanding of relationships and of the world and represents this mathematically and visually; see Kelly, 1955), although his own practice of psychotherapy was psychoanalytically oriented. By his own account, he found the descriptions of patients' problems using repertory grid data more precise and useful than descriptions using psychoanalytic concepts in defining research questions, and gradually he came to feel such descriptions were also more clinically useful.

Alongside his use of personal construct theory and psychoanalytic thinking, Ryle was also increasingly aware of developments taking place in cognitive and behavioural therapy. He felt that some integration of these approaches should be possible and one of his early papers on this theme (Ryle, 1978) was written with the intention of describing psychoanalytic concepts from the point of view of cognitive psychology.

Over the next few years Ryle concerned himself with modifications to brief focal psychotherapy using the integrated views and language that he was developing. He applied descriptions to patients' problems derived from psychoanalytic object relations and cognitive psychology concepts, mostly using cognitive terminology (Ryle, 1979, 1980), and also applied these descriptions (snags, traps and dilemmas – see below) clinically as the focus for brief psychotherapeutic interventions. Further developments and modifications by Ryle and his associates have led gradually to the formal brief psychotherapeutic approach described in this chapter. For a complete and detailed account of CAT see publications edited by Ryle (Ryle, 1990, 1995d, 1997; Ryle & Kerr, 2002).

This chapter will start by outlining some of the theoretical tenets and therapeutic innovations of CAT, and will then present some of the principles and techniques of therapy. Then there will be a demonstration of their application via a case history. Similarities and differences between psychoanalysis and cognitive therapy will be drawn out, and the specific example of borderline personality will be considered. Finally, current and future research evidence will be considered, as well as implications for the development of CAT in the future.

Theoretical development and therapeutic innovations

In 1982 Ryle outlined a procedural sequence model (PSM) as a description of human activity (Ryle, 1982). A procedural sequence (or more simply 'procedure') is described by Ryle as being a linked chain of mental processes and actions involved in carrying out aim-directed actions (Ryle, 1985). According to this model the person carrying out an aim-directed activity is constantly appraising the situation they perceive themselves to be in and considering the means to achieve their desired ends, while continuing to appraise such decisions, possible actions, and very importantly, the consequences of any actions. Emotions are central to the process, along with cognitions, perceptions and actions. Much, or sometimes most, of the process may be unconscious, and as more than one aim is likely to be pursued at any one time, conflicts between aims readily occur.

The central importance of human relationships means that the focus of aim-directed activity is frequently other people. The consequences of the activity are seen in the perceived responses of the other person. In normal circumstances, with well-functioning individuals, there is some revision of aims or procedures, or both, in the light of an accurate perception of the responses of the other person. Neurotic procedures are not self-adjusting in response to the behaviour of others, but follow a closed loop that is self-perpetuating.

Example 1
Emily was the fifth child in a family where the father was a heavy drinker and the mother worked for long hours. As a child she experienced this as an emotionally depriving situation, and as an adult would sometimes be excessively demanding of others' attention and complain of being neglected. As a consequence, others withdrew or were rejecting and she reacted to this situation with more demanding actions which further increased others' rejections. This self-perpetuating cycle continued through several unsatisfactory relationships and she seemed to have little insight into the possibility that she might be suffering as a consequence of her own behaviour.

Ryle reviewed the case notes of a number of his patients and felt that neurotic procedures fell into three typical patterns, which he called snags, traps and dilemmas (Ryle, 1979).

Snags

A procedure is a snag when the person presumes that they will be blocked or punished for their action. Reasonable personal needs may not be asserted if the person assumes that either retaliation or harm to others will be the inevitable consequence. The person will often not be aware of the part played by guilt in this procedure (see Example 2).

Example 2
Michael's mother had suffered from recurrent bouts of depression throughout his childhood. He had felt concerned for her and tried to avoid causing any problems at home. As an adult he found it very difficult to confide in others for fear of burdening them and as a result was unable to find emotional support when he had problems in his own marriage.

Traps

Here, the person proceeds on the basis of a negative assumption and the resulting behaviour ends up seeming to confirm that negative assumption. A common example is the 'trying to please' trap.

Example 3
Emily (referred to in Example 1 above) believed that if she pleased other people then they would be caring and considerate towards her. However, she found that the opposite was often the case and she felt frequently taken advantage of. The angry resentment that she then felt led to the angry demanding behaviour referred to above. The consequent rejections then seemed to confirm to her that she would only be wanted if she tried to please.

Dilemmas

A person in a dilemma believes that his or her choice of action is restricted to either of two opposite activities, neither of which is satisfactory (see Example 3).

Example 4
In her childhood, Susan often seemed to experience a situation in which her parents ridiculed her if she talked about problems at school and as a result she learned to keep these feelings to herself. This made her very unhappy and her schoolwork deteriorated. She grew up to feel, however, that she only had two choices: either keep her feelings bottled up or risk being humiliated.

Early in therapy the patient is asked to fill in a questionnaire called the psychotherapy file that describes typical snags, traps and dilemmas. Six specific traps are described, as are a number of dilemmas concerning a person's feelings about themselves, and about how the person feels they relate to others. Snags are described more generally, without giving a suggested list. Ryle suggests that in the neurotic individual, these self-reinforcing procedures are to some extent contained in a personality that retains a fair degree of integration between different procedural loops; there is the feeling that the different aspects of the person are available for the interaction.

In patients with personality disorders, however, there is a separation or splitting so that the different procedures seem to function without reference to each other and a switch from one procedure to another feels like a change of personality. The psychotherapy file therefore also includes a short questionnaire concerning unstable states of mind and possible shifts in state, for example 'how I feel about myself and others can be unstable, I can switch from one state to a completely different one'. This switching phenomenon is most obvious in the borderline personality (see later in this chapter). Clear examples of how procedures may operate in clinical cases can be found in Walsh, Hagan & Gamsu (2000) and Sheard *et al* (2000).

Reciprocal roles

The procedures described above refer to overt behaviour, rather than to the person using these procedures. In CAT the person is viewed as proceeding out of a role in relation to another person, usually without being aware of the way in which this is happening. The term 'role' is used in CAT to refer to a state of mind far more profound than the term often implies in other contexts, and is derived from psychoanalytic object relations theory with the term role replacing the concept of identification with an internal object.

Roles are gradually built into the individual's mind ('internalised' in psychoanalytic terminology, or developed into schemas, in cognitive therapy terms) from early on in childhood in relationships with the parents. In a close relationship with a caring mother the infant is enabled to feel secure and cared for. The infant's state of mind at this time is an early role 'secure and cared for' and is experienced in relation to mother's role 'caring and reliable'. This total situation is internalised in the infant's mind as two roles relating to each other with mutuality and reciprocity. An action by the infant may be responded to in mother's facial expression, which in return is responded to by the infant, giving a reciprocal role pair 'secure and cared for' ↔ 'caring and reliable'.

In CAT the term reciprocal role is used to describe this interrelationship. An important consequence of both sides of the reciprocal roles being internalised in a person's mind is that he or she may then identify with either role, at different times. It is uncomfortably instructive to hear a 3-year-old boy moralising in critical tones about his parents' misdemeanours, virtually in the same words as have been used to him when he has been naughty. In this situation the child is adopting the 'critical parent' role in relation to the 'naughty child' role – now the unfortunate parent. Similarly the little girl will take on a mothering role to her dolls, and at the same time will look for mothering for herself from her own mother. These examples illustrate the way in which a person's state of mind may be derived from either pole in a reciprocal role pair. It is noticeable that it is often easier to recognise in oneself the more benign pole of the pair.

Example 5

John seemed often to feel implicitly that he occupied the role 'abandoned, neglected' in relation to the role 'absent, self-preoccupied', the latter role being ascribed to the other person present at the time – friends, work colleagues, therapist. He was rarely aware of the times that he was the one who was 'absent and self-preoccupied', when he would induce the reciprocal role in the other.

Reciprocal roles are in a way unique to each person, but also fall broadly into familiar patterns to which the person's individual experiences add the colours and emphasis. It would be expected that a child would have significant experience of more than one kind of intimate relationship during their upbringing and commonly he or she will have internalised more than one important reciprocal role pair during their formative years. More than three reciprocal roles of importance would be less common and can often be traced to the differences in reciprocal roles being exaggerated by detail. Further clarification will usually make it clear that three or fewer reciprocal roles are in operation. An exception to this is the borderline personality where a number of quite distinct mental states will exist, each state having its own set of reciprocal roles.

A common example of a normal or neurotic personality structure might be the two pairs of reciprocal roles 'absent–neglected' and 'criticised–feeling bad and guilty', coming from the experiences of the two parents, for example an occasionally absenting mother and a somewhat critical father. Alternatively they may come from two aspects of the one person, for example a mother who was sometimes critical and sometimes absenting. The person who has internalised these reciprocal roles has therefore four roles to move between or identify with at different times and/or in different circumstances.

In object relations theory, objects (that is aspects of other people) are internalised, becoming the person's internal objects. The person's self relates to these internal objects either by identification, or in a way that is reciprocal to the internal objects' characteristics. Thus in relation to a harshly critical and punitive internal object the self feels severely criticised and attacked. It is also recognised that a person may identify with an internal object and become harshly critical and punitive towards another person. It is explicit that CAT has largely developed from psychoanalytic object relations theory in particular Ogden's (1983) work. Some of the differences between CAT and psychoanalysis will be described later in this chapter.

Procedural sequence object relations model

Originally Ryle referred to CAT making use of the procedural sequence model (PSM) (described above). As ways were found to translate and incorporate object relations theory into the CAT model in the form of reciprocal roles, the model was changed to the 'procedural sequence object relations model' (PSORM; Ryle, 1991). The combination of reciprocal roles and procedures (referred to as 'reciprocal role procedures') allows for a clearer conceptual framework linking internal feeling states with behaviour. When roles and procedures are accurately described using words conveying the depth of feeling involved, the person is less likely to think of themselves as an observer, outside of their experience.

Often the person (and indeed the inexperienced therapist) will find it relatively easy to recognise themselves in the role that seems to be on the receiving end of the destructive aspects of the reciprocal role pair, and find it much less easy to see themselves in the other role, as with the example of Emily above. As a consequence they lack important insights into their behaviour.

This common difficulty in psychotherapy of helping patients see themselves sometimes as provoking or attacking others may be more easily overcome if the patient can see the behaviour as a part of an overall picture in which their position is not fixed but alternates within a reciprocal role pair. Clinically in the therapy, this approach is supported by the therapist and patient first writing a brief account of the patient's life experiences (the prose reformulation) and following this by collaboratively drawing a schematic diagram which shows the reciprocal roles and associated procedural sequences. This is referred to as a sequential diagrammatic reformulation (SDR). An example is shown in Fig. 1 later in the chapter. The patient can then use these reformulations between sessions to help understand what is happening. The diagrammatic reformulation is also used within the therapy session to draw attention to, and aid understanding of, the therapeutic relationship and the transference.

In this way the SDR is seen as a tool of therapy, which takes us into some of the more theoretical aspects of CAT, the work of Vygotsky and action theory.

Tools, signs, and mediated joint activity

Lev Vygotsky (1896–1934) was born in Byelorussia, and for the last 10 years of his life worked as a psychologist studying how children learned. He was enthusiastic about the application of Marxist theory in the new Soviet Union and was drawn towards ideological questions on the differences between human beings and animals, particularly higher order primates. In this ideological background the importance of work and the use of tools by humans to alter the environment were regarded as discriminating features. In the laboratory and in the classroom Vygotsky studied the way in which the child's use of tools mediated between the child and his/her environment, making it possible for the child to undertake tasks, which previously would have been too difficult or impossible. The ability to use tools then allows the child to conceive of further possibilities that could not otherwise have been thought of. In this way tools become an essential and integral part of human activity, including thinking.

Vygotsky considered a tool as being not only concrete, such as using a chair to reach up to the top of a cupboard, but also being conceptual, such as the development of mnemonics to aid memory. Such tools expand the available environment and open up possibilities for the individual. Similarly, Vygotsky developed the concept of the sign, which also mediates between the individual and the environment. A sign, such as a knot in the handkerchief to aid memory, effectively expands memory. Language is a highly complex series of signs that expands the process of thought from pre-verbal patterns. Vygotsky described the evolution of signs as a gradual process, for example the gradual development of the gesture of pointing (a sign) as coming from an early simple attempt to grasp an object out of reach. The mother interprets this grasping attempt as a sign or gesture of 'pointing' and this view is gradually internalised by the child, who eventually then produces the gesture intentionally as a communication to the adult. This internalisation means that the concept of the gesture is carried forward by the child within the context of a relationship, as a communication. Eventually language itself develops, which in many instances replaces the gesture and itself becomes a 'tool'.

In the educational field Vygotsky introduced the notion of the zone of proximal development. He noted that a child of any given age could perform a task up to a certain level if left on its own. If the child is helped by an adult, their performance improves beyond that which they can achieve on their own, the degree of this improvement varying from child to child. Vygotsky called the difference between these two levels of performance the zone of proximal development and saw it as giving an indication of what further development might be expected of the child in the foreseeable future, 'What a child can do with assistance today, she will be able to do by herself tomorrow' (Vygotsky, 1978).

Vygotsky emphasised the child's active involvement in the learning process with the adult so that over time the interpersonal situation becomes internalised and intrapersonal.

An essential feature of learning is that it creates the zone of proximal development; that is, learning awakes a variety of internal developmental processes that are able to operate only when the child is interacting with people in his environment and in cooperation with his peers. Once these processes are internalised they become part of the child's independent developmental achievement. 'Learning is not development; however properly organised learning results in mental development' (Vygotsky, 1978).

These experimental results and theoretical formulations are seen as providing a further theoretical basis for CAT, in addition to that derived from psychoanalysis. The Prose Reformulation and Sequential Diagrammatic Formulation are seen as tools provided by the therapist for joint use to be taken away by the patient and used to make personal and environmental changes. These reformulations also have a sign function in that they signify, represent, and pattern behaviour and psychic structure, and make them available for further internal processing in therapist and patient. The joint work in the psychotherapy session where the patient is helped to understand and conceptualise at a level not at first possible on his or her own, takes place in the zone of proximal development. The patient's active participation in the process of therapy is seen as an essential prerequisite for internalisation of the higher psychological function of combined tool and sign mediated activity - the interpersonal process is gradually transformed into an intrapersonal one.

Most of the theoretical formulations surrounding CAT have been presented by Anthony Ryle and one of his associates, Michael Leiman (1992, 1994, 1997). Some of the ideas of Winnicott on the development of gestures have also been incorporated in relation to the use of signs – the gesture is a sign developed in the interpersonal world and gradually internalised. That is, it is essentially a communication to others, whether consciously or not. The notion of self has also evolved, such that it is now seen as essentially social, and as developing through communication. Hence the underlying perspective is dialogic, that is, the person is created through internal and external dialogue, and the self is seen as essentially permeable, and elaborated via shared language.

The contribution of cognitive theory and therapy

The cognitive approach of construct theory was an important component of early CAT, as was the contribution of many techniques from cognitive therapy. Currently the contribution of cognitive therapy to CAT can be seen most clearly in the importance placed on addressing and monitoring overt behaviour and cognitions, the emphasis on the collaborative, real relationship between therapist and patient, and the role given to assigned homework between sessions. Conceptually cognitive therapy has also contributed the notion of safety behaviours (whereby it can be observed, for example, that patients fail to address their anxieties by protecting themselves in a variety of neurotic ways); and the notion of automatic thoughts and underlying schemas which are understood to represent stored structures of rules, assumptions or beliefs such as 'I must succeed at everything'(see for example Clark & Fairburn, 1997).

In working with a patient, the CAT therapist may draw upon these notions to help to formulate or stimulate change in the procedures employed. In addition, use of monitoring sheets, written formulations and ratings of problem procedures are designed to focus both therapist and patient on the tasks of brief therapy and to encourage the 'portability' of what has been learned after termination of therapy. It is probably true to say that in practice CAT is often seen as a dynamic rather than a cognitive therapy, although this remains a controversial issue.

Principles of therapy

Cognitive analytic therapy is a semi-structured approach normally involving 16 weekly sessions of approximately 50 minutes each. An additional follow-up session is arranged 3 months after the end of therapy.

Cognitive analytic therapy literature contains many written case examples of both reasonably straightforward and also complex cases. The reader should refer to these accounts, virtually all of which are easy to follow and understand (for example see Ryle, 1997; Ryle & Spencer, 1992; Ryle & Beard, 1993).

Broadly speaking, a 16-session therapy would fall approximately into the following sequence:

- sessions 1–3; history taking, psychotherapy file (traps, snags, dilemmas), self-monitoring, awareness of the therapeutic relationship
- session 4; written prose reformulation with coping procedures, target problems (TPs) and target problem procedures (TPPs) spelled out, including their occurrence within the therapeutic relationship. The TPs are usually the problems that the patient has come for help with, while the TPPs are the recurring patterns of behaviour, which give rise to and maintain the target problems, in accordance with the PSORM. In the following weeks, the TPs and the TPPs are monitored on a rating sheet, first to note whether they are being recognised when they happen, and later to record changes
- sessions 5–12; sequential diagrammatic reformulation (SDR), recognition of TPPs using diary, identification of core feeling states and TPPs in homework diary and in therapeutic relationship, including the transference, work on exits from problem procedures. The SDR is drawn up collaboratively within a couple of sessions of the prose reformulation being agreed. The main task after this is for the patient and the therapist to become able to recognise the occurrence of reciprocal roles and TPPs in the patient's everyday life in between sessions, and also their occurrence within the session. The latter includes drawing attention to the transference as well as use of the counter-transference. These areas are explicitly discussed using the SDR, which typically will be placed on a low table beside the therapist and patient for both to refer to as a kind of map. The therapist should take care that too ready a use of the SDR may constitute a flight in him/herself away from painful feelings evoked by the patient; a similar tendency in the patient, if significant, should already be included in

the patient's TPPs. Early pressure to work on solutions to difficulties 'exits', should be treated with caution as this may again indicate a flight from psychic pain. Initially the emphasis should be on a firm understanding and recognition of the TPPs, following which the patient will often find their own natural exits without further help from the therapist. Sometimes further behavioural and cognitive work will be needed to help the patient overcome specific obstacles. An example might be using Socratic questioning to examine the beliefs of an adult who has survived abuse, despite being threatened and terrified by the abuser as a child, that she was entirely to blame for not telling another adult about her childhood abuse (see Llewelyn & Clarke, 2001)

- sessions 13–16; ending phase of therapy, review of therapy and exchange of goodbye letters, feelings about the end of therapy, arrangements for follow-up. During this phase therapist and patient continue to work using the SDR as necessary for recognition of TPPs and reciprocal role states. TPPs to do with feelings of loss, abandonment and rejection may come more to the fore and be available for discussion. Both therapist and patient write a goodbye letter to each other giving their own views on how the therapy has progressed, what has been learnt and what has not, and what work still needs to be done. These letters are exchanged during one of the final sessions and openly discussed

- follow-up; review of progress since the end of therapy. The patient may now be discharged or some further sessions arranged.

Most patients are discharged from therapy at this point. Occasionally a few booster sessions may be arranged to re-enforce what has already been learnt. If a need is perceived for work in the longer-term, then within the CAT model the preference is for a number of 16-session contacts, with breaks in-between.

What has been outlined is a fairly standard CAT that will suit most patients with neurosis and mild personality disorders. For some patient groups the timetable for therapy is quite different, either to take account of the circumstances of referral, for example those presenting with deliberate self-harm (Cowmeadow, 1994), the consequences of childhood sexual abuse (Pollock, 2001) or borderline personality disorder (BPD) (Ryle & Golynkina, 2000). In these cases up to 24 sessions may be offered.

Example 6

Jane was in her mid-30s when she was referred for psychotherapy following marital difficulties that had led to separation from her husband and impending divorce. She was angry and depressed about the circumstances of the separation, although also concerned about the part she had played and very worried about her husband's access to their three children.

The first three sessions were spent in gaining information and some understanding of the recent difficulties, and in taking a history. At the end of the third session the therapist agreed to write a brief account of the discussion and bring it to the next session. In the fourth session the therapist came with two copies, one for himself and one for Jane in the form of a letter, and read it aloud:

'Dear Jane

Over the past couple of weeks we have talked about how, when you were growing up, you felt strongly that nobody was interested in you for yourself. You always felt that your mother was more interested in organising you and telling other people about you. You were desperate for attention from your father, but he seemed indifferent and preoccupied with his work, which often took him away from home for long periods. The contrast in their relationships with your brother, who it felt to you was the favourite of both your parents, was very distressing. You concentrated on academic success at school and your musical studies, in a way hoping your parents would appreciate you, while always anxious that getting close emotionally would mean being controlled by your mother.

As you got older, particulary during your teens, you still had the memories of the conflicts you experienced in your relationship with your mother, and you rebelled by staying out all night and took to smoking cigarettes. You coped by maintaining a distance from your mother and insisting on independence, although inside you frequently felt overwhelmed with anger and sadness about the situation. The feelings of your mother's control over you were so strong that the lesson you learnt was that to confide and trust would inevitably lead to others taking advantage of you. You eventually decided that to gain your independence you should leave home and pursue your career. You met your husband while you were at college and when you married you were optimistic about the future, but you soon realised that you married a man who repeatedly withdrew from you and denied you the emotional and physical closeness that you wanted. At times the two of you got on well, especially when the children were young. More recently however your relationship deteriorated, as the feelings of rejection became more frightening and frequent. You responded to his behaviour by provoking him, trying to make him pay attention to you, but this only had the effect of pushing him further away.

In our meetings we have discussed how this scenario is like times from your past, when you felt others tried to control you so you backed away, except in this case with your husband the roles are reversed. Almost inevitably, you were left with the familiar feeling that nobody was interested in you.

From the psychotherapy file you described particularly the dilemmas of either 'holding your ground' but risking criticism, and being compliant but feeling mistreated. You also highlighted the conflicts of being close to others but feeling overwhelmed, or staying aloof but feeling lonely.

In our sessions to date we have observed your tendency to keep your distance to avoid the risk of being hurt by criticism from me, and we need to anticipate your need to feel in control and keep the intrusion of distressing feelings and realisations at arms length.

Your main target problems are, firstly, feelings of frustration that you experience when someone is withdrawn, which tends to lead you to become angry or withdrawn also. You have realised that both of these strategies can result in your feeling even further distanced from the other person. Second you are aware of a fear of being mistreated or controlled, to which you respond by 'digging in my heels' and fighting back. You now recognise that this often drives others away and reduces even more the chances of your needs being met. In both these target problems, in spite of your seeking out others' company, the result is that your own needs are not met and this seems to be a repeating pattern.

In coming into treatment you have acknowledged the possiblity that your inner feelings, outlook on others, and patterns of behaviour affect your relationships. In our meetings we have already seen that in spite of your fear that I too might be rejecting, or will try to control you, you have felt more able to risk showing your feelings and thereby allow the possibility that a new experience of mutual respect might occur.'

When this was read out to Jane, the therapist could see that she was struggling for several minutes to keep control of her feelings. It was apparent that she had been emotionally affected by the reformulation, but as she collected herself she started to correct some of the minor factual errors it contained. The therapist responded to this by drawing Jane's attention to her fear of not being completely in control in the session and worried about exposing her feelings and being vulnerable, as described in the reformulation. This led to some relaxation in the atmosphere of the session and they agreed to construct a diagram that would show simply Jane's problem procedures and emotional states that led to them. In the next session Jane and her therapist worked out the SDR showing the procedural sequences as well as the reciprocal roles that lay behind the procedures (Fig. 5.1). Target problems and TPPs were listed on the rating sheet.

For several sessions the task in therapy centred on recognising the operation of the problem procedures and labelling the feeling states that accompanied them. A homework diary was kept to record the situations in which Jane felt

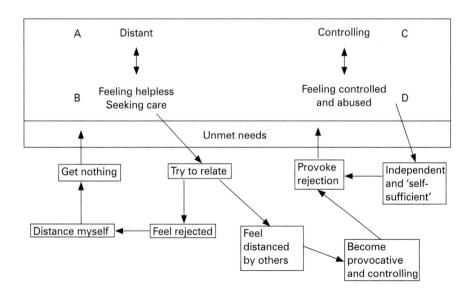

Fig. 5.1 Sequential diagrammatic reformulation showing procedural sequences and reciprocal roles

helpless, and times when she felt intruded upon. Recognition of TPs and TPPs was scored weekly on the rating sheet. For example, she related an incident where she and a friend had gone to meet two girlfriends for a night out, but the friends had not turned up. Although on closer examination it seemed that the arrangement had been quite casual, Jane was angered by it and spoke of going to find them to express some of her anger. Using the SDR it was possible to see how the women represented the role 'A', with Jane in the role 'B', and how she was now planning to carry out the procedure in which she became emotionally 'provocative and controlling'. In the session she was impressed by the pattern being so clearly visible in the diagram, together with the probable outcome, and could readily see that her plan was unlikely to produce a response that would meet her needs.

On another occasion, while trying to negotiate over the telephone with her husband for access arrangements for him to see their children, she began to feel quite angry about his apparent aloofness and could feel herself becoming more demanding. By this stage in the therapy she was becoming accustomed to thinking about the SDR or having it available to consult, and she quickly realised she was about to enter the 'provocative and controlling' procedure yet again. When she realised this, she decided she would not fall into this pattern of behaviour and so backed off, conveying to her husband that she would fit in with his arrangements on this occasion. Much to her surprise, it seemed that this led to a change in her husband's position, and by the end of the conversation they had agreed arrangements that she felt were better for herself and the children than she had hoped for at the start of the discussion.

In a similar way, she was able to carry through a visit to see her parents without feeling that at any moment she may be taken over by her mother. In fact she commented in the session following this visit (session 12) that she realised now that her mother was quite a frail old woman and that she had little to fear from her. With apparently new-found skill she managed to handle the situation without the confrontation that had always arisen in the past.

On several occasions the SDR was used to elucidate aspects of the therapeutic relationship. For example, Jane asked for a change in the time of one of the sessions and seemed reluctant to offer any explanation for the request. The therapist enquired if there might be a possibility that Jane was now being distant 'A' in the therapy to put the therapist in position 'B'. Jane's reply was that when a fortnight previously the therapist had rearranged the date of a session without explanation she had felt both irritated and also worried that the sessions might mean more to her than to the therapist (therapist 'A' v. Jane 'B'). There also seemed to be a threat in Jane's mind relating to her need to be in control, which was challenged by the earlier rearrangement (therapist 'C' to Jane 'D'). Jane's reaction had been to follow previous patterns of behaviour 'distance myself' and 'independent' rather than openly express her feelings, as she was now doing.

By session 12 it was clear that Jane was making good use of what she had learned in the therapy and was spontaneously applying it. She was keeping regular notes on her homework monitoring sheets of progress in recognising and challenging her unhelpful procedures. Whereas she had previously denied that termination would be an issue for her, she now came to realise that the therapy had been of great support to her and she feared slipping back after it ended. However, by virtue of the fact that she was speaking in this way about the ending, and did not at this point seem to be moving into a 'problem procedure', both she and the therapist felt that she would be unlikely to slip back and that new and more adaptive procedures were becoming more natural. She also reported that someone said she had become more open at work. She had allowed herself to disclose more of what she felt about work situations and found that others usually responded well to being told more and did not take advantage.

On session 13 goodbye letters were exchanged. In the therapist's letter, it was sympathetically pointed out that seeing others less in stereotyped roles, and more as whole people, considerably reduced her anxiety in social situations and led to her being more open and less confrontational. For example

'You have started saying more about your feelings and you found that others did not seem to use this as an opportunity to get the upper hand or control you. As a consequence you have been feeling better about yourself and more confident, and able to work in partnership with others when there are things to be done.'

The therapeutic relationship was also referred to:

'At one point early on in our meetings I suggested you seemed to feel inhibited about exposing your feelings in case it gave me the chance to get the better of you, which is what you experienced with your mother. We thought the underlying fear in our relationship was of a repeat of the reciprocal relationship with her, only with me as the controlling one in this situation. Of course, our discussion did not completely resolve your fears about showing feelings in our meetings but it did result in you feeling more relaxed about this. In particular it seems that outside of the therapy you now feel much more in touch with your feelings and able to express them.'

A final paragraph referred to the likelihood that old patterns would continue to emerge and that this is to be expected especially at times of stress. The importance of re-reading the reformulation and SDR and of continuing to use this was emphasised. Finally the appointment in 3 months' time to review progress was noted.

Jane also brought in a goodbye letter in which she commented on her increasing ability to reflect on the importance of her early experiences, particularly with her mother, and her understanding of how she had become locked into counterproductive ways of relating to others. She also commented that although she had not found therapy easy, all the major issues had been openly and honestly discussed, and moreover that the result had not been as painful as she had anticipated.

Jane forgot to turn up for the next session, and telephoned apologetically the following day. At the final session, the SDR was discussed, including how forgetting the previous session might have been her reaction to the impending ending, construed as 'distant 'A' v. seeking care 'B'', which she had dealt with by attempting to turn the tables and become the one who was 'distant'. In the course of this discussion Jane was able to acknowledge both angry and anxious feelings about the end.

At the 3-month follow-up appointment she had continued to make adjustments. Satisfactory arrangements were in place for her husband's access to his children; she had cautiously formed a new relationship with another man, and seemed to have little difficulty in allowing him freedom. She remained less concerned than previously about being controlled by others.

Contrasts and comparisons with psychoanalysis

There are a number of similarities and differences between CAT and psychoanalysis. Ryle has written on this subject in several articles as well as in his books (Ryle, 1992, 1993, 1994a, 1995c, 1996, 2001), which he describes as an ongoing attempt to question and clarify psychoanalytic assumptions and practices. For Ryle, psychoanalytic views on the importance of development and the way this affects one's personality, object relations theory, and the concepts of transference and countertransference are an essential part of CAT. However there are many differences, for example the perception that psychoanalysis may involve the analyst wielding power over the analysand, unlike the collaborative methods of CAT, and also that psychoanalysis places emphasis on innate drives as compared to the experience of the infant with its parents and others. Perhaps for this reason the work of Bowlby on human attachment has become, of late, more prominent in CAT literature, largely because of Bowlby's attention to observational studies of early infant relationships, and his view that attachment behaviour is innate. (Ryle, 1995a, 1995d). However, it must be noted that Ryle has drawn a distinction between the theoretical contributions of attachment theory and of CAT (Jellama, 1999), suggesting that attachment theory has not generated a coherent clinical method, and also that it is essentially 'cognitivist', not dialogically focused (Ryle, 2001).

The unconscious

The length of CAT does not allow the unfolding of deeply hidden unconscious material that takes place during the years of psychoanalysis. In Ryle's view this is usually irrelevant as the PSORM concentrates on overt behaviour, manifesting the unconscious at work in the patient's life, and shows what the patient has to deal with.

Drives

Drives are acknowledged in CAT as existing, but are not seen as explaining much about human differences, for which sociocultural explanations or traumatic life events are preferred. In particular, the idea of the internal world being dominated by anxiety and destructiveness that is innate is rejected. CAT emphasises intentional action.

Technique

The length of pychoanalytic treatment is seen as impractical and inappropriate for most NHS settings. It is also considered that in analysis there is insufficient linking between the interpersonal and the intrapersonal. Sitting behind the patient is seen as a non-collaborative activity and as refusing to offer a healthy reciprocating relationship.

Interpretation

Interpretation is seen as a relatively dangerous and usually unhelpful activity, regarded by Ryle as too often being theory driven and as persuading the patient to accept something they cannot know. Further, it is assumed that analytical interpretation is always directed to what the patient does not know and so does not facilitate the patient's learning to be reflective themselves. Interpretations made from a view that destructiveness is innate must seem critical, whereas close empathic tracking excites the patient's wish for a perfect relationship. 'CAT is primarily concerned with accurate description and non-collusion' (Ryle, 1995d).

Projective identification

Projective identification is seen as a special example of the general situation in which a patient attempts to enact a reciprocal role procedure, in order to elicit a required role from the other (Ryle 1994b). In a more disturbed patient, it implies a splitting in the personality of the kind referred to earlier in the chapter, and in the section (below) on BPD. The other person is pressured to take on a role that the patient is frightened to experience, and in Ryle's view, dependency and control are usually implied. Projective identification in infancy as a communication is seen as a way of enabling the infant to function in the zone of proximal development by helping the infant to contain emotional experience that would otherwise be overwhelming, and in CAT terms involves the joint creation and shaping of mediating signs. Therapeutic 'reverie' occurs when the therapist is available to receive projective identification, is able to recognise and name it, and integrate it by relating it to other aspects of the patient's functioning using the reformulation. Use of the SDR by the therapist is vital to prevent continued enactment by the therapist of the role assigned to him or her by the patient.

Contrasts and comparisons with cognitive therapy

As noted above, CAT has probably drawn more from the theoretical heritage of dynamic psychology than cognitive psychology, especially in recent years. Nevertheless, Ryle pays a considerable tribute to the work of George Kelly (1905–1967) (who can be described as an early cognitive psychologist) as being a major influence on the development of CAT. Grid methodology, developed by Kelly, is still widely used in CAT research, and the psychotherapy file uses language and concepts from construct theory. The use of structured formulations also parallels cognitive therapy. Ryle does however seek to distance CAT from constructivism, which he considers to be incompatible with philosophy of dialogism, that is, the self as defined and developed in relation to others. He contrasts the focus of CAT on general patterns of relationships, with that of the cognitive–behavioural therapy (CBT) focus on individual symptoms, behaviours and beliefs (see Ryle, 2001). Unlike CBT, formulations in CAT tend to demonstrate the circularity of procedures, and locate the sense of self as socially formed and multi-voiced, rather than unitary and individualised.

One specific application: borderline personality disorder

The most striking feature of BPD is the alternation between different states of mind in the one person, with apparently little connection between the states. As a result, the patient appears to become a different person when triggered in some way. A previously helpful patient will suddenly become furious and threaten to sue because of a word misunderstood or uttered out of place. Another patient will seem to be relaxed among company, but when on her own begins to feel she is falling apart and can only hold herself together by cutting her arms or burning herself with cigarettes.

In CAT these different states of mind, or self states, which are split from each other are each described and separately represented in the reformulation and SDR, with particular attention paid to the triggers which cause the movement between the states. Each self state will have its own reciprocal roles and procedures. The aim of the therapist using CAT is to help a patient to understand his or her apparently inexplicable fury when faced with apparent rejection (for example a friend failing to return a telephone call) as being the consequence of the fracturing effect of an emotionally depriving early environment in which the infant has been required to operate in and beyond the zone of proximal development without the help of a parent or carer. Feeling abandoned and abused most of the time, the patient has created in his mind an ideal world in which he is ideally cared for, only to be plunged back into despair and fury when the ideal carer appears to fail in any way (for example see Clarke & Llewelyn, 2001). CAT therapists have found the SDR of particular help with this group, describing the integrating effect of naming the various self states, and clearly documenting their interconnections. This allows the patient a chance to act as an observer, and to trace the confusing shifts in their feelings and movement from one self-state to another (Ryle & Beard, 1993; Ryle, 1995d). Perhaps not surprisingly CAT is now increasingly being used with this patient group.

Possibly one of the most helpful contributions of CAT to therapy with BPDs is in fact to help clinical staff to understand the behaviours and reaction of patients. The swings in mood and operation of different reciprocal roles within a patient can frequently lead to splitting within staff teams, if no understanding of the process is available. Having a model that contains and explains why some staff members have very different views of a patient from others (for example helpless victim versus manipulative perpetrator) can defuse potentially destructive situations for the benefit of patient and team alike (Dunn & Parry, 1997).

Research and CAT

There have been a number of studies pointing to CAT as being an effective therapy in a variety of situations. For example, in clinical studies, without randomised controls, CAT has been associated with a positive outcome in a community mental health centre population (Garyfallos *et al*, 1993); with adult survivors of childhood sexual abuse (Clarke & Llewelyn, 1994; Llewelyn & Clarke, 2001); in an intensive study of two women who stabbed their partners (Pollock & Kear-Colwell, 1994); in a further seven women who had been sexually abused in childhood and who had committed violent offences (assault, stabbing and shooting) against their partners (Pollock, 1996, 2001); and in out-patient groups (Duignan & Mitzman, 1994; Hagan & Gregory, 2001). Of note is the number of patients diagnosed as suffering from BPD in the above studies; not only as would be expected in Pollock (1996) but also in Garyfallos *et al* (1993), Duignan & Mitzman (1994) and Hagan & Gregory (2001). In these studies many of the patients obtained good outcomes. Ryle and a number of his colleagues have also been involved in a long-term study of BPD and CAT. Results so far have indicated a good success rate (Ryle & Golynkina, 2000) and data are still being collected.

A number of researchers have been working on the development of appropriate psychometric measures for an evaluation of CAT. For example Pollock (2001) describes research into the properties of the Personality Structure Questionnaire (PSQ) as a measure of identity disturbance. Such measures will undoubtedly assist in the empirical investigation of CAT, particularly with patients with personality disorder.

Turning to controlled trials, CAT has been found to be effective and produced equivalent symptomatic change to time-limited psychotherapy (Mann & Goldman, 1982), with CAT subjects improving significantly more on repertory grid measures, suggesting greater internal change (Brockman *et al*, 1987). CAT has also been found to be effective with non-compliant patients suffering from insulin-dependent diabetes (Fosbury, 1994; Ryle, 1995*d*) and with poor-complying asthmatic patients (Bosley *et al*, 1992). In a pilot study comparing CAT with educational behaviour therapy for out-patients with anorexia nervosa, Treasure *et al* (1995) found that CAT patients reported greater subjective, but not objective improvement. Other controlled trials are currently in progress; for example that led by Clarke (2001) for the treatment of BPD.

Lastly, a number of process studies have looked at the additional value of using a CAT model to investigate the psychological mechanisms inherent in various mental health problems and situations. Many of the above treatment studies have included an investigation of process. Studies have confirmed the usefulness and validity of the SDR, the concept of self-states, the impact of reformulation (Evans & Parry, 1996), and reciprocal role procedures (Clarke & Llewelyn, 1994; Pollock, 1996, 2001; Ryle, 1995*b*). Clarke & Pearson (2000) have looked at changes in personal constructs of males who have survived sexual abuse in group CAT, while Walsh (1996) has used CAT to investigate a dysfunctional staff group in a surgical unit.

Clearly the research base for CAT is at an early stage. The structure of CAT, with its explicit written documentation and time limits lends itself to empirical research. It is to be expected that more evidence will accumulate with time and as the number of practitioners increases.

Implications

Cognitive analytic therapy is indicated for a wide range of neurotic disorders and personality disorders. Patients suffering from severe phobic or obsessive–compulsive symptoms will probably need another form of treatment at least initially, as will intoxicated substance misusers. There is little evidence as yet to support the use of CAT in the psychoses. There are many other situations where CAT may be profitably employed, such as in medical patients not complying with treatment, and in organisational consultancy. It seems likely that CAT is most usefully used for the more difficult-to-treat individuals, such as those with BPDs, where clarity of thinking and good communication is particularly crucial.

Although CAT is an interesting new development in psychotherapy, it is not without its critics. Ryle's critiques of other psychotherapeutic work have provoked debate and a number of interesting points have been made in reply (Scott, 1993; Fonagy, 1995; Likierman, 1995; Jellama, 1999). First, there is the issue of the time frame; does CAT allow the time for 'working through'? Ryle explicitly acknowledges that CAT does not allow time for growth, but aims to do something about patients stopping themselves from growing. In reality what does this amount to; does the process simply inform or educate the patient about his or her problems and then leave them to get on and make the best of it on their own?

Second, doubts have been expressed about the degree of psychopathology that can be addressed with a treatment that seems to rely on the patient being able to think in symbolic terms. What of concrete-thinking individuals who may be unable to grasp the representational nature of what CAT is trying to teach, for example with the SDR? Is the apparent improvement in the case of BPD due to a temporary increase in self-esteem brought about by being treated by the therapist as a thinking individual?

Third, much is made of the power imbalance, for example in psychoanalysis, which allows the analyst to make interpretations about things the patient cannot know and yet have them accepted by the patient. Yet is CAT likely to be free of similar accusations when the therapist can produce a piece of writing and a diagram in the course of three or four meetings, which seems to sum up a patient's life experience? How likely is this to provoke envy or irritation in the patient that is nevertheless hidden behind a temporary compliance towards the therapist? How often is the understanding of a patient prematurely foreclosed so that he or she will fit into a CAT formulation?

Next, how focal is CAT? The reformulations are wide-ranging and may reflect profound aspects of the patient's personality and identity. How much can such central aspects of a person change in short-term work?

Last, what about the evidence base? As noted above, no randomised controlled trial has yet been carried out for CAT, which seriously affects its chances of widespread acceptance in many circles, especially given current emphasis on the evidence base within the NHS.

In response, Ryle and others address a number of these issues in the literature and point to the ethics and pragmatics of offering something psychotherapeutic to all referrals, as compared with long-term therapy to the privileged few. CAT can be seen as a first-line approach from which patients may go on to long-term work or group therapy if necessary. For others it may well be all that is needed to promote healthier development. Continued research and the accumulation of clinical experience should indicate over the next 10 years how helpful CAT will be, and for which patients.

References

Bosley, C. M., Fosbury, J., Parry, D. T., *et al* (1992) Psychological aspects of patient compliance in asthma. *European Respiratory Journal*, **5** (suppl. 15).

Brockman, B., Poynton, A., Ryle, A., *et al* (1987). Effectiveness of time-limited therapy carried out by trainees: comparison of two methods. *British Journal of Psychiatry*, **151**, 602–610.

Clark, D. & Fairburn, C. (eds) (1997) *Science and Practice of Cognitive Behaviour Therapy*. Oxford: Oxford University Press.

Clarke, S. (2001) A randomised trial of the efficacy of CAT for the treatment of personality disorder. *Association of Cognitive Analytic Therapy Newsletter*, **15**, 15.

Clarke, S. & Llewelyn, S. (1994) Personal constructs of survivors of childhood sexual abuse receiving cognitive analytic therapy. *British Journal of Medical Psychology*, **67**, 273–289.

Clarke, S. & Llewelyn, S. (2001) A case of borderline personality disorder. In *Cognitive Analytic Therapy and Adult Survivors of Childhood Abuse* (ed. P. Pollock), pp. 123–143. Chichester: Wiley.

Clarke, S. & Pearson, C. (2000) Personal constructs of male survivors of childhood sexual abuse receiving cognitive analytic therapy. *British Journal of Medical Psychology*, **73**, 169–178.

Cowmeadow, P. (1994) Deliberate self-harm and cognitive analytic therapy. *International Journal of Short-Term Psychotherapy*, **9**, 135–150.

Duignan, I. & Mitzman, S. (1994) Measuring individual change in patients receiving time-limited cognitive analytic therapy. *International Journal of Time-Limited Psychotherapy*, **9**, 151–160.

Dunn, M. & Parry, G. (1997). A formulated care plan approach to caring for people with borderline personality disorder in a community mental health service setting. *Clinical Psychology Forum*, **104**, 19–22.

Evans, J. & Parry, G. (1996) The impact of reformulation in cognitive analytic therapy with difficult-to-help clients. *Clinical Psychology and Psychotherapy*, **3**, 109–117.

Fonagy, P. (1995). Psychoanalysis, cognitive-analytic therapy, mind and self. British Journal of Psychotherapy Annual Lecture 1994. *British Journal of Psychotherapy*, **11**, 575–584.

Fosbury, J. A. (1994). Cognitive analytic therapy with poorly controlled insulin-dependent diabetic patients. In *Psychology and Diabetes Care* (ed. C. Coles), pp. 959–964. Chichester: PMH Productions.

Garyfallos, C., Adampoulou, M., Saitis, M., *et al* (1993) Evaluation of cognitive analytic therapy (CAT) outcome. *Neurologia Psychiatra*, **12**, 121–25.

Hagan, T. & Gregory, K. (2001). Group work with survivors of childhood sexual abuse. In *Cognitive Analytic Therapy and Adult Survivors of Childhood Abuse* (ed. P. Pollock) pp. 190–205. Chichester: Wiley.

Jellama, A. (1999) Cognitive analytic therapy: developing its theory and practice via attachment theory. *Clinical Psychology and Psychotherapy*, **6**, 16–28.

Kelly, G. A. (1955) *The Psychology of Personal Constructs. Vols 1 & 2*. Norton Press.

Leiman, M. (1992) The concept of sign in the work of Vygotsky, Winnicott and Bakhtin: further integration of object relations theory and activity theory. *British Journal of Medical Psychology*, **65**, 209–221.

Leiman, M. (1994) Projective identification as early joint action sequences: a Vygotskian addendum to the Procedural Sequence Object Relations Model. *British Journal of Medical Psychology*, **67**, 97–106.

Leiman, M. (1997) Procedures as dialogical sequences: a revised version of the fundamental concept in cognitive analytic therapy. *British Journal of Medical Psychology*, **70**, 193–207.

Likierman, M. (1995) Response to 'Defensive organisations or collusive interpretations?' by Anthony Ryle. *British Journal of Psychotherapy*, **12**, 69–72.

Llewelyn, S. & Clarke, S. (2001) Adult psychological problems and abuse. In *Cognitive Analytic Therapy and Adult Survivors of Childhood Abuse* (ed. P. Pollock), pp. 107–122. Chichester: Wiley.

Mann, J. & Goldman, R. (1982) *A Casebook of Time-Limited Psychotherapy*. New York: McGraw Hill.

Ogden, T. H. (1983) The concept of internal object relations. *International Journal of Psycho-Analysis*, **64**, 227–242.

Pollock, P. (1996) Clinical issues in the cognitive analytic therapy of sexually abused women who commit violent offences against their partners. *British Journal of Medical Psychology*, **69**, 117–127.

Pollock, P. (ed.) (2001) *Cognitive Analytic Therapy and Adult Survivors of Childhood Abuse*. Chichester: Wiley.

Pollock, P., & Kear-Colwell, J. (1994). Women who stab: a personal construct analysis of sexual victimisation and offending behaviour. *British Journal of Medical Psychology*, **67**, 13–22.

Ryle, A. (1978) A common language for the psychotherapies? *British Journal of Psychiatry*, **132**, 585–594.

Ryle, A. (1979) The focus in brief interpretive psychotherapy: dilemmas, traps and snags as target problems. *British Journal of Psychiatry*, **134**, 46–54.

Ryle, A. (1980) Some measures of goal attainment in focused integrated active psychotherapy: a study of fifteen cases. *British Journal of Psychiatry*, **137**, 475–486.

Ryle, A. (1982) *Psychotherapy: a cognitive integration of theory and practice*. London: Academic Press.

Ryle, A. (1985) Cognitive theory, object relations and the self. *British Journal of Medical Psychology*, **58**, 1–7.

Ryle, A (1990) *Cognitive Analytic Therapy: Active Participation in Change*. Chichester: Wiley.

Ryle, A. (1991) Object relations theory and activity theory: a proposed link by way of the procedural sequence model. *British Journal of Medical Psychology*, **64**, 307–316.

Ryle, A. (1992) Critique of a Kleinian case presentation. *British Journal of Medical Psychology*, **65**, 309–317.

Ryle, A. (1993) Addiction to the death instinct? A critical review of Joseph's paper 'Addiction to Near Death'. *British Journal of Psychotherapy*, **10**, 88–92.

Ryle, A. (1994a) Response. Psychoanalysis and cognitive analytic therapy. *British Journal of Psychotherapy*, **10**, 402–404.

Ryle, A. (1994b) Projective identification: a particular form of reciprocal role procedure. *British Journal of Medical Psychology*, **67**, 107–114.

Ryle, A. (1995a) Holmes on Bowlby and the future of psychotherapy: a response. *British Journal of Psychotherapy*, **11**, 3, 448–452.

Ryle, A. (1995b) Transference and counter-transference variations in the course of the cognitive-analytic therapy of two borderline patients: the relation to the diagrammatic reformulation of self-states. *British Journal of Medical Psychology*, **68**, 109–124.

Ryle, A. (1995c) Defensive organizations or collusive interpretations? A further critique of Kleinian theory and practice. *British Journal of Psychotherapy*, **12**, 6068.

Ryle, A. (ed.) (1995d) *Cognitive Analytic Therapy. Developments in Theory and Practice*. Chichester: Wiley.

Ryle, A. (1996) Ogden's autistic–contiguous position and the role of interpretation in psychoanalytic theory building. *British Journal of Medical Psychology*, **69**, 129–138.

Ryle, A. (1997) *Cognitive Analytic Therapy and Borderline Personality Disorder: The Model and the Method*. Chichester: Wiley.

Ryle, A. (2001) Constructivism and CAT. *Association of Cognitive Analytic Therapy Newsletter*, **15**, 23–25.

Ryle, A. & Beard, H. (1993) The integrative effect of reformulation: CAT with a patient with borderline personality disorder. *British Journal of Medical Psychology*, **66**, 249–258.

Ryle, A. & Golynkina, K. (2000) Effectiveness of time-limited cognitive analytic therapy of borderline personality disorder. *British Journal of Medical Psychology*, **73**, 197–210.

Ryle, A. & Kerr, I. (2002) *Introducing Cognitive Analytic Therapy*. Wiley.

Ryle, A. & Spencer, J. (1992) When less is more or at least enough. Two case examples of 16-session cognitive analytic therapy. *British Journal of Psychotherapy*, **8**, 401–412.

Sheard, T., Evans, J., Cash, D., *et al* (2000) A CAT-derived one to three session intervention for repeated deliberate self-harm: a description of the model and initial experience of trainee psychiatrists in using it. *British Journal of Medical Psychology*, **73**, 179–196.

Scott, A. (1993) Response to Anthony Ryle. *British Journal of Psychotherapy*, **10**, 93–95.

Treasure, J., Todd, G., Brolly, M., *et al* (1995). A pilot study of a randomised trial of cognitive analytic therapy vs. educational behavioural therapy for adult anorexia nervosa. *Behaviour Research and Therapy*, **33**, 363–367.

Vygotsky, L. (1978) *Mind in Society. The Development of Higher Psychological Processes.* (eds M. Cole, V. John-Steiner, S. Scribner, *et al*). Cambridge, MA: Harvard University Press.

Walsh, S. (1996) Adapting cognitive analytic therapy to make sense of psychologically harmful work environments. *British Journal of Medical Psychology*, **69**, 3–20.

Walsh, S., Hagan, T. & Gamsu, D. (2000). Rescuer and rescued: applying a cognitive analytic perspective to explore the 'mis-management' of asthma. *British Journal of Medical Psychology*, **73**, 51–168.

CHAPTER 6

Behavioural and cognitive theories

Lynne M. Drummond & Hilary Warwick

This chapter covers the main theoretical basis for the development of the behavioural and cognitive therapies, more commonly now referred to jointly as cognitive–behavioural therapy (CBT). It begins with a review of learning theory and how this was applied to development of behavioural treatments with patients. It then follows on to describe the development of cognitive theories and the subsequent expansion in the range of therapeutic applications that are then described in detail in the next chapter.

Learning theory

Classical conditioning

The famous experiments of Pavlov at the end of the 19th century, demonstrated the principles of classical conditioning. Dogs will usually salivate (an unconditioned response) in the presence of food (an unconditioned stimulus). The presentation of food to dogs was repeatedly paired with the sound of a bell, and eventually the sound of the bell alone would produce salivation in the absence of any food. So the dogs had been conditioned, or had learnt, to salivate (the conditioned response) to a new stimulus (the conditioned stimulus). It was also discovered that the conditioned response would fail to occur, or extinguish, if the conditioned stimulus was repeatedly presented without the unconditioned stimulus; eventually the dogs after time ceased to salivate to the sound of the bell if it was not followed immediately by food.

Operant conditioning

Skinner (1953) described operant conditioning, in which learning occurs by reinforcement. The law of effect states that 'behaviour which is followed by satisfying consequences will tend to be repeated, and behaviour which is followed by unpleasant consequences will occur less frequently'. Positive reinforcement is the situation where a behaviour occurs more frequently because it is followed by positive consequences. Similarly negative reinforcement describes the increase in frequency of a behaviour which occurs in the absence of an expected aversive event. If an aversive event is presented then the frequency of the behaviour decreases, i.e. punishment. If an expected reward does not occur the frequency of the preceding behaviour decreases, i.e. frustrative non-reward.

Subsequent experimental work with animals showed that conditioning could produce neurotic behaviour and that this behaviour showed all the characteristics of normal learning. Mowrer (1947) suggested a two-factor model to account for fear and avoidance, in which fears of specific stimuli were acquired through classical conditioning. As fear is an aversive experience, the animal learns to reduce it by avoiding the conditioned stimuli. This reduction in fear leads to reinforcement of the avoidance behaviour and its increase in frequency: avoidance is learnt as an operant. Mowrer's theory thus accounted for the aetiology and maintenance of the fear.

Applications of learning theory to human behaviour

Treatment principles that were derived from classical and operant conditioning were used in the first behaviour therapy, which started to be developed in the early 1950s. Behaviour therapy was first applied in two areas, the treatment of the behaviour of people with chronic psychiatric disorders and in the treatment of adult neurotic disorders.

Chronic psychiatric disorders

Long-term severe mental health problems were conceptualised in Skinnerian operant terms, in that the abnormal behaviours of the patients were thought to be the result of inappropriate conditioning. Normal behaviour could therefore be shaped by the use of appropriate reinforcement, hence appropriate responses were followed by reward and non-rewarding consequences followed inappropriate behaviours. These principles were applied to conditions such as chronic schizophrenia, autism and mental handicap (as it was termed then). Behaviour modification is the term currently used in the UK to describe treatment techniques derived from operant conditioning principles. Examples are contingency management, token economy, shaping and massed practice, and their clinical applications are described in Chapter 7.

Adult neurotic disorders

Neurotic conditions have been defined as 'persistent unadaptive learned habits, with anxiety as the foremost feature' (Wolpe, 1982). Rachman (1977) described a two-process model to account for the acquisition and maintenance of phobias. In phobic disorders, classical conditioning leads to anxiety in the presence of a stimulus that would not normally be regarded as dangerous. Escape from the feared stimulus leads to an immediate reduction in anxiety and this reduction reinforces the escape behaviour.

Future escape from and avoidance of the feared stimulus prevents extinction of the initial anxiety, as further exposure to the initial stimulus and hence habituation cannot occur and the phobic problem is maintained.

In obsessive–compulsive disorder, the initial intrusive phenomena, for example thought, image or impulse, is the conditioned stimulus and leads to anxiety. There is usually an associated urge to neutralise this anxiety and the discomfort it causes. Thus, the involuntary obsessional intrusion is followed by voluntary behaviours, known as compulsive rituals, which relieve the anxiety and discomfort by terminating exposure to the feared stimuli. Compulsive rituals can be covert thoughts as well as overt behaviour and their occurrence prevents extinction of the initial anxiety. The decrease in anxiety and discomfort experienced serves to reinforce the compulsive behaviour and its frequency increases, therefore maintaining the problem.

Avoidance of situations that trigger the obsessional intrusions is also learnt as an operant and is a further maintaining factor. A wide range of stimuli can lead to irrational fears, however prepotency theory (Marks, 1969) suggests that members of a species are more likely to respond to certain stimuli of particular evolutionary significance than others. For example it is relatively easy for a child to learn fear of spiders, whereas fear of trees is much rarer and normally preceded by an obvious aversive event associated with a tree (Ohman & Dimberg, 1984; Ohman et al, 1984).

Wolpe (1958) conducted important animal experiments in which neuroses were induced, and also developed fear reduction techniques. Fear was reduced by reintroducing the animal to the fear conditioning stimulus in a gradual way, providing the animal with food at intervals. Wolpe went on to develop the theory of reciprocal inhibition. This proposes that successful treatment of anxiety depends on repeated exposure to feared stimuli, along with the imposition of an incompatible response, which inhibits the fear. In humans, the gradual exposure to feared stimuli was carried out in the imagination and was paired with relaxation as the inhibition of fear. This important technique was known as systematic desensitisation.

Behaviour therapy for neuroses has gradually been refined and graded exposure in real life, without a fear inhibitor such as relaxation, is recognised as the treatment of choice for neuroses such as phobias and obsessive–compulsive disorder. As predicted from learning theory described above, successful exposure treatment leads to extinction of the conditioned fear response. This is achieved by elimination of operant behaviours that lead to premature termination of exposure to the conditioned stimulus. A patient with a phobia must stay in the situation that provokes his or her fear without escaping from it, and a patient with obsessive–compulsive disorder must be exposed to feared stimuli and must not be permitted to carry out compulsive rituals – response prevention. Exposure can then be of adequate duration for extinction to occur. Anxiety levels will initially be high, but will gradually fade, in the process known as habituation. A full account of clinical behaviour therapy for neuroses is given in the next chapter.

Learning theory does not take into account vicarious acquisition and informational acquisition that are also important in the aetiology of anxiety, therefore the need for a comprehensive new theory of fear and anxiety was noted (Rachman, 1977). In addition some people became dissatisfied with behaviour therapy during the 1970s and 1980s, as practitioners gave less importance to learning theory per se and treatments became more empirically based. This dissatisfaction helped to lead to the development of cognitive approaches.

Cognitive theories

Changing behaviour leads to a cognitive shift, so that when behaviour therapy teaches a patient to alter his behaviour his thinking also changes. Radical behaviourists did not attempt to manipulate cognitive variables directly. They found, however, that when the behavioural principles effective in the treatment of anxiety disorders and chronic psychiatric disorders were applied to depression, there was little success.

This led to examination of the cognitive component of depressive disorders, which commenced in the 1970s. Wolpe (1982) states that many non-neurotic fears, those relating to real threats, are cognitively based, having been acquired through information. Misinformation can bring about fears that are as powerful and enduring as those based on truth. In describing social learning theory, Bandura (1969) suggested that central mechanisms have an important role in learning, in addition to the more peripheral concept of behaviour. He stressed the importance of vicarious, symbolic and self-regulatory learning processes and argued that virtually all behaviour learned through direct experience can be learned from observation. Crucially he suggested that cognitive processes provide a link between external stimuli and overt behaviour.

Seligman (1970) observed that depressed patients often blame themselves when things go wrong, even when events are beyond their control. This learned helplessness theory of depression states that the basic cause is an expectation. The patient expects that bad events will occur and there is nothing he can do to prevent their occurrence. Evidence suggests that when patients fail at important tasks and make internal explanations for their failure, passivity appears and self-esteem drops. When individuals make external explanations for failure, passivity ensues but self-esteem stays high (Abramson *et al*, 1978).

According to Meichenbaum (1977) the persistence of many disorders is due to the fact that patients engage in unhelpful internal dialogues when faced with stressful situations, for example a patient in a train might say to himself 'if this train stops in a tunnel I shall go mad'. Cognitive therapy encourages the patient to change unhelpful internal dialogue.

The type of cognitive therapy advocated by Ellis (1962) is called rational–emotive therapy. Ellis suggests that if a disorder is caused by illogical premises or illogical ideas, patients can often be persuaded or taught to think more logically and hence overcome the disorder. He identified certain self-defeating ideas held by neurotic patients and tried to change them by rational argument designed to alter cognitions directly.

According to Beck (Beck *et al*, 1979), the emotional impact of an event is mediated through the meaning of the event, rather than the event itself. The meaning is accessed through conscious automatic negative thoughts and images. The marked mood swings that can be a feature of the patient who is depressed are brought on by idiosyncratic automatic thoughts and images. These thoughts take the form of negativistic ideas concerning the person in relation to his environment, which have been well rehearsed over a number of years. Beck suggests a cognitive triad, in which the patient holds negative views of him- or herself, the world and the future. The patient consistently makes a number of thinking errors, or cognitive distortions, which are prominent in the content of their negative automatic thoughts.

Examples of negative automatic thoughts:

- all or nothing thinking: a woman ruins a special dinner and thinks 'I am a complete failure'
- overgeneralising: a man attends an interview and does not get the job, 'I will never get a job, no one will ever take me on'
- disqualifying the positive: a man was thinking about his considerable recent successes at work, 'It was nothing, anyone could have done this better than me'
- jumping to conclusions: a man with indigestion after a large spicy meal, rushed to his doctor, 'I must have stomach cancer'
- magnification or minimisation: a girl made a minor error in an essay, 'My whole paper is ruined, it's a disaster'
- emotional reasoning: a woman held distressing beliefs based only on her emotions, rather than any objective evidence 'I feel useless, so I cannot be any good at anything'.

When a situation provokes negative automatic thoughts, a number of reactions follow. The person will experience a change in emotion, for example sadness or depression, changes in behaviour, such as social withdrawal, and physiological symptoms, such as heaviness in the abdomen.

It is suggested that negative automatic thoughts are produced when a stressful event activates unrealistic core beliefs. From our early childhood, all of us try to make sense of the environment and to organise our experiences in a coherent way, in order to function adaptively (Rosen, 1988). Interactions with the world and other people lead to certain beliefs about self, others and the world, which may vary in their accuracy and functionality (Beck & Emery, 1985). These beliefs are fundamental to all individuals and often not articulated by the person, just accepted as truths. Core beliefs are global, rigid and overgeneralised. From core beliefs the person develops a set of stable intermediate beliefs (i.e. assumptions, rules and attitudes) that govern their subsequent responses to events.

These core beliefs may be erroneous and if held along with assumptions, rules and attitudes, they will influence a person's vulnerability to experiencing a depressive response to subsequent events. It is suggested that individuals with depression may exhibit negative core beliefs in one or both of two main areas, helplessness and unloveability.

Most individuals who are non-depressed maintain relatively positive core beliefs, e.g. 'I can do most things competently', compared with 'I'm inadequate', which is typical of a patient with depression. An example of an intermediate attitude derived from the core belief of inadequacy is 'It's terrible to be inadequate', a rule – 'I should be great at everything I try' and an assumption 'If I don't work hard I will fail' (from Beck & Emery, 1985).

The cognitive therapy of depression derived from Beck's theory involves helping the patient to recognise his or her negative automatic thoughts and images and to replace them with more rational and appropriate alternative interpretations of situations. Recognition of cognitive errors and cognitive restructuring, involving reattribution and behavioural experiments, should lead to a resolution of depressed mood. It is essential, particularly in terms of relapse prevention, to identify and modify dysfunctional core and intermediate beliefs and schemata (see later in this chapter). Reattribution and behavioural experiments are again used and details of these techniques are given in the next chapter.

Cognitive therapy for depression has been thoroughly evaluated in controlled clinical trials and has been shown to be as effective as anti-depressant medication and possibly better in preventing relapse (Williams, 1997). In the light of this success, Beck's cognitive theory of depression has been modified for use in a number of other psychiatric disorders. The crux of the cognitive model remains unchanged, that distorted or dysfunctional thinking, which influences mood and behaviour, is common to all psychological disturbances.

In the cognitive theory of anxiety disorders (Beck & Emery, 1985) it is suggested that the patient has an enduring tendency to appraise situations as more threatening than they really are, and to underestimate their coping abilities. When faced with a situation that they feel constitutes a threat, the emotion will be of anxiety. This contrasts with depression, where the faulty appraisal is usually centred on the theme of loss, leading to associated lowering of mood.

When a person is anxious, but feels the threat is low and/or they are likely to be able to deal with the situation, then the behavioural response will be to confront the threat, the 'fight' response described in preparedness theory (Seligman, 1970). If the threat is perceived as high, and/or with inadequate coping abilities then the patient will try to escape from the threat ('flight'). In some circumstances the response will be to 'freeze', experienced by some in examinations, or the parasympathetically mediated fainting response, experienced in blood-injury phobia.

The preoccupation with threat is manifested by repeated negative automatic thoughts and images, in which typical cognitive errors occur, such as catastrophising and jumping to conclusions. A person's vulnerability to anxiety is also determined by the distortions in the core beliefs they hold. Anxious individuals also consistently overestimate the likelihood of harm. For example, a patient who believes that 'all strangers are out to do me harm' is much more likely to become alarmed by someone who asks them the time than someone who believes that 'strangers are generally harmless and not out to cause trouble'.

In the cognitive theory of panic disorder Clark (1986) states that panic attacks result from catastrophic misinterpretations of bodily sensations. Once established, these misinterpretations are then maintained by selective attention to bodily events, avoidance and safety seeking behaviours. Normal bodily sensations and anxiety sensations are typically misinterpreted. Typical negative automatic thoughts would be 'I am going to pass out and die', 'I am going to lose control' or 'I am going to go mad'. Such thoughts lead to feelings of panic that in turn lead to further autonomic symptoms and further misinterpretations, hence completing a vicious circle.

In hypochondriasis (Warwick & Salkovskis, 1990) innocuous physical symptoms are persistently misinterpreted as a threat to health, so the patient erroneously becomes convinced that they are physically ill and experiences health anxiety. The tendency to misinterpret symptoms occurs because the patients hold faulty beliefs relating to health, illness and medical interventions. Hypochondriacal patients typically carry out numerous behaviours designed to seek reassurance that they are not ill, such as reassurance and consultation seeking and bodily checking, which serve to maintain the health anxiety.

In hypochondriasis and anxiety disorders, the importance of safety seeking behaviours has been highlighted (Warwick *et al*, 1996). A logical link is described between anxiety-provoking threat-related cognitions and subsequent behaviours. Such behaviours are of importance in the maintenance of these disorders as they help to preserve the tendency to misinterpret, despite repeated episodes when the feared consequence does not occur. The belief tends to develop that the safety seeking behaviour has in itself prevented a disastrous event.

In obsessive–compulsive disorder, Salkovskis (1985, 1989) has proposed that the basic fault is an over-inflated idea of personal responsibility and that this needs to be modified if a successful outcome is to be achieved. The idea originally proposed by Rachman (1976) was that compulsive behaviours would be reduced if the patient did not feel responsible for a disastrous outcome. Salkovskis (1999) took this idea further. He suggests that the key problem in obsessive–compulsive disorder is the way in which intrusive thoughts, images and doubts are interpreted. There is a major problem when the patient believes that failure to perform compulsions will lead to harm to self and/or others, even when most people would not see themselves as responsible. For example, someone with inflated responsibility cognitions may telephone the gas supplier several times a day as they believe they may have smelled gas in the street.

Salkovskis (1999) argues that these heightened responsibility interpretations lead to increased neutralising behaviour, increased selective attention to any perceived threat and a depressed or negative mood. These effects themselves lead to more guilt and feeling of responsibility and thus a vicious circle is created.

Menzies and his coworkers in Australia (Menzies *et al*, 2000) have focused on an alternative cognitive mediator of danger expectancies. They looked at whether belief in the danger of an obsessional thought was related to the performance of anxiolytic rituals. Danger ideation was more highly correlated to rituals than measures of responsibility, self-efficacy, perfectionism or anticipated anxiety (Jones & Menzies, 1997). Experimentally increasing danger expectancies also led to an increase in symptoms in obsessive–compulsive washing (Jones & Menzies, 1998).

In a review article Rachman (2002) examined the various cognitive theories and proposed that both over-inflated sense of personal responsibility, as well as over-estimation of danger, had a role to play in those who compulsively check. Although CBT has been advocated for obsessive–compulsive disorder, there is no clear evidence that in general it produces any better results than simple exposure and response prevention (James & Blackburn, 1995; Cottraux *et al*, 2001; McLean *et al*, 2001).

Cognitive–behavioural models have been developed for a number of other disorders, and treatment strategies derived from these models have been used successfully and evaluated in controlled outcome studies, for example generalised anxiety disorder (Butler *et al*,1991), social phobia (Clark & Wells, 1995), eating disorders (Fairburn *et al*, 1991) marital disorders (Jacobson & Follette, 1985) and hypochondriasis (Warwick *et al*, 1996). Applications of cognitive theory are being evaluated in other disorders, such as psychotic illnesses, personality disorders and chronic pain.

Cognitive psychology

Teasdale (1993) states that 'the development of cognitive therapy for depression has proceeded largely in isolation from basic cognitive science' and draws attention to a number of problems in the conceptualisations involved in Beck's cognitive therapy. Cognitive therapy works within a narrow definition of cognition and the emphasis is on the modification of consciously experienced thoughts and images, whereas in cognitive psychology it is assumed that the majority of cognitive processing is not experienced as consciously accessible thoughts or images.

Teasdale further challenges the basic assumption made in Beck's cognitive therapy for depression, that certain types of cognition lead to emotional reactions, and points out that sometimes cognition appears to be a consequence of the emotional state. Patterns of negative thinking in depressed patients largely disappear when their mood improves following treatments not directly related to modification of cognitions, such as antidepressant medication.

It is suggested that there may be a reciprocal relationship between cognition and emotion. Some negative thoughts are antecedents to emotional states, which in turn increase the likelihood of those same cognitions. Further concerns expressed by Teasdale are that there has been a failure to demonstrate the persistence of dysfunctional attitudes in vulnerable people after their depression has remitted, that many patients experience emotional reactions without being able to identify proportionate negative thoughts, that rational argument is frequently ineffective in changing the emotions and that cognitive therapy is too often ineffective.

Teasdale & Barnard (1993) have developed a comprehensive theoretical framework that accommodates the knowledge of cognitive science and clinical cognitive theory, the interacting cognitive subsystems framework. This complex scheme proposes the existence of nine types of information, each representing a different aspect of experience. They propose that there are mental codes relating to two levels of meaning. The propositional code represents specific meaning and the implicational code represents generic and holistic levels of meaning. These codes are said to be directly linked to emotion and the implicational code is most important in emotional experiences. It is suggested that the central goal of therapy should be to replace implicational code patterns related to depressive schematic models with alternative patterns related to more adaptive higher level meanings.

Schema-based approaches to cognitive therapy

These are based on the original ideas of Beck (Beck & Emery, 1985). The theory of cognitive therapy is that early life experience produces a number of patterns of thoughts or schemata. These are habitual ways of thinking that are semi-conscious and are used as a short cut when evaluating events and situations. These schemata result in underlying assumptions and from these the negative automatic thoughts. Many schemata may lie dormant but can be activated by a critical incident.

Example 1

Joanna, a 35-year-old married, legal secretary with 2 children, had led an active and fulfilling life. However, when her father died suddenly she developed a severe depression.

Assessment of her problems showed that she had excessive guilt feelings that she should have been able to save him. He had died at a family gathering when he suddenly collapsed with a massive myocardial infarction. Joanna had tried to apply cardiopulmonary resuscitation but to no avail. Negative automatic thoughts were for example 'I should have tried harder and he would still be alive'; 'If I had gone to the refresher course in first aid I might have saved him'.

Underlying assumptions were that she should always be able to help everyone she cared for and that she was ultimately solely responsible for her family. The self-critical and over-inflated responsibilty schema seemed to have dated from a time when her mother had been admitted to hospital when Joanna was 6-years-old. She had been told by a relative that she would have to take care of her father and 2-year-old sister and that if she was good, God would ensure that her mother returned safe and well.

A schema is thus a pattern of unconditional beliefs that are hard to access and are self-maintaining. These schemata are maintained by three main cognitive processes, see below (Young & Klosko, 1993; Young, 1999; Young *et al*, 2003).

Schema surrender

This is the way in which a patient will always seek evidence that supports the beliefs and dismiss evidence that contradicts the beliefs, for example a woman who believes she is ugly will focus on any minor negative comment, but will ignore compliments as 'they are just saying that to make me feel better and probably would not feel the need if they did not realise that I am ugly'.

Schema compensation

This refers to primary avoidance of emotional arousal by developing strategies that enforce the beliefs, for example a man who has core beliefs that he will be abandoned by everyone due to his unlovable nature may be excessively self-sacrificing to his friends and family.

Schema avoidance

These are a group of blocking behaviours that help avoid emotional arousal, for example binge eating may temporarily reduce the emptiness and social isolation experienced by the woman who had been neglected as a child. This is known as secondary avoidance of emotional arousal.

In most clinical situations, cognitive therapy aimed at examining the negative automatic thoughts and underlying assumptions will be sufficient to produce lasting change. However, for patients with personality disorders, the unhealthy and damaging schemata can be so pervasive that longer-term therapy is necessary to try and alter these belief-systems. Such therapy will often be conducted over 50 or even 75 sessions rather than the short-term therapy more usually associated with cognitive and behavioural approaches.

There are some self-help books for patients with deeply entrenched and negative beliefs, but these do tend to require a high level of education and motivation (Young & Klosko, 1993). Other workers have examined the way in which schemata may change during therapy and developed therapeutic tools that may be used to aid this process (Padesky, 1994).

Clinical applications of cognitive–behavioural theory

Cognitive–behavioural theories continue to evolve and develop. There continues to be some controversy over the separation between behavioural and cognitive theories, and some of these issues have yet to be resolved.

There is now little argument in the clinical setting, however. It is accepted that some belief change is necessary for behavioural change and similarly it is recognised that demonstrable changes in behaviour are an especially powerful way of changing beliefs. Treatment strategies developed from behavioural and cognitive–behavioural theories have now been rigorously evaluated in many disorders. Clinical applications are fully described in the following chapter.

References and further reading

Abramson, L. Y., Seligman, M. E. P. & Teasdale, J. (1978) Learned helplessness in humans: critique and reformulation. *Journal of Abnormal Psychology*, **87**, 32–48.

Bandura, A. (1969) *Principles of Behaviour Modification*. New York: Holt, Rinehart & Winston.

Beck, A. T., Rush, A. J., Shaw, B. F., *et al* (1979) *Cognitive Therapy of Depression*. New York: Guilford Press.

Beck, A. T. & Emery, G. (1985) *Anxiety Disorders and Phobias: A Cognitive Perspective*. New York: Basic Books.

Butler, G., Fennell, M., Robson, P., *et al* (1991) Comparison of behaviour therapy and cognitive behaviour therapy in the treatment of generalised anxiety disorder. *Journal of Consulting and Clinical Psychology*, **59**, 167–175.

Clark, D. M. (1986) A cognitive approach to panic. *Behaviour Research and Therapy*, **24**, 461–470.

Clark, D.M. & Fairburn, C.G. (1977) *Science and Practice of Cognitive Behaviour Therapy*. Oxford: Oxford University Press.

Clark, D. M. & Wells, A. (1995) A cognitive model of social phobia. In *Social Phobia: Diagnosis, Assessment and Treatment* (eds R. Heimburg, M. Liebowitz, D. A. Hope, *et al*), pp. 69–93. New York: Guilford Press.

Cottraux, J., Note, I., Yao, S. N., *et al* (2001) A randomized controlled trial of cognitive therapy versus intensive behaviour therapy in obsessive–compulsive disorder. *Psychotherapy and Psychosomatics*, **70**, 288–297.

Ellis, A. (1962) *Reason and Emotion in Psychotherapy*. New York: Lyle-Stuart.

Fairburn, C.G., Jones, R., Peveler, R., *et al* (1991) Three psychological treatments for bulimia nervosa: a comparative trial. *Archives of General Psychiatry*, **48**, 463–469.

Gray, J.A. (1971) *The Psychology of Fear and Stress*. Cambridge: Cambridge University Press.

Marks, I.M. (1987) *Fears, Phobias and Rituals*. New York: Oxford University Press.

Jacobson, S. M. & Follette, W. C. (1985) Clinical significance of improvement resulting from two behavioural marital therapy components. *Behaviour Therapy*, **16**, 249–262.

James, I. A. & Blackburn, I. M. (1995) Cognitive therapy with obsessive–compulsive disorder. *British Journal of Psychiatry*, **166**, 444–450.

Jones, M. K. & Menzies, R. G. (1997) The cognitive mediation of obsessive–compulsive handwashing. *Behaviour Research and Therapy*, **36**,959–970.

Jones, M. K. & Menzies, R. G. (1998) The role of perceived danger in the mediation of obsessive–compulsive washing. *Depression and Anxiety*, **8**, 121–125.

Marks, I. M. (1969) *Fears and Phobias*. New York: Academic Press.

McLean, P. D., Whittal, M. L., Thordarson, D. S., *et al* (2001) Cognitive versus behaviour therapy in group treatment to obsessive–compulsive disorder. *Consulting and Clinical Psychology*, **69**, 205–214.

Meichenbaum, D. (1977) *Cognitive Behaviour Modification: An Integrative Approach*. New York: Plenum Press.

Menzies, R. G., Harris, L. M., Cumming, S. R., *et al* (2000) The relationship between inflated personal responsibility and exaggerated danger expectancies in obsessive–compulsive concerns. *Behaviour Research and Therapy*, **38**, 1029–1037.

Mowrer, O. H. (1947) On the dual nature of learning – a reinterpretation of 'conditioning' and 'problem-solving'. *Harvard Educational Review*, **17**, 102–148.

Ohman, A. & Dimberg, U. (1984) An evolutionary perspective on human social behaviour. In *Sociopsychology* (ed. W. M. Waid). New York: Springer.

Ohman, A., Dimberg, U. & Ost, L.-G. (1984) Animal and social phobias: biological constraints on learned fear responses. In *Theoretical Issues in Behavior Therapy* (eds R. Heimburg, M. Liebowitz., D. A. Hope *et al*), pp. 123–178. New York: Academic Press.

Padesky, C. (1994) Schema change processes in cognitive therapy. *Clinical Psychology and Psychotherapy*, **1**, 267–278.

Rachman (1977) The conditioning theory of fear acquisition: a critical examination. *Behaviour Research and Therapy*, **15**, 375–387.

Rachman, S. (2002) A cognitive theory of checking. *Behaviour Research and Therapy*, **40**, 625–639.

Rosen, H. (1988) The constructivist–development paradigm. In *Paradigms of Clinical Social Work* (ed. R. A. Dorfman), pp. 317–355. New York: Brunner/Mazel.

Rachman, S. (1976) Obsessional–compulsive checking. *Behaviour Research and Therapy*, **14**, 269–277.

Salkovskis, P. M. (1985) Obsessional–compulsive problems: a cognitive–behavioural analysis. *Behaviour Research and Therapy*, **25**, 571–583.

Salkovskis, P. M. (1989) Cognitive–behavioural factors and the persistence of intrusive thoughts in obsessional problems. *Behaviour Research and Therapy*, **27**, 677–682.

Salkovskis, P. M. (1999) Understanding and treating obsessive–compulsive disorder. *Behaviour Research and Therapy*, **37** (suppl. 1), 29–52.

Seligman, M. E. P. (1970) On the generality of the laws of learning. *Psychological Review*, **77**, 406–418.

Skinner, B. F. (1953) *Science and Human Behaviour*. New York: Macmillan.

Teasdale, J. D. (1993) Emotion and two kinds of meaning: cognitive therapy and applied cognitive science. *Behaviour Research and Therapy*, **31**, 339–354.

Teasdale, J. D. & Barnard, P. J. (1993) *Affect, Cognition and Change: Re-modelling Depressive Thought*. Hove: Erlbaum.

Warwick, H. M. C. & Salkovskis P. M. (1990) Hypochondriasis. *Behaviour Research & Therapy*, **28**, 105–18.

Warwick, H. M., Clark, D. M., Cobb, A. M., *et al* (1996) A controlled trial of cognitive–behavioural treatment of hypochondriasis. *British Journal of Psychiatry*, **169**, 189–195.

Williams, J. M. G. (1997) Depression. In *Science and Practice of Cognitive Behaviour Therapy* (eds D. M. Clark, & C. G. Fairburn), pp. 259–283. Oxford: Oxford University Press.

Wolpe, J. (1958) *Psychotherapy by Reciprocal Inhibition*. Stanford, CA: Stanford University Press.

Wolpe, J. (1982) *The Practice of Behaviour Therapy* (3rd edn). New York: Pergamon.

Young, J. E. (1999). *Cognitive Therapy for Personality Disorders: A Schema Focused Approach* (3rd edn). Sarasota, FL: Professional Resource Exchange.

Young, J. E., & Klosko, J. S. (1993). *Reinventing Your Life*. New York: Plume Publishers.

Young, J. E., Klosko, J. S., & Weishaar, M. E. (2003). *Schema Therapy: A Practitioner's Guide*. New York: Guilford.

CHAPTER 7

Behavioural and cognitive therapies

Lynne M. Drummond & Hilary Warwick

Modern behavioural–cognitive psychotherapy can be used in the treatment of a large number of conditions found in psychiatric practice. It can also be used as an adjunct to other types of therapy. Over recent years a wide range of increasingly sophisticated techniques has been developed. Some of the treatments widely applicable in psychiatric practice such as exposure, cognitive therapy and operant techniques have been particularly selected for this chapter. Social skills training, behavioural marital therapy, sex therapy and the expanding area of behavioural medicine and behavioural liaison psychiatry have been largely omitted. Conditions as varied as phobias, obsessive–compulsive disorder, depression, generalised anxiety, alternative sexual practices and schizophrenia are discussed in detail. Brief mention is also made of more recent applications of behavioural–cognitive therapy such as in post-traumatic stress disorder and hypochondriasis.

This chapter is not intended to be a comprehensive review of the subject nor is it a handbook for therapy, rather it is intended to give an introduction into the field and an idea of the range of techniques available and their use in clinical practice.

Exposure treatment

Exposure treatment has been shown to be effective in 66% of individuals with agoraphobia (Mathews *et al*, 1981); between 75 and 85% of individuals with obsessive–compulsive disorder (Foa & Goldstein, 1978; Rachman *et al*, 1979) and highly effective in individuals with a variety of specific and social phobias (Marks, 1981).

There is often fear of using exposure treatment outside specialist centres. This appears to arise from erroneous views about its applicability, its success rates, the time commitment required by the therapist and also fear of the unknown. In fact, graduated exposure is a remarkably quick and cost-efficient treatment that can be easily applied in many general practice and hospital settings (Marks, 1981, 1986; Stern & Drummond, 1991). Although some basic training is required, this can easily be obtained by reading about clinical techniques (Hawton *et al*, 1989; Stern & Drummond, 1991) and by obtaining supervision from a trained behavioural psychotherapist.

The most effective exposure has been shown to be:

- prolonged rather than of short duration (Stern & Marks, 1973)
- in real life rather than in fantasy (Emmelkamp & Wessels, 1975)
- regularly practised with self-exposure homework tasks (McDonald *et al*, 1978).

Self-exposure treatment

One of the concerns about exposure treatment has been that it requires considerable professional input to accompany an anxious individual into fear-provoking situations.

Fortunately, it has been demonstrated that instruction in self-exposure techniques can be all that is required for many individuals with phobic anxiety and obsessive–compulsive disorder (Ghosh *et al*, 1988; Marks *et al*, 1988). The efficacy of self-exposure has led to the development of a number of self-help manuals. However, few individuals can successfully complete a treatment programme without some professional guidance. The individual needs to be seen initially for education about anxiety and its treatment and for help in devising treatment targets. Subsequent meetings are required to monitor progress, give encouragement and advise on any difficulties that may arise (Ghosh *et al*, 1988).

Treatment of agoraphobia with graduated self-exposure

Example

Jane, a 42-year-old housewife, had a 7-year history of fear of travelling alone. She was able to visit nearby relatives only when accompanied by her 8-year-old son. If accompanied by her sister she would travel in a bus but always insisted on sitting close to the door. Train travel was impossible. Her husband had to drive her to the supermarket for the weekly shopping trip. Once there she would insist that they did the shopping as quickly as possible. If there was a queue at the checkout, Jane would return to the car while her husband paid for the goods.

Jane's problems had begun after the birth of her son. She had suffered from post-natal depression and had spent 3 months housebound. Once her depression lifted she had tried to go out but found that she felt extremely anxious. She feared that she might get so anxious that she would collapse.

After a comprehensive behavioural assessment had been carried out, she was educated about anxiety and its treatment. The possible physical and emotional symptoms of anxiety were explained to her. She was then advised how avoidance of feared situations would lead to further avoidance.

Next she was given the following rules about exposure treatment:

- anxiety is unpleasant but does no harm; it was explained that anxiety does not result in death, serious physical harm or madness
- anxiety does eventually reduce; prolonged exposure to the feared situation results in habituation of the anxiety. This usually takes between 1 and 2 hours

- practice makes perfect; regular practice of the exposure task is needed until little anxiety is experienced.

Targets of treatment were then defined with Jane. She identified 4 specific tasks that she would like to be able to perform by the end of treatment. If successful this would demonstrate to both herself and her doctor that she had improved. The tasks were to:

- go to the local shops with her son and remain there for 2 hours
- travel by bus into town on her own and do some browsing and shopping
- drive herself to the supermarket and do the weekly shopping alone
- travel on the bus and train to Southampton to visit friends.

Jane was then asked to think of a number of tasks which would be stages towards achieving these targets. She was also asked to rate the anxiety that each of the tasks would cause her using a 9-point scale (where $0 =$ no anxiety; $2 =$ mild anxiety; $4 =$ moderate anxiety; $6 =$ severe anxiety; $8 =$ panic).

Jane and her therapist decided that it would be easiest for Jane to start treatment by walking in her local area on her own. She agreed to go out for at least an hour every day and visit local shops and parks. The details of her exposure tasks were to be recorded in a diary together with a record of her anxiety levels at the beginning, middle and towards the end of the task.

The following week Jane was delighted with her progress and had found that her anxiety had reduced considerably. She felt able to progress to the next item on her fear hierarchy. Over the next 12 weeks, Jane managed to perform all her treatment targets. Throughout this time she met weekly with the therapist whose role was to praise and encourage progress and to discuss any difficulties.

Her husband attended some sessions and was able to assist in some of the exposure tasks. For example, as Jane had not travelled on a train for 7 years and was too fearful to travel alone, he initially travelled with her. As her anxiety reduced, he moved to a different part of the carriage. Later he sat in a different carriage and eventually, she gained sufficient confidence to make a train journey alone.

Although Jane progressed extremely well in treatment, some weeks she was able to see the results of her efforts clearly, whereas other weeks there seemed to be little improvement. The therapist also checked the precise way in which she was performing the exposure tasks, ensuring that she was concentrating on the task and not using any avoidance strategies such as reading a magazine. This is a form of avoidance as the patient tries to 'escape' from their situation and surroundings by becoming absorbed in something else. Other frequently used forms of avoidance include listening to music on a personal stereo and wearing sunglasses even when the light is not bright.

Treatment of social phobia

A careful assessment must be made to see if the patient possesses adequate social skills. It may be that the patient has learnt social skills but has become too anxious to use these skills adequately. However, some patients have longstanding social skills deficits and will require social skills training prior to any exposure to social situations. Assessment will elicit the specific deficits, for example lack of eye-contact and lack of conversational skills.

Role-play can be helpful to identify the problems. The patient can then be taught appropriate alternative behaviours, which are initially modelled by the therapist. The patient practises by role-play in the therapy sessions initially, followed by homework tasks in a structured series of real-life tasks. Social skills training often takes place in group settings.

Treatment of obsessive–compulsive disorder

Although exposure is still the cornerstone of treatment for obsessive–compulsive disorder, it needs to be combined with another technique known as response prevention, which helps the patient not to ritualise. Rituals are overt behaviours or internal thought patterns that are used to counteract the obsessional fears. Rituals can usually be prevented or substantially reduced by demonstrating to the patient how they interfere with exposure. In exposure treatment, the aim is to produce prolonged periods of contact with the feared situation until the anxiety reduces (habituation). Compulsions or rituals reduce the anxiety and this serves to reinforce the ritual. However, the reduction in anxiety produced by a ritual tends to be small and the effect temporary. In effect, rituals prevent therapeutic exposure and instead increase the tendency to ritualise further.

Self-exposure treatment of obsessive–compulsive disorder

Example

Anne was an 18-year-old unemployed typist who lived at home with her family. She presented with a 6-month history of fear of contamination by dirt and 'germs', which had led to her losing her job.

The problem had been precipitated by her watching a television programme about hepatitis. She had become nervous that she might contract and spread hepatitis to other people.

Although she recognised that her fear was exaggerated, she felt unable to prevent herself from taking elaborate precautions to prevent 'contamination'. These precautions included washing her hands at least 40 times a day, bathing for 3 hours nightly and avoiding touching door handles or other objects which had been handled by people unknown to her or only touching these items using paper tissues. Any clothes which she had worn were placed in a plastic bag immediately following removal and were not allowed to come into contact with 'clean' clothes.

Following assessment and educating both Anne and her mother about the rationale of behavioural treatment, Anne agreed to start an exposure programme at home with her mother acting as co-therapist. The targets for the first week were that, with the help of her mother, she was to touch her 'dirty' clothes and then systematically 'contaminate' all her clean clothes and to sleep every night in her bed even if she did not feel perfectly clean. The following week, Anne returned with her mother to report on her success. Initially she had been tearful and very anxious when attempting the tasks. Her mother had firmly but kindly reminded her of the rationale for treatment and eventually Anne had appeared more settled and agreed to take the risk of touching her external clothing and then the outside of her wardrobe and chest of drawers where her clean clothes were kept. During this exposure, she was noticeably tremulous and tearful but had managed to continue. Once she had finished this contamination exercise, she agreed to try and touch all her clean clothes. She was surprised to find that her anxiety did reduce as she continued, although she remained concerned that her fear might escalate later. Before completing the session, Anne volunteered to 'contaminate' the bedclothes of her clean bed.

She continued to make progress and reported that once she had 'taken the plunge' and found that her anxiety did eventually reduce, it was possible for her to continue and increase the difficulty of the exposure tasks. Over the next 6 weeks she practised exposing herself to situations of increasing difficulty and eventually reintroduced 'normal' washing activities. Returning to work was her final target, which she achieved 2 months after commencing treatment.

A recent disturbing trend has been for therapists to concentrate on cognitive therapies instead of behavioural treatments in phobias and obsessive–compulsive disorder.

Emmelkamp et al (1988) found rational emotive therapy (RET) as effective as exposure and response prevention, while Van Oppen et al (1995) found cognitive therapy with almost no exposure to be at least as effective as exposure and response prevention. Further evaluation of the efficacy of cognitive therapy in obsessive–compulsive disorder is needed and in straightforward cases it is better to use exposure and response prevention unless there are specific contraindications or the behavioural–cognitive assessment suggests that this will not work.

Cognitive approaches may well have a role where exposure-based behaviour therapy is not effective, for example in individuals with obsessive–compulsive disorder who refuse behavioural treatment or drop out. Cognitive treatment may also have a role in those who fail to respond to behaviour treatment such as patients with overvalued ideation (see Salkovskis & Warwick, 1985). Freeston et al (1997) describe a controlled study in which 29 individuals with obsessive–compulsive disorder who did not have overt compulsive rituals were randomly assigned to waiting list control or cognitive–behavioural treatment. Results indicate that cognitive–behavioural therapy is effective in treatment of individuals with obsessive thoughts, a group often considered resistant to treatment.

A pragmatic approach is to treat the majority of patients with exposure therapy combined with response prevention but to consider other therapy in the small group of patients who fail with this approach. In the patients who fail, detailed analysis of the problem may then suggest the correct treatment (see Table 7.1) (Drummond, 1993).

Salkovskis (1985, 1989) developed a new model and treatment for obsessive–compulsive disorder using cognitive methods. Despite the numerous studies in this area, there is no clear evidence that cognitive therapy gives any better results than simple exposure and response prevention (James & Blackburn, 1995; Cottraux et al, 2001; McLean et al, 2001).

Table 7.1 Pragmatic approach to obsessive–compulsive disorder (adapted from Drummond, 1993)

Possible explanation of previous failure	Action
Lack of motivation to change	Consider cognitive, family or psychodynamic therapy; educate patient about the problem and discharge (can be re-referred if motivation changes)
Inappropriate previous treatment	Exposure and response prevention
Treatment in hospital/clinic has not generalised to home	Home-based treatment or treatment in hospital with weekend leave and domiciliary treatment
Cognitive rituals	Education plus either audiotape of anxiogenic obsessions (Salkovskis, 1983; Headland & McDonald, 1987) or high-intensity exposure and response prevention
Major depressive illness	Antidepressant drug followed by exposure and response prevention; cognitive therapy for depression as necessary
Overvalued ideation that obsessions are realistic	High-intensity exposure and response-prevention or cognitive restructuring (Salkovskis & Warwick, 1985) followed by exposure and response prevention

It should be noted that poorly carried out cognitive therapy can worsen problems of obsessive–compulsive disorder by teaching the individual new ways of performing cognitive rituals.

However Menzies and his co-workers in Australia have focused on an alternative cognitive mediator of danger expectancies (Jones & Menzies, 1997a, Jones & Menzies, 1998a; Menzies *et al*, 2000).

Based on their research they have developed the new treatment of danger ideation reduction therapy (DIRT) that has been used with some success on patients with obsessive–compulsive contamination fears who have failed more conventional treatments (Jones & Menzies, 1997b; Jones & Menzies, 1998b; Menzies *et al*, 2000).

Danger ideation reduction therapy consists of 6 main stages that are applied at different times, dependent on the patient's clinical state. These stages are:

1. cognitive restructuring; based on the techniques of rational emotive therapy (Ellis, 1962), the individual is taught to identify unrealistic thoughts about contamination and then to re-evaluate these
2. filmed interviews; these consist of a number of filmed interviews with people who work in situations commonly feared by those with obsessive–compulsive disorder

3. corrective information; the individual is asked to view a list of facts about their feared contaminant. For example, the number of healthcare workers who have contracted HIV through their work. The individuals are also given information about the deleterious effects of overzealous hand-washing; this is a report that discusses how excessive hand-washing can break the skin's natural barrier to infection

4. microbiological experiments; results of microbiological experiments which were undertaken at the University of Sydney are discussed with the individual. In these experiments subjects were asked to touch frequently feared contaminants such as money or toilet door handles with one hand while keeping the other hand 'clean'. Fingerprints from both hands were then imprinted on blood agar plates. Normal commensal flora were found after culture and no pathogens found despite subjects having touched such contaminants as dogs' hair and toilet doors

5. probability of catastrophe; individuals are asked to estimate the probability of catastrophe occurring in different situations. They are then asked to break down this scenario into its component parts and estimate the likelihood of the feared consequence at each stage. This is then computed and compared with the original probability estimate

6. attentional focusing; this is a form of meditation. Individuals are taught to focus the mind away from the danger-related intrusive thoughts and onto benign, non-threatening stimuli.

Danger ideation reduction therapy has been applied in a controlled way in Australia, although there are reports (at the time of writing) that will shortly be available in the UK, with a case report (Govender *et al*, 2006) and a controlled trial studying the usage in severe, chronic, resistant obsessive–compulsive disorder (further details available from author upon request).

Cognitive therapy for depression

Cognitive therapy for depression is a relatively brief treatment that is focused on present symptoms, collaborative, goal-oriented and makes use of homework. (Cognitive–behavioural therapy for depression is also discussed in Chapter 8.) Treatment encourages the individual to recognise negative automatic thoughts and images and to challenge their validity, using cognitive restructuring and behavioural techniques. The emphasis in treatment is on the use of Socratic questioning, in which the therapist does not tell the individual that their thoughts are right or wrong, but develops a collaborative relationship with the individual to help challenge these beliefs and assess their validity. The individual is asked a number of questions to help them construct more rational alternatives to their negative thoughts and beliefs. Three of the most commonly used questions are:

• what is the evidence for these thoughts?

- is there another way of looking at this?
- would it be better to look at this in a different way?

Example

Susan is a nurse who is being treated for a depressive illness.

Therapist I have your automatic thought record from last week, and it seems that you became particularly depressed at work. Can you tell me more about that?

Susan Well it started when I forgot to order a special diet for one of the patients I am nursing, and this was pointed out to me by the ward sister, in front of my colleagues. I felt really down, and I don't want to go back to work.

Therapist Can you tell me what was going through your mind when she pointed out your error?

Susan I thought 'She has found out how useless I am. She knows I am not fit to be a nurse.' Afterwards I couldn't get it out of my mind I kept thinking that the other nurses were thinking I am useless. To me it shows that I will never make a good nurse.

Therapist So let me just make sure I have understood the situation properly. You forgot to order the diet and the sister informed you of that in the ward meeting, and you think that she and all your colleagues feel you are a bad nurse. Also you feel you will never make a good nurse, and you don't want to go back to work. Is that right?

Susan Yes that's it.

Therapist How strongly do you believe that your colleagues are thinking that you are a bad nurse, from 0 to 100?

Susan I know that is true, 100%.

Therapist Can I check if you have any real evidence for that belief, what did they say to you about it afterwards?

Susan Well no one mentioned it at all.

Therapist So you have no factual evidence. It is just what you thought they thought about you.

Susan I suppose so.

Therapist Well, what was the ward sister like with you about it?

Susan Well she wasn't angry, she just asked me to get it done, and she didn't mention it again. But this doesn't mean anything, everyone was too busy to mention it again anyway, and I bet they all just feel so disgusted with me that they kept quiet.

Therapist I can see that you might think that, but is there another way of looking at this situation? What has the ward sister done in the past if she has been annoyed with you?

Susan She has never been annoyed with me, all my assessments have been fine. She was angry with a student last week though, and she arranged a meeting to discuss the problem with her.

Therapist Would she have arranged to see you if she was angry?

Susan I suppose so, I know she takes her training role very seriously. But what about all the others?

Therapist Let's see, what did you think about that student who had the problem last week, did you think she was a bad nurse?

Susan	No, she had just made a mistake, she will learn.
Therapist	Is there a chance your colleagues might think that way about you?
Susan	(Smiling) Yes, you could be right there, they would probably think like that. But that doesn't help, I still forgot to order the diet, I'm still a lousy nurse.
Therapist	So you forgot to order one diet, you're a lousy nurse. Could you look at this in a different way? How would you look at this if someone else had done it?
Susan	Well I suppose everyone makes mistakes, and I didn't harm the patient in any way.
Therapist	Can you learn anything from that error?
Susan	Oh yes, I have already changed the way I do things so that will not happen again.
Therapist	So to sum up. You made an error that did not cause any harm. Your ward sister was not angry, she has not discussed it with you and you know she always talks to nurses who have difficulties with their work. You have no evidence that your colleagues think you are a lousy nurse, you really know that they will just think you made a mistake. Your previous assessments have been very good, and you have learnt from and rectified this error. How much do you believe now that you will never be a good nurse?
Susan	When you put it like that, maybe only 10%.

Patients are also taught to identify and challenge particular cognitive errors, of which the following are examples.

The first example also illustrates how patients are taught to regard their beliefs and attitudes as though they were hypotheses that can be abandoned if they are found to be inadequate and in favour of alternative more adaptive beliefs.

Arbitrary inference

Example: 'being a bad mother'

Therapist	Do you think you are the only mother of two young children to shout at them?
Patient	I suppose not ... but I don't hear other mothers shrieking all the time like I do.
Therapist	Fine, that may be so. Maybe you could test out how many other mothers of young children shout at them. How do you think you might do that?
Patient	Well, I suppose I could go to the mothers and toddlers group coffee mornings and see if they shout at their kids. I could also ask my best friend if she shouts at her children.
Therapist	Good, I would like you to put that into practice before our next session so we can discuss it then.

At the next session the patient reported that she shouted about half as much as most other mothers. This evidence served to change her idea about being a bad mother.

Selective abstraction

Example: 'her husband did not care for her'

Therapist What is the evidence that your husband does not care for you?

Patient He does not seem to be interested when I tell him things.

Therapist OK, I can see you are disappointed in that, but let us suppose for the sake of argument that you are putting too much store by that. To support this argument can you tell me anything else he does which might mean he cares?

Patient He usually brings me flowers, and I get a kiss on the cheek when he comes in from work.

Therapist Now that sounds to me as if you are not really paying attention to his behaviour overall.

She was then given the homework task of trying to think as much as possible about the evidence for her husband loving her during the next week, and to write down such activity when it occurred and bring the list to the next session. She reported that this served to reduce the time spent thinking about his lack of conversational attention.

Overgeneralisation

Example: 'she was a born failure'

This patient had recently failed her driving test, and this served to confirm her hypothesis that she was a failure.

Therapist Do you think everyone passes their driving test first time?

Patient No, I suppose not, but my husband did.

Therapist So if you cannot compete with him this means you are a failure?

Patient I see what you mean. If I compare myself with him I am bound to look pathetic especially in areas where he excels; he has an advanced drivers certificate. The woman next door has failed her test four times, but I just assume I will fail again on the next attempt so I might as well give up now.

Therapist Have you heard of any other people failing their test first time?

Patient Yes, now I come to think of it there is Mrs B and also Mrs C.

Therapist So in fact lots of people fail the test first time. What is the evidence that you will fail next time?

Patient Well there isn't any. My instructor is hopeful, and was surprised when I failed last time.

Magnification

Example: 'a burnt meal becomes a disaster'

Therapist What did you say to yourself when you burnt the meal?

Patient That is it...I can't cope with another thing...my husband will really think me pathetic...give up...I even thought of killing myself though I know that's ridiculous.

Therapist What did your husband actually say?

Patient Let us see if we can get a baby-sitter and go out to eat. But we could not get one, so that was it as far as I was concerned. He tried to persuade me that he could bring in some take-away food, but I just felt it was too hopeless.

Therapist	What do you feel about it now?
Patient	I can see that I made a mountain out of a molehill. I should not have let things get out-of-hand.
Therapist	The important thing is to learn from this experience, and the next time small things get out of proportion, could you try and remember this session?

Dysfunctional core beliefs and assumptions are also challenged.

Example

A patient believed that if anything bad was going to happen, it would happen to her. 'Nothing good ever happens to me, I'm Mrs Jinx'. This led to her consistently misinterpreting experiences, concentrating on any negative events and ignoring the positive aspects. It also led to her avoiding various activities, such as driving the car for fear of an accident.

She was asked to carry out two homework tasks to test out this assumption. First she was asked to make a list of all the good and bad things that had happened to her during the past 5 years. She was also asked to keep a record of events as they occurred over the next week, classing them as good or bad. At review she was amazed to find that on both lists the good events outnumbered the bad ones considerably. She went on to test out her assumption further by ceasing to avoid events, and showing herself that bad things did not happen to her all the time.

Modification of imagery

In cognitive therapy it is important not to neglect the importance of imagery. Negative intrusions that take the form of images can be highly aversive and result in a marked change in affect. Patients are taught how to deal with such images.

The first step is to ask the patient to try to conjure up the image as vividly as possible. The patient and therapist then work together to think of a similar image that has a positive outcome. For example, a patient had a persistent image of standing up to give a lecture and being unable to utter a word. After a few seconds his boss got up and told the audience that the patient was useless, could not do his job and should be sacked. The patient noted feeling depressed whenever this image occurred. The alternative positive image was of the same lecture room, the patient in the same clothes, standing before the same audience. The image continued with him successfully giving the lecture and receiving applause. He was instructed to practise the positive image regularly, and to switch to the positive ending every time the original image recurred.

Cognitive treatment of panic

In the cognitive theory of panic (Clark, 1986) it is suggested that the central feature is the catastrophic misinterpretation of bodily sensations, usually the autonomic symptoms of anxiety. Typical negative automatic thoughts would be 'I am going to pass out and die', 'I am going to lose control' or 'I am going to go mad'. Such thoughts lead to feelings of panic, which in turn causes more autonomic symptoms and misinterpretation, hence completing a vicious circle. Treatment consists of helping the patient to construct alternative non-threatening interpretations of their sensations, using cognitive restructuring and behavioural experiments. For example, hyperventilation is a common cause of unpleasant physical sensations in panic. This can be easily demonstrated to the patient by a simple provocation test and the patient can then be informed of the causes of hyperventilation and the fact that it is harmless. Such treatment has been shown to be effective in controlled studies (for example Beck *et al*, 1992).

Behavioural–cognitive treatment of generalised anxiety

Whereas an acute anxiety state following a traumatic life event will generally reduce and abate after a few weeks or months, many individuals have chronic problems. As drug treatment of chronic anxiety problems is no longer acceptable because of well-known dependence problems, more attention has recently been paid to psychological treatments.

Durham & Allan (1993) considered the results of the studies of psychological treatments of generalised anxiety that have been carried out since 1980. They conclude that psychological treatment is associated with moderate improvement, with 50% reduction in severity of somatic symptoms, 25% reduction in trait anxiety and 50% of individuals attaining normal functioning. Their review suggests that best results are likely to be obtained with cognitive therapy, although they stress the treatment strategies used in the various studies may have differed. A study by Butler *et al* (1987) showed that most individuals with chronic severe anxiety symptoms were helped by an anxiety management package. The main elements of the package were cognitive restructuring, exposure, distraction and relaxation.

In practice, a comprehensive behavioural analysis should be completed. This will enable the therapist to identify relevant factors that contribute to anxiety and can be modified, such as alcohol intake or work stress. It will enable the therapist to construct a treatment package using the most appropriate strategies from those listed above.

Example

Mark's case shows how lifestyle can bring about anxiety symptoms. He worked in a smoke-filled office and contributed to this by chain-smoking himself. He worked excessively long hours and then tried to relax after work by drinking with his friends. When he did eventually return home to his long-suffering wife he was usually too exhausted to have sexual intercourse. He would sit up drinking black coffee, and then wonder why he could not sleep. In addition Mark took no regular exercise, and was considerably overweight. Treatment included giving him information and helping him to schedule his activities.

Giving information is a simple step that is often ignored. The link between the lifestyle and anxiety was easy to make; Mark complained of various anxiety symptoms, such as insomnia, lack of energy, difficulty in making decisions and impotence. It was pointed out to him that these were symptoms of anxiety and steps to reduce his indulgence in cigarettes, alcohol and coffee were undertaken.

Activity scheduling was a way to ensure that first he did one thing at a time, as at present he was trying to do several things at once, which increased his perceived time pressure. He was also encouraged to take short breaks between tasks as this reduces fatigue. As he said that there was never enough time in the day to do all that he needed at work, he was asked to make a list of priorities to be done in a sequential order. He also agreed on a reasonable time to leave work, and, after a session in which he was seen along with his wife, agreed that drinking after work should not happen more than an agreed frequency (once a week). It also came out in discussion that his insomnia was related to excessive drinking, as well as too much coffee and he was able to sleep when these, and other causes for anxiety were removed.

Behaviour modification

Reduction of undesirable behaviour

The previous sections have concentrated on altering maladaptive fear responses using the exposure principle and on cognitive therapy techniques. Other maladaptive habits or behaviours may develop in response to stimuli unrelated to fear and in these cases alternative strategies may be needed.

In these cases the therapist has the option of:

- eliminating the behaviour using aversive stimuli (only indicated if the behaviour is life-threatening or a severe public nuisance) for example covert sensitisation
- modifying the stimulus resulting in the response, for example orgasmic reconditioning
- modifying the response to the stimulus, for example stimulus control techniques
- replacing the problem behaviour with alternative adaptive responses, for example habit reversal
- reducing the desirability of the problem behaviour, for example mass practice; response cost.

These 5 categories are not mutually exclusive and any therapist who tries to eliminate a particular behaviour without helping the individual to develop alternative strategies is doomed to failure.

Alternative sexual practices

There are now very few indications for aversion therapy. It is little used because its efficacy is uncertain, and because of the obvious ethical problems involved. Ethical problems include ensuring that the individual gives fully informed consent or that the nature of the problem is severe enough to pose a threat to the life of the individual or others. In some cases antisocial sexual behaviour causing a public nuisance requires immediate action to prevent harm and arrest. In these cases, rapid treatment to suppress deviant sexual urges based on aversion therapy may be justified. The form of aversion generally used is covert sensitisation. This involves asking the individual, almost always male, to describe 2 or 3 aversive scenes and to rate their aversiveness. Scripts are then written describing arousing and aversive scenes. The individual is asked to relax and is asked to imagine in detail an arousing scene talking the therapist through their fantasy. Before the individual arrives at the culmination of the fantasy the therapist asks them to change to an aversive scene, which they are also asked to describe in detail. This procedure is repeated 5 or 6 times per treatment session. The individual is then asked to read through the scripts in a similar manner at home. Alternatively, the scripts can be read by the individual onto an audio tape and played back at home. It is important to check frequently the anxiety level caused by the aversive scene, as habituation can occur rendering it useless in therapy. It is therefore useful to substitute different aversive scenes to try and prevent this habituation. As the therapy progresses the aversive scene is introduced progressively earlier in the arousing scene until as soon as the individual thinks about his deviant fantasy, anxiety is caused. This method can be successful but clearly requires the individual to be well motivated. Even in such cases, a successful treatment plan must incorporate other elements to increase general levels of social functioning.

If an individual has a sexual preference which worries them and is a cause of concern to his or her sexual partner but is not in itself dangerous or causing a public nuisance, then less radical treatments should be used. Orgasmic reconditioning, originally described by Marquis (1970), is a technique frequently used in these cases. In this treatment, the individual is asked to masturbate regularly to their troublesome deviant fantasies but, at the point of orgasmic inevitability, to switch to the desired 'non-deviant' fantasy. As treatment progresses the non-deviant stimulus is introduced earlier and earlier in the arousal process until masturbation is achieved without deviant fantasy. Following this further sexual or social skills training is usually needed to ensure that the arousal to non-deviant stimuli is maintained.

When dealing with troublesome sexual urges it is important to set realistic goals with the patient. Whereas a bisexual individual who wishes to become exclusively heterosexual may be helped by appropriate orgasmic reconditioning and sexual skills training, it is not possible to change the orientation of an exclusively homosexual individual. In the latter case counselling to help the individual accept their sexual preference may be needed. Similarly, if a homosexual paedophile is referred for treatment, it would be unrealistic to set the goal of adult heterosexual contact but adult homosexual orientation is more likely to be achievable.

Addictive behaviour

Addictive behaviour can be modified using a number of techniques that modify the stimulus, the response and the reinforcers of the response. The main difference between problems such as drug and alcohol misuse and obesity is that frequently total abstinence is the desired goal, whereas total avoidance of food is not a reasonable goal for the obese patient.

Treatment of alcohol misuse

Example

John, a 55-year-old unemployed Glaswegian labourer, had a 40-year history of excessive drinking. This problem had resulted in the loss of numerous jobs, separation from his wife and children and social and financial deterioration. When referred he had already undergone a detoxification regimen but, as relapse had been a frequent occurrence in recent years, attended to see if we could 'improve my will power'. His physical health had been greatly affected by his drinking behaviour. His liver function tests were grossly abnormal and he had a history of duodenal ulceration and haematemesis. Previous treatment had included referral to self-help groups and a 6-month attendance at an out-patient clinic for supportive psychotherapy.

Behavioural analysis of John's problem demonstrated that, although he had achieved abstinence in the past for several days and weeks, if he once took a drink he felt that he had lost control and would then continue to drink until he passed out or his money ran out. He would previously drink at any time of the night or day and whether he was alone or in company. Previous periods of abstinence had broken down when he had received his social security benefit and had then seen friends going into a pub or off-licence.

Treatment commenced with the therapist discussing ways in which John could avoid some of the stimuli that precipitated a drinking bout or to control his access to alcohol once he had started drinking. Plans were made with him to move into a hostel and to attend Alcoholics Anonymous, to try to increase his social contacts with people who were abstemious. He also agreed to only carry a maximum of £5 at any time, changing his habits by collecting his benefit from a post office that was adjacent to a branch of his bank.

John did not achieve permanent avoidance of alcohol. Generally he was able to reduce his drinking but, at times of stress, would go on a drinking binge. These binges have occurred at a frequency of approximately 3-month intervals. Four years after starting therapy, John has considerably reduced his drinking but has not achieved the goal of abstinence. His drinking is sporadic but of a 'binge' and out-of-control pattern. Attempts to introduce controlled drinking have failed. On the positive side, however, he is now working as a night watchman and has held this job for 2 years. His employers have been tolerant of his occasional absenteeism due to alcohol. The general physicians are less worried about his physical health but would still wish him to be alcohol-free.

Habit disorders

Problem behaviours may also take the form of bad habits that have been learnt in response to a whole range of stimuli. Azrin & Nunn (1973) pioneered the treatment of habit reversal, which has been used to treat a range of nervous habits including multiple and facial tics, nail-biting and neurodermatitis. This treatment has four components:

- awareness training
- competing response training
- habit control motivation
- generalisation training.

Treatment of tics

Example

Peter was referred to the clinic with a 14-year history of unsightly and embarrassing facial tics. The onset had occurred at puberty but was not related to any particular life event. Over the years he had received treatment with a variety of medication including haloperidol and benzodiazepine drugs with no effect. The tics occurred at any time but were more frequent if he was anxious or bored. Close observation of the movements revealed that it commenced with screwing up both eyes followed by crinkling his nose and then making a sharp downward movement of his chin and opening his mouth. What Peter was asked to do was to record the frequency of his tics over a few days. This awareness training is useful as many people with habit disorders are oblivious of some of the times when they perform the undesirable behaviour. He was asked to divide each page of a notebook into columns which represented a 1-hour period. Every time he performed the tic, he was asked to place a mark in the appropriate column and to record his activity at each hourly interval. This diary was a baseline measure of the problem and was maintained throughout treatment to monitor progress. Another assessment measure was the recording of the interview on videotape for a 20-minute period. During the interview, the therapist asked a series of 'neutral' questions about his job and hobbies and some more emotive questions about the effect of the tic on his life. The mean number of tics per minute during the 'neutral' and 'emotive' discussion was then calculated and this procedure was repeated at the end of treatment with the therapist asking identical questions. The baseline measures showed that Peter performed the tic an average of 300 times a day or approximately 0.5 tics per minute.

At the second session the principle of competing response practice was explained. The therapist said:

'One of the problems with a longstanding habit is that you have built up and strengthened the muscles of your face which are involved in the tic at the expense of the opposing muscles. What I will be asking you to do is to perform some exercises to strengthen these opposing muscles. The start of every tic begins with you screwing up both your eyes. As soon as you feel that you are going to tic, I want you to raise your eyebrows, wrinkling your forehead. You may find this easier to do if you place your thumb and index finger of one hand under each of your eyebrows. I then want you to hold this position to the count of 20 or until the urge to tic passes, whichever is the longer time. At the same time as doing this I would like you to clench you teeth together very tightly and likewise to maintain this position'. Following this description, the therapist asked him to practise the competing response in the session. The therapist then asked Peter to list all the deleterious effects of having a tic and the advantages of being tic-free. He was asked to write this list down and to read it through whenever he felt bored or disheartened by the treatment (habit control motivation). Finally, ways in which he could incorporate the competing response movements into everyday life without looking conspicuous were discussed. Peter suggested that if he were outside, he could place his hand under his eyebrows as if shielding his eyes from the sun. If he was inside and sitting at a desk or table, he could use his hand under his eyebrows to support his head (generalisation training).

When Peter was seen a week later, the frequency of tics had already reduced to less than 10% of the baseline level. Six weeks after the initial appointment, Peter was discharged from active treatment. The frequency of tics was less than 1%, which was acceptable to him. This improvement was maintained at 1-year post-treatment follow-up.

Although habit reversal is a very rapid and effective treatment for many individuals with habit disorders, some individuals fail to respond. Mass practice can sometimes be used for individuals in whom habit reversal has failed or is inappropriate.

Treatment of an irritating habit using mass practice

Example

Michael had been treated for pneumonia 3 years previously. Since then he had developed the habit of repeatedly clearing his throat despite having no phlegm to move. This habit occurred 60–80 times an hour and was causing some marital problems as it greatly irritated his wife. Treatment with habit reversal had been unsuccessful as it was difficult to find an effective competing response. The therapist then decided to use mass practice. Michael was first asked to find 3 half-hour periods in the day when he could retire to his room alone and would not be heard by his family. He was then told that during these times he was to repeatedly clear his throat for the entire 30-minute period. At other times of the day, he was to try not to clear his throat but to 'save it up' to his next throat clearing session. The week after this instruction was given, he reported that he had complied with the instructions for the first 3 days but that since that time the thought of clearing his throat was so aversive to him that he had not been able to do it at all. His wife was delighted with his improvement. He was asked to continue monitoring his throat-clearing and to reintroduce mass practice if the frequency increased to more than 5 times a day.

Applying operant techniques to chronic problems

In patients with chronic behaviour problems, treatment techniques based on operant conditioning (or in other words sticks and carrots) are used. These principles are not always obvious to apply, as one man's stick may be another man's carrot or vice versa. Premack's (1959) principle addresses this finding by observing that high-frequency preferred activity can be used to reinforce lower-frequency, non-preferred activity. In other words, if a child spends most of his/her time playing with toy racing cars, this high-frequency preferred activity could be used to reinforce the lower frequency non-preferred activity of tidying his/her bedroom.

The role of this type of treatment aimed at reducing undesired behaviours and increasing socially acceptable behaviour has increased in the past few years with the increasing closure of many of the older psychiatric institutions and a move towards community care. Discharge to the community or even admission into a psychiatric unit of a district general hospital often means that bizarre or socially unacceptable behaviour is not tolerated as well as in the old 'asylums'. Different problems are also presented by those individuals who were resident in 'old-style' long-term institutions ('old' long-stay patients) and those individuals who are in long-stay care today ('new' long-stay patients).

By far the most commonly applied form of reinforcement to be used is positive reinforcement. Negative reinforcement or even punishment are rarely used in clinical practice and usually only in dangerous or life-threatening situations. The ethical problems with negative reinforcement and punishment are obvious but clear ethical dilemmas may also arise with positive reinforcers, particularly if necessary items such as food are used as reinforcers and the patient has not 'earned' a meal that day. The types of reinforcers are given in Table 7.2.

Reinforcers that increase specified activities

Positive reinforcers

- social approval, for example therapist's approval in an individual with a phobia who has complied with exposure task
- feedback reinforcement, for example social skills group
- food reinforcers (difficulty with withholding meals and problems with obesity if use sweets and biscuits etc.)
- higher-frequency preferred activities (with some 'old' long-stay patients this may amount to cigarettes, with resultant ethical dilemma of possible increasing consumption)
- tokens, awarded for certain activities, which can be 'spent' on a number of reinforcers.

Negative reinforcers

This means the removal of an aversive event after a specific response is obtained, i.e. aversive relief and this has little place in treatment today. If used, then covertly, for example a man with sexual deviancy who has been trained to have aversive images following arousing deviant images can gain relief from these aversive experiences by switching to neutral thoughts.

Reinforcers that reduce specified activities

1. Punishment
   - Time out, i.e. removal of the individual from reinforcing environment for up to 3 minutes. For example a child who is aggressive to other children during a game may be removed from the room for a few minutes.
   - Overcorrection, for example a patient smashes his cup to the floor, he is asked not only to clear up the mess but then to wash the entire ward floor.
   - Positive punishment, for example a child puts its finger towards an electric socket and receives a sharp slap on the hand.

169

Table 7.2 Types of reinforcement

++ Positive (i.e. apply a positive stimulus)	+ − Punishment (i.e. apply a negative stimulus)
− − Negative (i.e. remove a negative stimulus)	− + Response cost (i.e. remove a positive stimulus)

2. Response cost
   - Penalty involving some time and effort in response to certain behaviours, for example a disruptive child at school has to write out 100 times 'I must make every effort to be silent in class'.
   - A positive reinforcer is removed if certain non-desired activities are indulged in.

Positive reinforcement programme

Example

Flora, an 82-year-old woman, had suffered from a cerebrovascular accident two years earlier, which had resulted in moderate intellectual impairment. She had spent these past 2 years living in a geriatric hospital, where her problem of incontinence was a problem to the staff who were required to change her incontinence pad 8 or 9 times daily. This incontinence was not felt to be organic in origin but attempts to regularly 'toilet' Flora had not produced any obvious success. Despite this, it was noted with interest that Flora was rarely incontinent overnight.

The therapist arranged to spend 2 days on the ward. The first day was spent observing Flora and obtaining baseline measures. What rapidly became clear was how tired the staff were with Flora's problem and how they had little or no interaction with her except when she was incontinent. The nurses were very busy but were inadvertently reinforcing Flora's incontinence. It would have been unproductive for an outsider to impart this information to the nursing staff after only being on the ward for a few hours and would have been unlikely to engage staff cooperation. The therapist therefore decided to check how frequently Flora was incontinent by examining her incontinence pad every 30 minutes. In addition, she was taken to the toilet by the nursing staff 5 times a day as usual. The first day's data revealed that Flora passed small amounts of urine every hour although this was not noticed on every occasion by the nursing staff.

The next day the therapist explained to the staff that Flora was going to be taken to the toilet every 30 minutes. Smiles, praise and social reinforcement would be used whenever she managed to pass water. If she did not urinate, she would be taken back to the day room after 5 minutes on the toilet without any further communication.

The therapist started this programme as described. At first Flora did not appear to listen to praise when given. This unfamiliarity with social reinforcement was overcome by the therapist looking Flora in the face while smiling and praising at the same time as gently stroking her hand. After 4 hours of this programme, Flora seemed to understand what she was required to do. She began passing water on almost every visit to the toilet. If wet at other times, this was ignored until her pad was changed at her next toilet visit.

The nursing staff were asked to continue this programme for the next week. Their initial reaction was that they were much to busy to take her to the toilet so often. When it was pointed out that the time previously spent in changing Flora's incontinence pad and the bed on frequent occasions when overflow occurred was also time-consuming, they agreed to give it a trial.

When the therapist arrived on the ward a week later, the staff were noticeably more enthusiastic about Flora's programme. The nurses reported that they had recorded that Flora had not been incontinent for 3 days but was passing water on each occasion that she was taken to the toilet. The therapist, therefore suggested that they should reduce the frequency of toileting to hourly and to continue monitoring when her pad was dry and wet and when she used the lavatory. Only if her pad was wet on >50% of occasions for 2 days should they increase the frequency of toileting to every 45 minutes.

Treatment of schizophrenia and other psychoses

The management and treatment of patients suffering from schizophrenia is one of the most important challenges to modern mental health services. Modern drugs have altered the course of schizophrenia and allowed the large asylums to be closed. However, the drugs have side-effects and variable effects on symptoms. Behavioural and cognitive treatments have been used in a variety of ways to tackle the symptoms of schizophrenia and its social effects.

These therapies are too extensive to be fully covered in this chapter and are discussed in more detail in Chapter 8. In addition, a review of this topic has been published elsewhere (Drummond & Duggal, 1997). They will be discussed here briefly under three headings as follows.

Acute symptoms

Reinforcement techniques have been used since the 1960s to try and reduce the frequency and intensity of delusions and hallucinations (for example Rickard, Digman & Horner, 1960, Rutner & Bugle, 1969). The problem with these techniques is that it is difficult to demonstrate whether the patient really does have a reduction in hallucinations and delusions following reinforcement or whether there is purely less discussion by the patient about the symptomatology. Second, these techniques often do not generalise into the community.

Cognitive techniques have also been tried over the past 30 years. Initially these took the form of the patient learning to think verbal commands to themselves to 'be logical' or 'be coherent'. This procedure was called self-instructional training (Meichenbaum & Cameron, 1973).

Recently, cognitive therapy based on the work of A. T. Beck has been used successfully in some individuals with schizophrenia. Using the approach of collaborative empiricism, described earlier in this chapter, abnormal beliefs are identified and challenged by testing their validity (Alford & Beck, 1994). This approach is contrary to traditional psychiatric thinking as delusions have previously been thought to be unshakeable. Kingdon, Turkington & John (1994) also used cognitive therapy with individuals with schizophrenia to help them distinguish real and hallucinatory experiences.

Coping strategy enhancement (CSE) is another treatment that aims to decrease acute symptoms by teaching the patient to cope with and control the cues and reactions to symptoms (Tarrier, 1992; Tarrier *et al*, 1990).

Chronic symptoms

These have mainly been approached using the operant programmes described earlier in this chapter. These have either been applied individually or in token economy systems as described by Ayllon & Azrin (1968). The efficacy of the token economy system as opposed to a positive, encouraging and reinforcing environment was not demonstrated by the large controlled trial of token economy performed in the UK (Hall, Baker & Hutchinson, 1977).

Social skills deficits often found in individuals with chronic schizophrenia have also been treated using the standard techniques described earlier in this chapter. These programmes have generally been shown in controlled trials to be beneficial to these patients (for example Eckman *et al*, 1992).

Relapse prevention and integrative programmes

Although antipsychotic medication reduces the number of individuals with schizophrenia who relapse, approximately one-third of individuals do still relapse. Environmental stress and high expressed emotion in relatives and carers has been demonstrated to be associated with acute relapse (Brown *et al*, 1972; Leff & Vaughn, 1985; Tarrier & Barrowclough, 1990).

Behavioural–cognitive approaches include family interventions (Falloon, 1992; Lam, 1991), training in illness self-management (Eckman *et al*, 1992) and training in coping strategies (Tarrier *et al*, 1993), and all of these have been shown to be successful in reducing relapse and morbidity.

Family interventions consist of focusing on the strengths and weaknesses in the family; education of relatives including cognitive restructuring for faulty beliefs about schizophrenia; prescribing of regular structured contact between relatives and the individual with schizophrenia; setting of behavioural tasks and goals in the family; communication skills training and problem-solving techniques. Family intervention in schizophrenia has been found not only to reduce relapse but also to improve individuals' social adjustment including employment status and family adjustment (Falloon *et al*, 1985; 1987).

A recent randomised controlled trial of intensive behavioural and cognitive therapy comprising coping strategy enhancement, training in problem-solving and training in strategies to reduce risk of relapse was found to be significantly superior in terms of number and intensity of positive symptoms to routine care or supportive counselling and routine care (Tarrier *et al*, 1998).

New developments in behavioural and cognitive psychotherapies

Behavioural and cognitive treatment techniques are now being tried in a number of other conditions, and outcome data from more extensive controlled treatment trials are awaited.

Hypochondriasis

In primary hypochondriasis, a number of workers have suggested cognitive–behavioural formulations of the disorder (see Warwick & Salkovskis, 1990). From case-reports (Salkovskis & Warwick, 1986) and an uncontrolled trial of group treatment (Stern & Fernandez, 1991) it appears that cognitive–behavioural treatment derived from such an approach may be effective. Results of a controlled trial found that cognitive–behavioural treatment of hypochondriasis was significantly more effective than a no treatment waiting-list control in 32 patients randomly allocated to receive either 16 sessions of cognitive–behavioural therapy or no treatment control (Warwick *et al*, 1996).

Example

Janet, a 43-year-old married woman, was convinced she had throat cancer. She spent a great deal of time checking her throat for lumps and looking down it with a dental mirror for any signs of cancer. She repeatedly checked the functioning of her throat, by swallowing deliberately up to a hundred times per day, and by singing to herself repeatedly. She also asked her husband to examine her throat and asked him repeatedly for reassurance that she did not have cancer. Whenever she became aware of any change in feeling in her throat, or thought that the appearance had altered in any way, she would think 'That's it, I have it now, there is no hope for me', believing she had cancer 100%. She would then visit her doctor for examination as soon as possible.

Treatment started by constructing with Janet a simple version of the cognitive–behavioural formulation of her problem. In this, she was shown how her negative automatic thoughts, such as the one given above, caused her to feel anxious about her health. This health anxiety led to a number of factors, which maintained her health fears, such as bodily checking, reassurance-seeking and selective attention to health. Her attitudes to health and illness in general were also examined, and it became apparent that she held a number of erroneous, dysfunctional attitudes, such as 'I'm a generally unlucky person, I'm bound to get ill', and 'physical symptoms must mean that I have a serious illness'. Cognitive–behavioural treatment involved identification and modification of negative automatic thoughts about health, and behavioural techniques such as response-prevention to deal with maintaining factors. Her dysfunctional attitudes were also corrected using cognitive techniques. On completion of a 16-session course of cognitive–behavioural treatment, Janet's health anxiety had resolved, and she no longer believed that she had cancer.

Post-traumatic phobias (post-traumatic stress disorder)

Recently, attention has focused on the prevalence and severity of psychological sequelae following a traumatic life-event or disaster. Individuals with post-traumatic stress disorder (PTSD) may often present with a phobia that dates back to the time of the disaster or shortly afterwards. In addition, they often suffer from irritability, tension, startle, depression, insomnia, nightmares and flashbacks as well as fear and avoidance of objects or situations that remind them of the disaster (see Marks, 1987).

Treatment involves graduated exposure to the avoided fear-provoking cues. This often involves fantasy exposure to thinking about the traumatic event itself. This exposure must be sufficiently prolonged to allow anxiety to reduce. As this can be a time-consuming and emotionally testing treatment for the therapist, severe cases are best treated by a specialist behavioural–cognitive psychotherapist.

There have been extensive case reports that demonstrate the efficacy of exposure combined with cognitive therapy for these individuals and some controlled trials (for example, Foa, Hearst-Ikeda & Perry, 1995). One recent controlled trial showed that while both exposure and cognitive restructuring were both equally effective in treating PTSD, a combination of exposure and cognitive therapy showed no advantage over the other treatment on their own (Marks *et al*,1998).

Conclusion

Overall, behavioural and cognitive psychotherapy has come a long way since the days when it was used for purely phobic and obsessive–compulsive disorders. It is now used, and has been shown to have proven benefit, in the whole spectrum of psychiatric disorders. The addition of cognitive techniques to behavioural treatment has greatly increased the range of patients who can benefit from the approach.

A worrying development, however, is for therapists with little or no training to attempt to treat individuals using these techniques. This can have disastrous results. Any individual referred for behavioural–cognitive psychotherapy needs to have a full psychiatric and physical assessment as well as a properly conducted behavioural–cognitive analysis to ensure that the correct diagnosis has been made and that an appropriate treatment package is to be implemented. Appropriate contingency plans need to be available if things do not go according to plan.

Acknowledgement

The authors are grateful to Cambridge University Press for permission to reproduce extracts from Stern & Drummond (1991).

References and further reading

Alford, B. A. & Beck, A. T. (1994) Cognitive therapy of delusional beliefs. *Behaviour Research and Therapy*, **12**, 369–380.

Ayllon, T. & Azrin, N. (1968) *The Token Economy*. New York: Appleton Century Crofts.

Azrin, N. H. & Nunn, R. G. (1973) Habit reversal: a method of eliminating nervous habits and tics. *Behaviour Research and Therapy*, **11**, 619–628.

Beck, A. T., Rush, A. J., Shaw, B. F., *et al* (1979) *Cognitive Therapy of Depression*. New York: Guilford.

Beck, A. T., Sokol, L., Clark, D. A., *et al* (1992) Focused cognitive therapy of panic disorder: a cross over design and one-year follow-up. *American Journal of Psychiatry*, **147**, 778–783.

Brown, G. W., Birley, J. L. T. & Wing, J. K. (1972). Influence of family life on the course of schizophrenia disorders: replication. *British Journal of Psychiatry*, **121**, 241–258.

Butler, G., Cullington, A., Hibbert, G., *et al* (1987) Anxiety management for persistent generalised anxiety. *British Journal of Psychiatry*, **151**, 535–542.

Clark, D. M. (1986) A cognitive approach to panic. *Behaviour Research and Therapy*, **24**, 461–470.

Cottraux, J., Note, I., Yao, S. N., *et al* (2001) A randomized controlled trial of cognitive therapy versus intensive behaviour therapy in obsessive–compulsive disorder. *Psychotherapy and Psychosomatics*, **70**, 288–297.

Drummond, L.M. (1993) The treatment of severe, chronic, resistant obsessive–compulsive disorder: an evaluation of an in-patient programme using behavioural psychotherapy in combination with other treatments. *British Journal of Psychiatry*, **163**, 223–229.

Drummond, L. M. & Duggal, A. (1997) Behavioural cognitive approaches to psychosis. In *The Psychotherapy of Psychosis* (eds C. Mace & F. Margison), pp. 93–114. London: Royal College of Psychiatrists.

Durham, R. C. & Allan, T. (1993) Psychological treatment of generalized anxiety disorder. A review of the clinical significance of results on outcome studies since 1980. *British Journal of Psychiatry*, **183**, 19–26.

Eckman, T. A., Wirshing, W. C., Marder, S. R., *et al* (1992) Technique for training schizophrenic patients in illness self-management: a controlled trial. *American Journal of Psychiatry*, **149**, 1549–1555.

Ellis, A. (1962) *Reason and Emotion in Psychotherapy*. New York: Lyle Stuart.

Emmelkamp, P. M. G. & Wessels, H. (1975) Flooding in imagination *v.* flooding *in vivo* in agoraphobics. *Behaviour Research and Therapy*, **13**, 7–15.

Emmelkamp, P. M. G., Visser, S. & Hoekstra, R. J. (1988) Cognitive therapy versus exposure *in vivo* in the treatment of obsessive–compulsives. *Cognitive Therapy and Research*, **12**, 103–114.

Falloon, I. R. H., Boyd, J. L., McGill, C. W., *et al* (1985) Family management in the prevention of morbidity of schizophrenia. Clinical outcome of a two-year longitudinal study. *Archives of General Psychiatry*, **42**, 887–896.

Falloon, I. R. H., McGill, C. W., Boyd, J. L., *et al* (1987) Family management in the prevention of morbidity of schizophrenia: social outcome of a two-year longitudinal study. *Psychological Medicine*, **17**, 59–66.

Falloon, I. R. H. (1992). Psychotherapy of schizophrenia. *British Journal of Hospital Medicine*, **48**, 3–4, 164–170.

Foa, E. B. & Goldstein, A. (1978) Continuous exposure and complete response prevention in the treatment of obsessive–compulsive neurosis. *Behavior Therapy*, **9**, 821–829.

Foa, E. B., Hearst-Ikeda, D. & Perry, K. J. (1995) Evaluation of a brief cognitive–behavioral program for the prevention of chronic PTSD in recent assault victims. *Journal of Consulting and Clinical Psychology*, **63**, 948–955.

Freeston, M. H., Ladouceur, R., Gagnon, F., *et al* (1997) Cognitive–behavioural treatment of obsessive thoughts: a controlled study. *Journal of Consulting and Clinical Psychology*, **65**, 405–413.

Ghosh, A., Marks, I. M. & Carr, A. C. (1988) Therapist contact and outcome of self-exposure treatment for phobias: a controlled study. *British Journal of Psychiatry*, **152**, 234–238.

Govender, S., Drummond, L. M., & Menzies, R. A. (2006) Danger ideation reduction therapy for the treatment of severe, chronic and resistant obsessive–compulsive disorder. *Behavioural and Cognitive Psychotherapy*, **34**, 1–4.

Hall, J. N., Baker, R. D. & Hutchinson, K. (1977) A controlled evaluation of token economy procedures with chronic schizophrenic patients. *Behaviour Research and Therapy*, **15**, 261–283.

Hawton, K., Salkovskis, P. M., Kirk, J. & Clark, D. M. (1989) *Cognitive Behaviour Therapy for Psychiatric Problems: A Practical Guide*. Oxford: Oxford University Press.

Hollon, S. D., Shelton, R. C. & Loosen, P. T. (1991) Cognitive therapy and pharmacotherapy for depression. *Journal of Consulting and Clinical Psychology*, **59**, 88–99.

James, I. A. & Blackburn, I. M. (1995) Cognitive therapy with obsessive–compulsive disorder. *British Journal of Psychiatry*, **166**, 444–450.

Jones, M. K. & Menzies, R. G. (1997a) The cognitive mediation of obsessive–compulsive handwashing. *Behaviour Research and Therapy*, **36**, 959–970.

Jones, M. K. & Menzies, R. G. (1997b) Danger ideation reduction therapy (DIRT): preliminary findings with three obsessive–compulsive washers. *Behaviour Research and Therapy*, **35**, 955–960

Jones, M. K. & Menzies, R. G. (1998a) The role of perceived danger in the mediation of obsessive–compulsive washing. *Depression and Anxiety*, **8**, 121–125.

Jones, M. K. & Menzies, R. G. (1998b) Danger Ideation reduction Therapy for obsessive–compulsive washers. A controlled trial. *Behaviour Research and Therapy*, **8**, 121–125.

Kingdon, D., Turkington, D. & John, C. (1994) Cognitive behaviour therapy of schizophrenia: the amenability of delusions and hallucinations to reasoning. *British Journal of Psychiatry*, **164**, 581–587.

Lam, D. H. (1991) Psychosocial family intervention in schizophrenia: a review of empirical studies. *Psychological Medicine*, **21**, 423–441.

Leff, J. P. & Vaughn, C. (1985) *Expressed Emotion in Families*. New York: Guilford Press.

Marks, I. M. (1981) *Cure and Care of Neurosis: Theory and Practice of Behavioural Psychotherapy*. New York: Wiley.

Marks, I. M., Gray, S., Cohen, D., *et al* (1983) Imipramine and brief therapist-aided exposure in agoraphobics having self-exposure homework. *Archives of General Psychiatry*, **40**, 153–162.

Marks, I. M. (1986) *Behavioural Psychotherapy. Maudsley Pocketbook of Clinical Management*. Bristol: Wright.

Marks, I. M. (1987) *Fears, Phobias and Rituals*. New York: Oxford University Press.

Marks, I. M., Lelliot, P., Basoglu, M., *et al* (1988) Clomipramine, self-exposure and therapist-aided exposure for obsessive–compulsive rituals. *British Journal of Psychiatry*, **152**, 522–534.

Marks, I. M., Lovell, K., Noshirvani, H., *et al* (1998) Treatment of post-traumatic stress disorder by exposure and/or cognitive restructuring. A controlled study. *Archives of General Psychiatry*, **55**, 317–325.

Marquis, J. N. (1970) Orgasmic reconditioning: changing sexual object choice through controlling masturbation fantasies. *Journal of Behaviour Therapy and Experimental Psychiatry*, **1**, 263–270.

Mathews, A. M., Gelder, M. G. & Johnston, D. W. (1981) *Agoraphobia: Nature and Treatment*. New York: Guilford Press.

McDonald, R., Sartory, G., Grey, S. J., *et al* (1978) Effects of self-exposure instructions on agoraphobic outpatients. *Behaviour Research and Therapy*, **17**, 83–85.

McLean, P. D., Whittal, M. L., Thordarson, D. S., *et al* (2001) Cognitive versus behaviour therapy in group treatment to obsessive–compulsive disorder. *Consulting and Clinical Psychology*, **69**, 205–214.

Meichenbaum, D. & Cameron, R. (1973) Training schizophrenics to talk to themselves: a means of developing attentional controls. *Behavior Therapy*, **4**, 515–534.

Menzies, R. G., Harris, L. M., Cumming, S. R., *et al* (2000) The relationship between inflated personal responsibility and exaggerated danger expectancies in obsessive–compulsive concerns. *Behaviour Research and Therapy*, **38**, 1029–1037.

Premack, D. (1959) Toward empirical behavior laws: 1. Positive reinforcement. *Psychological Review*, **66**, 219–233.

Rachman, S. J., Cobb, J., Grey, S., *et al* (1979) The behavioural treatment of obsessive–compulsive disorders with and without clomipramine. *Behaviour Research and Therapy*, **17**, 462–478.

Rickard, H. C., Digman, P. J. & Horner, R. F. (1960) Verbal manipulation in a psychotherapeutic relationship. *Journal of Clinical Psychology*, **16**, 364–367.

Rutner, I. T. & Bugle, C. (1969) An experimental procedure for the modification of psychotic behavior. *Journal of Consulting and Clinical Psychology*, **33**, 651–653.

Salkovskis, P. M. (1989) Cognitive-behavioural factors and the persistence of intrusive thoughts in obsessional problems. *Behaviour Research and Therapy*, **27**, 677–682.

Salkovskis, P. M. & Warwick, H. M. C. (1985) Cognitive therapy of obsessive–compulsive disorder – treating treatment failures. *Behaviour Research and Therapy*, **13**, 243–255.

Salkovskis, P. M. & Warwick, H. M. C. (1986) Morbid preoccupations, health anxiety, and reassurance: a cognitive–behavioural approach to hypochondriasis. *Behaviour Research and Therapy*, **24**, 597–609.

Shalev, A. Y., Bonne, O & Eth, S. (1996) Treatment of posttraumatic stress disorder: a review. *Psychosomatic Medicine*, **58**, 165–182.

Stern, R. S. & Marks, I. M. (1973) Brief and prolonged flooding: a comparison in agoraphobic patients. *Archives of General Psychiatry*, **28**, 270–276.

Stern, R. S. & Drummond, L. M. (1991) *The Practice of Behavioural and Cognitive Psychotherapy*. Cambridge: Cambridge University Press.

Stern, R. S. & Fernandez, M. (1991) Group cognitive and behavioural treatment for hypochondriasis. *BMJ*, **303**, 1229–1231.

Stuart, R. B. (1967) Behavioural control of overeating. *Behaviour Research and Therapy*, **1**, 357–365.

Tarrier, N., Harwood, S., Yusopoff, L., *et al* (1990) Coping strategy enhancement: a method of treating residual schizophrenic symptoms. *Behavioral Psychotherapy*, **18**, 283–293.

Tarrier, N. & Barrowclough, C. (1990) Family interventions for schizophrenia. *Behavior Modification*, **14**, 408–440.

Tarrier, N. (1992) Management and modification of residual psychotic symptoms. In *Innovations in the Psychological Management of Schizophrenia* (eds M. Birchwood & N. Tarrier). Chichester: Wiley.

Tarrier, N., Beckett, R., Harwood, S., *et al* (1993) A trial of two cognitive–behavioural methods of treating drug-resistant residual psychotic symptoms in schizophrenic patients: 1. Outcome. *British Journal of Psychiatry*, **162**, 524–532.

Tarrier, N., Yusupoff, L., Kinney, C., *et al.* (1998) Randomised controlled trial of intensive cognitive behaviour therapy for patients with chronic schizophrenia. *BMJ*, **317**, 303–307.

Van Oppen, P., de Haan, E., van Balkow, N. J., *et al* (1995) Cognitive therapy and exposure in the treatment of obsessive compulsive disorder. *Behaviour Research and Therapy*, **33**, 379–390.

Warwick, H. M. C. & Salkovskis, P. M. (1990) Hypochondriasis. *Behaviour Research and Therapy*, **28**, 105–117.

Warwick, H. M., Clark, D. M., Cobb, A. M., *et al* (1996) A controlled trial of cognitive-behavioural treatment of hypochondriasis. *British Journal of Psychiatry*, **169**, 189–195.

CHAPTER 8

Cognitive therapy for severe mental disorders

Jan Scott

This chapter will explore the role of cognitive therapy for individuals with severe mental disorders.

Until recently, severe mental disorders were widely regarded as biological illnesses best treated with medications (Prien & Potter, 1990; Scott, 1995a; Sensky et al, 2000). This approach is gradually changing for two reasons. First, in the past three decades, there has been a greater emphasis on stress–diathesis models. This has led to the development of new aetiological theories of severe mental disorders that emphasise psychological and social aspects of vulnerability and risk. It has also increased the acceptance of brief psychological therapies, such as cognitive therapy, as an adjunct to medication for individuals with medication refractory schizophrenia, and severe and chronic affective disorders (Scott & Wright, 1997). Second, there is a significant efficacy–effectiveness gap for pharmacological treatments for severe mental disorders. For example, mood stabiliser prophylaxis protects about 60% of individuals against relapse in research settings, but protects only 25–40% of individuals against further episodes in clinical settings (Dickson & Kendell, 1986). Similarly, despite research evidence of significant benefits of pharmacotherapy, 30% of individuals with depressive disorder are still symptomatic after 2 years of treatment with antidepressant medication and 50% of individuals with schizophrenia experience a further relapse over a 5-year period. The introduction of newer medications has not improved prognosis (Scott, 1995a). This less impressive symptomatic and functional outcome in day-to-day practice has increased interest in non-pharmacological treatment approaches.

This chapter explores the utility of cognitive therapy for chronic depressive disorders, bipolar disorders and schizophrenia. It will first outline the applicability of cognitive therapy, review adaptations of the basic cognitive therapy model that are required when working with severe mental disorders and highlight the different ways in which cognitive therapy may be incorporated into the overall treatment package. The use of cognitive therapy with severe mental disorders is essentially as an adjunct to medication, it is only exceptionally used as an alternative to pharmacotherapy in this client population. Finally, rather than review the considerable literature from randomised controlled trials, the reader will be directed to relevant meta-analyses or selected treatment trials of the use of cognitive therapy in severe mental diosrders.

The applicability of cognitive therapy

Beck's model of cognitive therapy (Beck, 1976) is the most widely tested short-term psychotherapy for any psychological problem and offers a robust, empirically based approach (Scott 1995b). In addition to its well-known use for patients with mild to moderately severe affective disorders, cognitive therapy is also applicable to patients with anxiety disorders (including post-traumatic stress disorder; PTSD), substance misuse problems, personality disorders, and can be used to help adjustment to cancer or chronic medical disorders (for examples Beck, 1996; Hawton *et al*, 1989) (see also Chapter 7). All of these problems may be part of the clinical picture in severe mental disorders.

Cognitive therapy may also be used in a wide variety of formats such as alone or in combination with medication; in individual, couples, or family therapy; or in out-patient or in-patient settings (Scott *et al*, 1991). This flexibility is important because individuals with severe mental disorder have heterogeneous and complex problems. Beck's approach (Beck *et al*, 1979) allows a consistent model to be applied to a broad spectrum of difficulties presented by such individuals in a variety of clinical settings, thus reducing the risk of confused messages about the treatment rationale being communicated to the individual and their significant others.

Cognitive therapy has specific characteristics that may benefit individuals with severe mental disorders. Its collaborative, educational style and its use of a step-by-step approach and of guided discovery make it acceptable to individuals who wish to take an equal and active role in their therapy (Beck *et al*, 1979; Scott, 1995a). Many individuals with severe disorders resist and challenge a didactic approach to treatment (Miklowitz & Goldstein, 1990). Because the individual plays an active role in developing the formulation of their own beliefs and problems, the interventions used appear rational and logical, giving cognitive therapy a sense of coherence. The structured approach to each session with agenda setting, prioritisation of problems for discussion and joint development of homework tasks, enables patients to retain their focus on specific topics or issues even when exhibiting psychotic symptoms (Kingdon & Turkington, 1994). The structure enables individuals with hypomania to retain their focus on the session despite being distractible (Scott, 2001). Clients with chronic depression also cope better with a structured approach as this tends to contain their sense of hopelessness and helplessness that might otherwise lead to such overwhelming levels of anxiety that the individual is unable to engage in therapy (Scott *et al*, 1991). Cognitive therapy can also encourage skills development and an increased sense of self-efficacy and control. These features of cognitive therapy may be particularly helpful to individuals who experience low self-esteem and perceive a loss of identity because they are viewed as a person with a severe or chronic mental disorder.

Cognitive models of severe mental disorders

Basic elements of the cognitive model

Beck's original cognitive model (now referred to as the linear processing model) suggests that emotional responses to events are determined by the conscious meaning that individual gives to that experience (Beck, 1976). This notion differs from the psychoanalytic approach, which emphasises subconscious drives and the behavioural model of environmental determinism. Beck hypothesised that cognitive vulnerability to emotional disorders centres on prepotent dysfunctional underlying beliefs (for example 'I am inadequate') that develop from early learning experiences, and drive thinking and behaviour. Life events that have a specific meaning for that individual may activate these beliefs. For example, an individual who experiences neglect or abuse in childhood may hold a belief that 'I'm unlovable'. As such, they may later experience depressed mood in the face of rejection by a significant other. Beck's model (Beck, 1976) also suggests that mood states are accentuated by patterns of thinking that amplify the initial mood shift. If an individual becomes depressed they then become more negative in how they see themselves, their world and their future (called the negative cognitive triad). Their immediate thoughts show a number of key information processing biases, and they jump to negative conclusions, overgeneralise from one event to another, interpret situations in all-or-nothing terms, and self-blame to an excessive degree. This further depresses their mood and leads to a further cascade of negative thoughts (the vicious cycle). Finally, the changes in behaviour that are recognised as symptoms of mental disorders (such as avoidance of social interaction, inactivity, hypervigilance etc.) may be regarded as a cause or a consequence of mood shifts and dysfunctional thinking.

Beck's later publications on cognitive models (including the descriptions of modes and the interacting cognitive subsystems model) highlight two other important aspects (Beck, 1996). First, there is an acknowledgement of the importance of biological vulnerability and biological change as an initial precipitant of mood change. Thus suggesting that changes in thoughts, mood and behaviour may play a role in the maintenance rather than the onset of some mental disorders. Second, he identifies the constructs of 'sociotropy' and 'autonomy' (Beck, 1983). These are defined as relatively enduring personality traits that may be relevant in establishing links between cognitive constructs of self-worth, life events and the onset of disorder. It is argued that sociotropy describes individuals whose sense of worth is defined in terms of interpersonal relatedness. In contrast, autonomy describes individuals whose sense of worth is defined in terms of attainment of personal goals, maintenance of independence and sense of freedom. It is proposed that a sociotropic individual is more likely to experience disorder as a result of an interpersonal life event, while an autonomous individual is likely to experience disorder as the result of a life event that thwarts goal attainment or limits personal freedom. There is empirical evidence that sociotropic individuals are at high risk of developing psychological problems in response to interpersonal life events, but only limited data about the role of autonomy (Hammen *et al*, 1989).

From the above description it is possible to define three ways in which cognitive therapy may be incorporated into the treatment of an individual with severe mental disorder:

- relapse prevention
- cognitive restructuring
- formulation.

Cognitive therapy targeted at relapse prevention would focus on the individual's personality style (i.e. sociotropic, autonomous) and the types of life events that may increase the risk of developing further illness episodes. The cognitive therapy would be used to modify the degree of sociotropy or autonomy accordingly. This type of brief intervention has been used successfully in relapse prevention in bipolar disorders.

Cognitive therapy might also be used to explore and modify the impact of the individual's underlying beliefs on the cognitive representation of the disorder and their engagement with treatment. For example, modifying perfectionist beliefs that may impede adherence to medication because the individual wants to get better on their own without the 'crutch' of drugs. This approach has much in common with cognitive models that are used to aid adjustment to physical disorders, and has been applied successfully with schizophrenia and more recently with individuals with bipolar disorder.

Lastly, cognitive therapy may be used to develop a specific and unique formulation of that individual's problems and the cognitive, behavioural, and emotional changes are seen as the core symptoms and psychopathology of the severe mental disorder. This model essentially mirrors the traditional cognitive therapy approach to common mental disorders. In reality, interventions focused on relapse prevention rarely focus only on personality style, but also explore maladaptive beliefs that influence the cognitive representation of illness. Likewise, a course of cognitive therapy based on a specific cognitive formulation of a particular severe mental disorder usually incorporates all the approaches just outlined.

These models are described below.

The 'cognitive representation of illness' model

Horne (1997) provides a useful review of health belief models, including the one promulgated by Leventhal *et al*, (1992). A diagram of the core elements of the model is shown in Fig. 8.1. Leventhal and colleagues suggest that beliefs about illness will influence the types of coping strategies individuals will employ to deal with symptoms or manage their treatment. The individual will then appraise the benefits of that strategy and either modify their coping technique or continue to use it according to their appraisal. This model can be used to understand why some individuals attempt to alleviate symptoms through unexpected or unreliable methods, for example trying to self-regulate mood shifts through alcohol use, or taking medication erratically by adhering with treatment when symptoms are present, but omitting it on other days (whether or not the drug half-life suggests the medication is beneficial when used in this way). Furthermore, Adams & Scott (1999) demonstrated that an individual's adjustment to and engagement with treatment in severe mental disorders will be influenced by their general attitudes and beliefs about themselves and their world (including attributional style), their perception of their own susceptibility to relapse, their views of the likely consequences for them of a relapse, and whether the benefits they see from treatment (e.g. reduced symptoms) overcome the perceived barriers to engaging with treatment (e.g. ideas such as 'taking medication means I'm defective'). Many patients describe certain cues, such as someone else becoming unwell or reading a negative article about treatment that may prompt them to re-engage or disengage from treatment in the short-term.

This cognitive model offers the opportunity for the clinician and patient to construct an accurate, coherent representation of severe mental disorder in the patient's mind that incorporates an understanding of the likely impact of severe mental disorder on that individual and the potential benefits of treatment. Evidence shows that although the content of an individual's

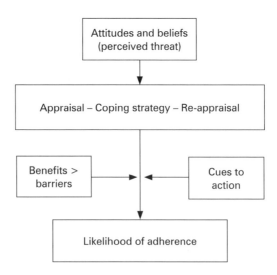

Fig. 8.1 Cognitive representation of illness model

> **Box 8.1**   Key themes in an individual's view of their disorder
>
> - Identity   What is it?
> - Cause   What caused it?
> - Time-line   How long will it last?
> - Consequences   How will it/has it affected me?
> - Cure   Can it be controlled or cured?

cognitive representation of their problem in their mind varies across different demographic and illness groups, the structure of this representation remains constant (Skelton & Croyle, 1991).

A person's views and ideas about their disorder usually relate to five key themes as shown in Box 8.1.

From the patient's perspective, any coping strategy they choose to employ in dealing with their symptoms will be based on their personal beliefs and the cognitive representation of the disorder that they have developed. As such, the general aims for employing cognitive therapy are to understand the beliefs that impact on the individual's adjustment to the severe mental disorder or their engagement with treatment, to increase or enhance effective and adaptive coping skills, to enhance adherence to treatment, and to help the individual recognise and manage psychosocial stressors. Improvements in adherence with medication and modifications to lifestyle are most likely to occur if there is coherence between the patient's abstract ideas about the severe mental disorder, their concrete experience of the symptoms and the rationale and information put forward by the therapist (Horne, 1997). Beliefs that influence the patient's view of their disorder and its treatment may be unique to the severe mental disorder (for example, chronic depression is a personality flaw not an illness, therefore medication is not required, I should just 'pull myself together') or the proposed treatment (for example, 'antipsychotic medication does people more harm than good'), or may reflect the general rules or assumptions that impact on many aspects of the individual's life (for example 'I must always be in control'; 'I must be perfect in everything I do'). Classic cognitive approaches may be beneficial whether the beliefs are specific to health issues or generic rules for living (Scott, 1999). Even a brief psychoeducation package that uses the five key topic areas of the cognitive representation may facilitate adjustment (Scott, 1999). Simply tackling negative thoughts that act as barriers to medication adherence may also be very effective.

Example
Michael was a businessman with a history of bipolar disorder. He noted that when he travelled away from home he often did not take a supply of mood stabilisers with him. At first, he and his therapist thought he may simply be forgetful and instituted a behavioural strategy, namely he tried to overcome

183

this problem by keeping an additional bottle of lithium tablets in his travel bag at all times. However, he reported that despite this he was still at high risk of non-adherence when he travelled to business meetings.

By monitoring this problem Michael and his therapist were able to identify some important cognitive barriers to adherence. Michael produced the following information:

- Situation and mood: 'Sitting in my hotel room on the morning of an important meeting about a contract for a new piece of work for my company. Taking the pill box out of my travel bag. Feeling anxious.'
- Recognise and record automatic thought: Thoughts included: 'This is an important job, my boss stressed it was important that I did this well, I really must be on the ball'.
  - Specific negative automatic thought: 'The tablets might slow me down and then I'll make a hash of this'.
  - Belief in specific thought: 85%
  - Anxiety level: 75%.

With the therapist, Michael evaluated the automatic thought:

- Review: evidence for and against thoughts about the negative effects of medication:
  - For: 'I read somewhere that lithium can slow people's thinking and that it can make you confused'
  - Against: 'I've been on lithium for 13 months and I don't feel slowed down. I've not messed up a previous meeting. My work has been of a high standard even while I've been taking lithium. The only meeting that went really badly occurred on a day when I didn't take my lithium! Confusion only usually occurs if the blood level is in the toxic range, my last test was fine.'
  - Alternatives include: 'I may just be putting all my worries onto the tablets, when really I'm just worried that the meeting goes well' and 'I could ask my doctor to assess if there is any evidence that I have been slowed down by the lithium. If it really is true, maybe he could recommend another mood stabliser'
  - Advantages and disadvantages include: Focusing on this thought is not advantageous to me at this minute. I need to be planning my meetings
- Response:
  - Belief in original automatic thought: 40%
  - Mood: less anxious: down to 45%
  - Homework action plan: 'I will read the MDF leaflet [MDF (Manic Depression Fellowship) Bipolar Organisation patient leaflets] on lithium and its side-effects when I get home and if I'm still concerned I will contact Dr — [the prescriber] and ask to discuss my worries at our next appointment.'

This brief model of cognitive therapy intervention may help adjustment and adherence in individuals with uncomplicated severe mental disorders. It can be delivered by a health professional in primary or secondary mental health services. However, for individuals with multiple problems or treatment refractory symptoms a more sophisticated course of cognitive therapy will probably be required.

A generic cognitive model of severe mental disorders

At a specific level, in order to understand severe mental disorder and its impact on the individual, a conceptualisation that encompasses cognitive (thoughts, images and beliefs), behavioural, affective, biological and environmental areas of the individual's life is required.

The generic approach described by Greenberger & Padesky (1996), with its clear acknowledgement of biology, is particularly useful in working with individuals with severe mental disorder as it allows the therapist to emphasise a stress–diathesis model that may also include neuroendocrine, neurotransmitter or other physical factors as precipitants of symptom shift (see Fig. 8.2). In order to use this approach in severe mental disorder, the therapist first asks the individual to describe their own views about the causes of the disorder and their problems (i.e. exploring their cognitive representation). As the individual talks about their own 'theory' about how the disorder evolved, their ideas and explanations are incorporated within the framework of the model. Links between four aspects of the individual (cognitions, behaviour, mood and biology) and the interaction between these aspects and the environment are stressed (past experience such as childhood adversity would be included here, as well as descriptions of contemporary events or experiences; environment may refer to living situation, family or community). The therapist then explains that small changes in one of these five areas may lead to small changes in another area. This rationale is used to engage the patient in cognitive therapy through monitoring and linking changes in thoughts, behaviours, feelings and the biological symptoms of bipolar disorder. Many will have been given a 'biological' explanation of severe mental disorder prior to coming to cognitive therapy sessions. When the connections between the biological and other aspects of their experience are exposed, the individual is able to understand the rationale for the use of cognitive therapy (alone or in combination with other treatments) without having to totally reject other causal models. This establishes the coherence

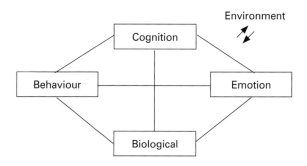

Fig. 8.2 Model of severe mental disorders

within their cognitive representation of the disorder and allows an inroad into exploring attitudes towards use of and adherence to medication and the individual's likely engagement with cognitive therapy.

The above approach is generally well received, particularly in the early stages of cognitive therapy when someone is trying to make sense of their disorder and the proposed treatment. Virtually all aetiological 'theories' proposed by the individual can be incorporated in the model outlined and so they gain confidence that the therapist is listening to their views about their problems and trying to help make sense of them.

Example

Jean was a woman of 43 years who presented with an 8-year history of chronic depressive disorder. In the early discussions with the cognitive therapist, however, Jean most wanted to talk about her childhood (as she spoke the therapist pointed to the word environment on the model). She said that from a very early age her family home was not a happy place. Her parents had constantly argued with each other and her father left to live elsewhere for periods of 3–12 months on several occasions. Each time her father left, she described that she had no idea why her father had gone nor whether he would return (later in life she discovered he had a series of extra-marital affairs). Neither of her parents discussed these departures or any other issues with her and as an only child she felt she had nowhere else to turn. At times she herself had been shouted at, ignored and/or neglected by her parents, but she never felt she had been able to predict when or how her parents would behave towards her.

Using the diagram, the therapist asked Jean how she reacted to this experience as a child, looking at cognitive, behavioural and emotional links. In addition, the focus on childhood experiences afforded an early opportunity to explore possible underlying beliefs.

At this stage, given that Jean may not have been aware of her own beliefs, the therapist took care not to explore these issues too directly. Instead the therapist reflected the story back to Jean and asked her 'if you were told this story about another child, what sorts of beliefs do you think that child would develop about themselves, what beliefs would they have about other people or the world around them?'

Without any knowledge of the cognitive therapy model of core maladaptive beliefs, nor any real awareness of her own underlying beliefs Jean was able to answer with minimal prompting that the sorts of beliefs (or themes reflected in the beliefs) about the self might include: 'It's my fault', 'I'm not important', or 'I'm unlovable'; beliefs about other people may include 'people will leave me' or even 'people cannot be trusted'.

The therapist then asked a question linking past experience, underlying beliefs and the recent life events reported by Jean, and said 'if as an adult that person was left by their husband for another woman and then found out he had also left them with significant financial debts, how do you think they might react?'

This question offered a bridge between the past and the present and then allowed further exploration of the links between events, thoughts, feelings, biological symptoms and behaviour.

Although this general model can be used to help the individual with severe mental disorder explore the origins of their problems, there are specific aspects of each disorder that need to be highlighted when working with different patient populations. An overview of key elements of the approach to chronic depression, bipolar disorders and schizophrenia is therefore described below.

Chronic depressive disorders

All professionals working with people experiencing chronic and refractory depressions are psychologically important to those individuals. Those suffering from persistent symptoms have usually experienced significant disappointments and demoralisation following the failure of several previous treatment regimens and they often describe perceived or actual rejection by the clinicians offering those treatments. Not surprisingly, the individual and those close to them may become increasingly sceptical or lose hope entirely about the possibility of remission. They may begin to doubt or reject the causal model of the disorder promoted by the psychiatrist and subsequently become ambivalent about adhering to the agreed treatment regimen.

A clinician who views their role as the intermittent assessment of the individual's mental state and the prescription of sophisticated combinations of medication will rarely achieve good outcomes with this population. At the very least the clinical management plan needs to include offering the individual information, education, advice, realistic hope and psychological support throughout the course of pharmacotherapy. However, for many individuals this clinical management package is inadequate and a formal course of psychotherapy is advised. There is good evidence for the benefits of cognitive therapy in chronic depression. The approach includes all the elements of cognitive therapy for acute depression, but there are important modifications that help address the specific problems of this client group. The most obvious one is that 20–30 sessions of cognitive therapy may be a more realistic course of therapy than the 8–16 used in other common mental disorders. Other adaptations are briefly outlined below.

The first issue to take into account is that an individual with persistent depression may be feeling hopeless and helpless as well as depressed and as such the therapist must work hard to engage the individual in cognitive therapy. The therapist needs to encourage healthy scepticism about the benefits of cognitive therapy, rather than allowing the client to engage in rigid predictions that, like all their previous treatments, cognitive therapy will fail. Offering a trial of 4–5 sessions of cognitive therapy with an agreement that the therapist and patient will then jointly review the pros and cons of continuing is a useful way forward.

Second, chronic depression is the final common pathway for many different types of problem; as such, cognitive therapists need to employ considerable flexibility in developing a customised case conceptualisation and treatment plan for each individual. In the treatment of dysthymia or mild depressions superimposed on a pre-existing personality disorder, the therapist may introduce intensive work on restructuring underlying dysfunctional attitudes and beliefs at an early stage of the therapy process. This may entail an increased interpersonal focus, to explore how maladaptive beliefs influence the therapeutic relationship and increased use of graded behavioural experiments specifically designed to test whether adopting more adaptive beliefs has a positive influence on the individual's well-being.

In severe chronic depressive disorders, cognitive and behavioural techniques may be used to provide rapid symptom relief from the first session and key problems such as high levels of agitation, insomnia, difficulties with concentration, or profound hopelessness may be targeted. Only later, when the person is less distressed will formulation-driven interventions be aimed at modifying underlying beliefs. In addition, sessions may be reduced in length but held more frequently, or brief telephone sessions may be alternated with face-to-face meetings. Scott *et al* (1991) recommend that 'overlearning' (repetition of behavioural assignments in different situations) during the initial stages of cognitive therapy might be important particularly with in-patients. More complex cognitive interventions (such as identifying and modifying dysfunctional underlying beliefs) may be delayed until the patient is better able to concentrate on and address psychological issues. It should be emphasised, however, that severely depressed people could often do at least some cognitive restructuring early in treatment (Scott & Wright, 1997). For example, someone with marked sleep problems not fully responsive to pharmacotherapy might be taught relaxation and imagery procedures and methods of reducing intrusive negative thoughts. This early use of methods to tackle negative cognitive bias is very important as two of the most significant features of severe or chronic depressive disorders are hopelessness and suicidal ideation, as such cognitive interventions to curb hopelessness and reduce the risk of self-harm are often needed at the outset of treatment.

As individuals with chronic depression often present with complex difficulties, it may not be possible to arrive at a clear conceptualisation until therapy has extended over 10 or so sessions. This is particularly likely in chronic depression as it is often difficult to disentangle antecedents and consequences of depression and because the individual may develop 'secondary maladaptive assumptions' about themselves during the course of a prolonged illness (for example, 'I must be a fraud, depressed people respond to antidepressants'). Early sessions may thus focus on teaching cognitive and behavioural strategies for tackling specific symptoms and building up skill levels, and identifying and modifying these secondary assumptions while constantly revising and re-visiting the formulation hoping that the 'noise in the system' is gradually being reduced. However, the goal for the therapist and patient is always to develop a clear formulation that guides interventions, as failure to modify maladaptive beliefs will leave the patient at high risk of relapse. Also, it should be borne in mind that, in the early stages of cognitive therapy, individuals with chronic depression are certain that their negative predictions will come true. As therapy proceeds, this certainty is gradually undermined and replaced by uncertainty about what will happen to them, so those with chronic depression invariably go through an extended period of anxiety on the road to recovery. The therapist should not assume they had misdiagnosed the problem or failed to identify a comorbid disorder, but they do need to be able to combine cognitive therapy for depression with relevant strategies for overcoming this emerging anxiety.

Although the therapist strives to develop an individual conceptualisation of why a particular person has developed persistent depression, it is important that the therapist draws on research data about the common characteristics of this disorder as it may help guide their investigations and interventions. For example, reviews of unipolar depression suggest that lack of social support, poor marital or family relationships or a preponderance of negative life events (particularly interpersonal loss), after the onset of the index depressive episode, may all be associated with chronicity (Paykel, 1994; Scott, 1988; Scott, 2000). Bothwell & Scott (1997) demonstrated that severely depressed in-patients who reported a strong need for approval by others and low trait self-esteem at admission to hospital were most likely to be depressed at a 2-year follow-up. Teasdale (1988) also describes how 'getting depressed about being depressed' may lead to persistence of depression. High levels of sociotropy, overgeneralisation, poor problem-solving strategies and/or avoidant coping style are also highly prevalent in those with chronic or partially remitted mood disorders (Krantz & Moos, 1988; Scott & Wright, 1997). A simple model to allow the therapist and patient to begin to formulate the patient's chronic depression is given in Fig. 8.3.

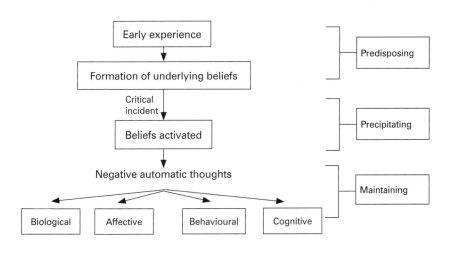

Fig. 8.3 Models of depression

Bipolar disorders

Research on cognitive theories of bipolar disorders is in its infancy, and as yet there is no adequate psychological model of the development of manic relapse, nor of what types of life events may precipitate mania as opposed to depression in a vulnerable individual. Nevertheless, there is evidence that, in comparison with healthy controls, individuals at high risk of bipolar relapse often show certain patterns of dysfunctional beliefs such as high levels of perfectionism, need for social approval and desire to be in control (Scott *et al*, 2000). Furthermore, individuals with bipolar disorders show unstable self-esteem, overgeneral memory, poor problem-solving skills, avoidant coping style and a tendency to overestimate the benefits and underestimate the risks of their actions.

These elements mean that it is feasible to develop individual cognitive formulations of onset and recurrence of manic and depressive episodes and to design appropriate cognitive and behavioural interventions. Although each individual will report a specific set of problems the common themes that need to be addressed in cognitive therapy for individuals with bipolar disorders are to:

- facilitate adjustment to the disorder and its treatment
- improve self-esteem and self-image
- reduce maladaptive or high-risk behaviours
- recognise and modify psychobiosocial factors that destabilise the individual's day-to-day functioning and mood state
- help the individual recognise and manage psychosocial stressors and interpersonal problems
- teach strategies to cope with the symptoms of depression, hypomania, and any cognitive and behavioural problems
- teach early recognition of relapse symptoms and develop effective coping techniques
- identify and modify dysfunctional automatic thoughts (negative or positive) and underlying maladaptive beliefs
- improve self-management through homework assignments.

Which goals are addressed first will depend on whether the client is euthymic, depressed or hypomanic.

If the client is euthymic, cognitive therapy may progress in an orderly manner as described below. Depression requires urgent attention and symptom reduction may be prioritised over formulation. Likewise if the individual is hypomanic, the sessions will focus on rehearsing specific simple behavioural strategies that enable the individual to manage basic day-to-day tasks and that keep them safe (Scott, 2001).

At the first cognitive therapy session, if possible, the individual is encouraged to tell their story and to identify problem areas through the use of a life chart. The most recent episode of mania and then of depression are explored in detail to look at the cognitive–behavioural cycle of change (see

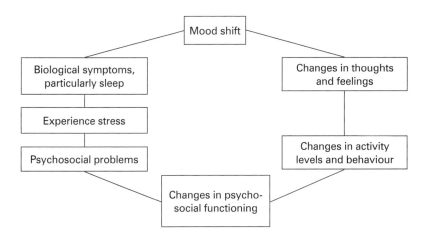

Fig. 8.4   Model of bipolar disorder

Fig. 8.4). The therapist and client use the diagram to identify key features of the episode and how these changes in functioning influence relationships. An example is given below.

Example

Duncan was a 42-year-old businessman. His business was struggling financially (stress). Duncan was worrying about this and was not sleeping (physical symptom). However, with this reduction in sleep he noticed he was feeling rather better in his mood (mood change), he became optimistic that he could solve the problems of the company by increasing the cash flow through a few 'quick deals and creative thinking'. He thought he was 'a genius' as his plan was to use some money to invest in a mink farm (changes in thoughts and behaviours). He would cover this venture by 'generating' some additional resources from his family income. He would use his own salary to place bets at the local casino. Duncan became increasingly preoccupied with these schemes and spent less and less time at home. His wife was frustrated that he was not around and that when he was he seemed 'distracted' (change in psychosocial functioning). He decided not to tell his wife about the casino as he decided she would 'worry too much' and 'put the dampers on my master plan'. The mink farm scheme failed, and Duncan lost increasing amounts of money at the casino. His mood shifted from elation to irritability, and one of his employees took out a complaint against him because he had been rude and angry with her during a meeting. His problems were compounded when his wife confronted him with the household bank statement; they had a large overdraft and the bank manager wished to see them (psychosocial difficulties). As the tensions at work and at home continued and the financial problems of his company and his personal overdraft got worse, Duncan began to feel tense, worried and depressed (stress and distress).

Having used the descriptions of recent episodes and explored any current difficulties, the client's problems are then classified under three broad headings:

- intrapersonal (for example, low self-esteem, cognitive processing biases)
- interpersonal (for example, lack of social network)
- basic problems (for example, symptom severity, difficulties coping with work).

These issues are explored in about 20–25 sessions of cognitive therapy. The last few sessions are offered 1 month and then 3 months after regular therapy has ended. These 'booster sessions' are used to review the skills and techniques learned.

Therapy begins with an exploration of the individual's understanding of bipolar disorder and a detailed discussion of all past illness episodes particularly focusing on the identification of prodromal signs, events or stressors associated with their onset, typical cognitive and behavioural concomitants of both manic and depressive episodes and an exploration of interpersonal functioning (for example, family interactions).

Early sessions include development of an understanding of key issues identified in the life chart, education about bipolar disorder, facilitation of adjustment to the disorder by identifying and challenging negative automatic thoughts, and developing behavioural experiments particularly focused on ideas about stigmatisation and fragile self-esteem.

Using information gathered previously, sessions are then used to help the individual to learn self-monitoring and self-regulation techniques, which enhance self-management of depressive and hypomanic symptoms, and to explore skills for coping with depression and mania. For example, this involves establishing regular activity patterns, daily routines, regular sleep patterns, developing coping skills, time management, use of support, and recognising and tackling dysfunctional automatic thoughts about self, world and future using automatic thought diaries. It often includes 'harm reduction' approaches to drug or alcohol use to try and reduce the use of substances to change or stabilise mood states.

Problems with adherence to medication and other aspects of treatment are tackled, for example, through exploration of barriers (challenging automatic thoughts about drugs; beliefs about bipolar disorder, excessive self-reliance; or exploring attitudes to authority and control) and using behavioural and cognitive techniques to enhance treatment adherence (Scott, 1999). This and data from previous sessions are used to help the patient identify their maladaptive assumptions and underlying core beliefs, and to commence work on modifying these beliefs. Further work is then undertaken on recognition of early signs of relapse and coping techniques (fortnightly sessions). For example, developing self-monitoring of symptoms, identifying possible prodromal features (the 'relapse signature'), developing a list of 'at risk situations' (for example, exposure to situations that activate specific personal beliefs), high-risk behaviours (for example, increased alcohol intake), combined with a hierarchy of coping strategies for each; identifying strategies for managing medication intake and obtaining advice regarding it; and planning how to cope and self-manage problems after discharge from cognitive therapy. Sessions also include typical cognitive therapy approaches to the modification of maladaptive beliefs that may otherwise increase vulnerability to relapse.

The use of cognitive therapy in bipolar disorders is a big challenge for therapists. The potential for rapid changes in mental state often means that the therapist and the individual with bipolar disorder cannot simply work on the conceptualisation in a systematic way. Individuals may arrive mildly hypomanic one week and significantly depressed a few weeks later. The therapist has to be able to cope with these changes and will often need to abandon the planned session in order to use crisis intervention techniques. Individuals with bipolar disorders are also more interpersonally demanding than many other individuals with severe mental disorder (Miklowitz & Goldstein, 1990) and in general it is more appropriate for expert therapists to work with this group.

Schizophrenia

Cognitive therapy for individuals with schizophrenia starts by helping the person come to terms with his or her current experiences. Discussing events that the patient finds perplexing is a useful way in which to begin to develop the therapeutic relationship (Morrison, 2002). As the individual with schizophrenia begins to trust the therapist, it is possible to start to jointly explore negative automatic thoughts and to develop hypotheses regarding idiosyncratic underlying beliefs. Identifying these beliefs may help to make sense of the specific content of delusions and hallucinations (Scott et al, 1993).

As in the cognitive therapy of other severe mental disorders, to make appropriate interventions to modify positive symptoms, the therapist must first undertake a collaborative assessment. For delusions, four dimensions are evaluated: conviction, accommodation (i.e. the degree to which the delusion can be modified), persuasiveness, and level of encapsulation (Kingdon & Turkington, 1994).

Research suggests that individuals who experience delusions 'jump to conclusions' when drawing inferences, underutilise disconfirming data, and tend to attribute negative events to external causes (Morrison, 2002). The classical cognitive characteristics of a delusion are that it is a culturally unacceptable explanation of an experience that attributes the cause of the experience outwith the individual (Morrison, 2002). Delusions should therefore be amenable to structured reasoning and behavioural approaches (Scott et al, 1993; Kingdon & Turkington, 1994). However, it is important that the therapist does not to proceed too rapidly with reality testing of

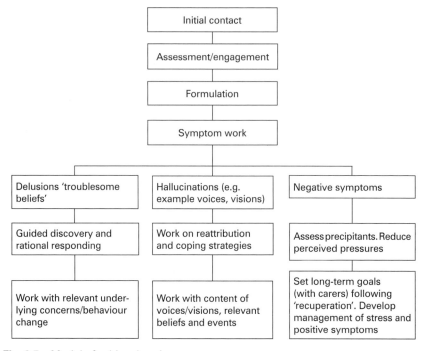

Fig. 8.5   Model of schizophrenia

these symptoms. It is usually better initially to deal with anxiety, panic, or depressive symptoms and then to move gradually toward interventions targeting positive symptoms (see Fig. 8.5). An example of working with delusions is given below.

Example

Mr H., a 43-year-old-man with a 10-year history of schizophrenia, believed a leading member of the Mafia was following him and that his life was in great danger. Initially, Mr H. and the therapist investigated the approximate time of onset of the delusions and why his past or present experiences may have led him to attach significance to a specific event. Mr H. had held this belief for about 8 years. A man with dark hair and brown eyes who Mr H. said, 'looked Italian' had attacked him in the street. The next day he had seen some graffiti on a garage wall in a local street stating 'Newcastle United Mafia rules OK'. Since that time, Mr H. was constantly on his guard. He also believed that a man in a raincoat followed him persistently.

The therapist gently used Socratic questioning to help identify inconsistencies in the data being presented by Mr H. Every piece of evidence identified as supporting his delusional belief was placed in rank order. First, the therapist asked Mr H. to describe the person he thought was following him in great detail. Next, the graffiti on the wall was recorded on the list. Additional evidence offered by Mr H. included 'being jostled on the bus when I travelled to town, people talking in the street, and car doors being slammed at night'. This supporting evidence was then examined in inverse order (starting with the least convincing data, 'car doors slamming') with a reality-testing approach.

Inconsistencies were initially explored through homework assignments, and alternative explanations were established that car doors were not being slammed on his street every night and that not everyone shutting car doors at night slammed them. Mr H. was also able to recognise that Newcastle United was the name of a local soccer team and that a group of the team's supporters had named themselves the 'local Mafia'. Mr H. was thus able to generate an alternative explanation for the graffiti he had observed. Lastly, Mr H. kept a detailed diary regarding his view that he was being followed. He compiled a detailed document that demonstrated that there was no evidence that a man in a raincoat who 'looked Italian' was following him. Mr H. noted that a number of people regularly travelled on the same buses but that none of them looked Italian nor fitted his original description. Mr H.'s conviction in this delusion was significantly reduced, but he occasionally became worried when it rained and lots of people wore raincoats. To try to maintain his improvement, Mr H. and the therapist developed a flash card for him (a credit card sized aide memoir that he could carry around) to refer to whenever he began to think that 'someone for the Mafia is following me'. This read as follows:

> When I think 'They're going to get me' I should 'Stop and think'
> Am I jumping to conclusions? Maybe it's not true
> I need to explore: What's the evidence?
> What are the alternatives?
> How sure am I?

The assessment of hallucinations in cognitive therapy is directed at the content, degree of variability, presence of antecedents or triggers, and any exacerbating or maintaining factors. All the techniques for exploring delusions can also be used to explore individuals' beliefs about their hallucinations. Guided discovery can be used to help the individual generate hypotheses regarding the origin of their hallucinations. Individuals who experience auditory hallucinations are believed to misattribute their own thoughts to external sources; as such techniques used to reduce distress related to other automatic thoughts (such as intrusive obsessions) can be applied here (Morrison, 1998). An example is given of this approach.

Example

Ms J., a 28-year old university graduate, was employed as a senior clerk with a national bank. Ms J. reported hearing voices telling her 'unless you follow our instructions, the economy will collapse'. The therapist and Ms J. first explored when she heard the voices. These usually occurred when she was alone in her apartment in the evenings, but there were some less-frequent occurrences in the staff restaurant at lunchtime. Socratic questioning was used to get Ms J. to evaluate possible reasons for the occurrence of the voices. Two hypotheses were generated: first that the voices were 'messages relayed by the government' and second, that the voices were 'symptoms of my illness and come from inside my head'. Ms J.'s belief that the voices were from the government was partly undermined by the fact that she was unable to explain to her own satisfaction how messages were relayed to her without others in the staff restaurant hearing them. Ms J. agreed to keep a diary about the voices. This revealed that the voices occurred more frequently when she was under stress (for example, at the end of the financial year). After evaluating the evidence for the alternatives, Ms J. began to believe that the most likely explanation of the voices was that they were internally generated symptoms of her illness.

The therapist then informed Ms J. that successful cognitive therapy interventions for hallucinations often involved the use of distraction techniques and stress management. Ms J. found that the most effective distractions from the hallucinations were reading aloud or engaging in mental activities such as doing crossword puzzles or solving mathematical puzzles. 'Personal stereo therapy' was also beneficial; Ms J. played music tapes of her choice whenever auditory hallucinations were particularly prominent. An additional strategy that proved helpful was for the client to record on an audiotape her rational responses to the comments made by the 'voices' and to play this tape during symptom exacerbation.

The anxiety associated with the auditory hallucinations was initially reduced with relaxation and breathing exercises. In addition, Ms J. decided to lower her use of caffeine. She found these approaches helpful, but still expressed anxiety when experiencing 'breakthrough' auditory hallucinations. Her fear that the national economy might suffer if she did not respond to the voices again became prominent. The therapist and client designed behavioural experiments to monitor what happened if Ms J. did not obey the voices. The therapist and Ms J. agreed that if stock prices did not fall by 10% and there was no news of a sudden downturn in the economy when Ms J. 'disobeyed orders' they would be able to conclude that she did not have to respond to the demands of the voices. Monitoring over a period of 3 months demonstrated that on only two occasions out of 15 did Ms J.'s refusal to comply with the demands of the voices coincide with the national press's reporting of new difficulties in the economy, and on no occasion did the share prices fall by 10%. On the basis of this evidence, Ms J. was able to conclude that she was not responsible for the nation's economic performance, and her emotional investment in the hallucinations was significantly reduced.

The pace of cognitive therapy in schizophrenia is usually dictated by the individual's ability to tolerate the process of guided discovery and the therapy may last considerably longer (for example, 9 months) than in non-psychotic disorders (Kingdon & Turkington, 1994). Unless the patient can place substantial trust in the therapist, any attempts at collaborative exploration of positive symptoms may be misconstrued as a challenge or confrontation. However, if therapist and patient have a good working relationship, it is usually possible to begin a gentle examination of these beliefs or to negotiate a withdrawal from the exploration of positive symptoms and to recommence this later, when this process is less threatening. It is also important to emphasise that cognitive therapy may also be used to treat negative symptoms.

Outcome research

There is considerable evidence that cognitive therapy has short-term benefits for individuals with severe mental disorder, and it also leads to sustained health gains over 12–48-month follow-up. The following references offer a selection of the key papers. There have been two large-scale randomised controlled trials of cognitive therapy in chronic depressive disorders (Keller *et al*, 2000; Paykel *et al*, 1999). In addition, DeRubeis *et al* (1999) and Thase *et al* (1997) offer important meta-analyses of the use of combined pharmacotherapy and cognitive therapy in severe and chronic depressions.

Outcome studies of cognitive therapy in bipolar disorders began with Cochran's (1984) small-scale randomised trial that used brief cognitive therapy to improve lithium adherence. Since then Perry *et al* (1999) have published a study using cognitive therapy to prevent relapse and Lam *et al* (2000) and Scott *et al* (2001) have published pilot studies of more formal courses of cognitive therapy on 25 and 42 subjects respectively. Large-scale studies in the UK and USA have been undertaken (for a review see Scott & Colom, 2005). In the last decade, a substantial number of randomised controlled trials have been published (for example Tarrier *et al*, 1993; Sensky *et al*, 2000) and Rector & Beck (2002) have published a meta-analysis.

Conclusions

The aims of treatment in severe mental disorder are to alleviate acute symptoms, restore psychosocial functioning, and prevent relapse and recurrence. The recognition that individual vulnerability, in association with internal or external stressors, plays a critical role in the onset, maintenance, and relapse or recurrence of severe mental disorder has increased the acceptance of combined pharmacotherapy and cognitive therapy approaches. This chapter illustrates that cognitive therapy may be an effective approach to the treatment of severe mental disorder, but there are gaps in our knowledge. More research on common underlying beliefs in individuals at risk of different types of severe mental disorder and on attitudes toward the disorder and views about its treatment could aid our understanding of adjustment difficulties. It will also be important to differentiate between specific and non-specific benefits of cognitive therapy and the mechanisms by which change is achieved. Ultimately, we will wish to know not only if the use of cognitive therapy is indicated for the patient with severe mental disorder but also whether, if indicated, it is effective because it enhances medication adherence, leads to the development of compensatory skills, or reduces vulnerability to relapse through change in core maladaptive beliefs. We will also wish to establish whether similar outcomes are obtained through the use of other evidence-based manualised approaches such as interpersonal psychotherapy and behavioural family therapy.

Outcome studies on the use of cognitive therapy in severe mental disorder are extremely encouraging. However, such research must not be accepted without question and should be viewed in the context of the realities of day-to-day clinical practice. Research has established that the skilfulness of a therapist may contribute 20–30% of the variance in client outcome and that level of expertise in cognitive therapy is particularly important when treating individuals with chronic and severe disorders (Roth & Fonagy, 1996; Scott, 2000). Furthermore, individuals treated by an expert cognitive therapist are less likely to drop out of therapy and significantly more likely to report symptomatic improvement than those treated by novice therapists (Burns & Nolen-Hoeksema, 1992).

The decision about whether to offer cognitive therapy to an individual with severe mental disorder will be influenced by the availability of an experienced therapist who is trained in the use of cognitive therapy in that particular disorder (Scott, 2000). The importance of the latter should not be underestimated. A pharmacotherapist would not consider a trial of medication to be adequate unless the appropriate drug had been given in an adequate dose for an adequate period of time. However, this should not mean that no psychotherapy is offered to those who may benefit from it. This chapter highlights that brief cognitive therapy may be utilised to modify personal coping styles or to modify cognitive representations of severe mental disorder. These interventions might be offered more widely, with a formal course of cognitive therapy being reserved for complex cases. This stepped-care approach to the delivery of cognitive therapy in severe mental disorder may offer a useful model of how to target scarce therapy resources according to need.

References

Adams, J. & Scott, J. (1999) Predicting medication non-adherence in severe mental disorders. *Acta Psychiatrica Scandinavica*, **101**, 119–124.

Basco, M. & Rush, A. J. (1995) *Cognitive Behaviour Therapy for Bipolar Disorders*. New York: Guilford Press.

Beck, A. T. (1976) *Cognitive Therapy and the Emotional Disorders*. Madison: International Universities Press.

Beck, A. T. (1983) Cognitive therapy for depression: new perspectives. In *Treatment of Depression: Old Controversies and New Approaches* (eds P. J. Clayton & J. E. Barrett). New York: Raven Press.

Beck, A. T. (1996) Beyond belief: a theory of modes, personality and psychopathology. In *Frontiers of Cognitive Therapy* (ed. P. Salkovskis), pp. 39–57. London: Guilford Press.

Beck, A. T., Rush, A. J., Shaw, B. F., *et al* (1979) *Cognitive Therapy of Depression*. New York: Guilford Press.

Bothwell, R. & Scott, J. (1997) The influence of cognitive variables on recovery in depressed inpatients. *Journal of Affective Disorders*, **43**, 207–212.

Burns, D. & Nolen-Hoeksema, S. (1992) Therapeutic empathy and recovery from depression in cognitive–behavioural therapy: a structural equation model. *Journal of Consulting and Clinical Psychology*, **60**, 441–449.

Cochran, S. (1984) Preventing medical non-adherence in the outpatient treatment of bipolar affective disorder. *Journal of Consulting and Clinical Psychology*, **52**, 873–878.

DeRubeis, R. J., Gelfand, L. A., Tang, T. Z., *et al* (1999) Medications versus cognitive behaviour therapy for severely depressed outpatients: mega-analysis of four randomised comparisons. *American Journal of Psychiatry*, **156**, 1007–1013.

Dickson, W. E. & Kendell, R. E. (1986) Does maintenance lithium therapy prevent recurrences of mania under ordinary clinical conditions? *Psychological Medicine*, **16**, 521–530.

Greenberger, D. & Padesky, C. (1996) *Mind Over Mood: A Cognitive Therapy Treatment Manual for Clients*. New York: Guilford Press.

Hammen, C., Ellicott, A., Gitlin, M., *et al* (1989) Sociotropy/ autonomy and vulnerability to specific life events in patients with unipolar depression and bipolar disorders. *Journal of Abnormal Psychology*, **98**, 154–160.

Hawton, K., Salkovskis, P., Kirk, J., *et al* (1989) *Cognitive Behaviour Therapy for Psychiatric Problems*. Oxford: Oxford University Press.

Horne, R. (1997) Representations of medication and treatment: Advances in theory and measurement. In *Perceptions of Health and Illness* (eds K. Petrie & J. Weinman), pp. 112–135. Harwood Academic Publishers.

Keller, M., McCullough, J., Klein, D., *et al* (2000) The acute treatment of chronic depression: A comparison of nefazadone, cognitive–behavioural analysis system of psychotherapy, and their combination. *New England Journal of Medicine*, **342**, 1462–1470.

Kingdon, D. & Turkington, D. (1994) *Cognitive Behavioural Therapy of Schizophrenia*. London: Guilford Press.

Krantz, S. & Moos, R. (1988) Risk factors at intake predict non-remission among depressed patients. *Journal of Consulting and Clinical Psychology*, **56**, 863–869.

Lam, D. H., Bright, J., Jones, S., *et al* (2000) Cognitive therapy for bipolar illness – a pilot study of relapse prevention. *Cognitive Therapy and Research*, **24**, 503–520.

Leventhal, H., Diefenbach, M. & Leventhal, E. (1992) Illness cognition: using common sense to understand treatment adherence and affect cognition interactions. *Cognitive Therapy and Research*, **16**, 143–163.

Miklowitz, D. & Goldstein, M. (1990) Behavioural family treatment for patients with bipolar affective disorder. *Behaviour Modification*, **14**, 457–489.

Morrison, T. (1998) Cognitive behaviour therapy for psychotic symptoms in schizophrenia. In *Treating Complex Cases* (eds N. Tarrier, A. Wells & G. Haddock), pp. 63–90. London: Wiley.

Morrison, T. (2002) *A Casebook of Cognitive Therapy in Psychosis*. London: Wiley.

Paykel, E. (1994) Epidemiology of refractory depression. In *Treatment Refractory Depression*. (eds W. Nolen, J. Zohar, S. Roose, *et al*), pp. 3–18. London: Wiley.

Paykel, E., Scott. J., Teasdale. J., *et al* (1999) Prevention of relapse in residual depression by cognitive therapy: a controlled trial. *Archives of General Psychiatry*, **56**, 829–835.

Perry, A., Tarrier, N., Morriss, R., *et al* (1999) Randomized controlled trial of efficacy of teaching patients with bipolar disorder to identify early symptoms of relapse and obtain treatment. *BMJ*, **318**, 149–153.

Prien, R. & Potter, W. (1990) NIMH workshop report on the treatment of bipolar disorders. *Psychopharmacology Bulletin*, **26**, 409–427.

Rector, N. A. & Beck, A. T. (2002) Cognitive therapy for schizophrenia: from conceptualization to intervention. *Canadian Journal of Psychiatry*, **47**, 39–48.

Roth, A. & Fonagy, P. (1996) *What Works for Whom? A Critical Review of Psychotherapy Research*. London: Guilford Press.

Scott, J. (1988) Chronic depression. *British Journal of Psychiatry*, **153**, 287–97.

Scott, J. (1995a) Psychotherapy for bipolar disorder: an unmet need? *British Journal of Psychiatry*, **167**: 581–588.

Scott, J. (1995b) Psychological treatments of depression: An update. *British Journal of Psychiatry*, **167**, 289–292.

Scott, J. (1999) Cognitive and behavioural approaches to medication adherence. *Advances in Psychiatric Treatment*, **5**, 338–347.

Scott, J. (2000) New evidence in the treatment of chronic depression. *New England Journal of Medicine*, **342**, 1518–1520.

Scott, J. (2001) *Overcoming Mood Swings: A Self-help Guide Using Cognitive and Behavioural Techniques*. New York: University Press, London: Constable Robinson.

Scott, J. & Colom, F. (2005) Psychosocial treatments for bipolar disorders. *Psychiatric Clinics of North America*, **28**, 371–384.

Scott, J., Byers, S. & Turkington, D. (1993) The chronic patient. In *Cognitive Therapy with Inpatients* (eds J. Wright, M. Thase, A. T. Beck, *et al*), pp. 179–198. New York: Guilford Press.

Scott, J., Cole, A. & Eccleston, D. (1991) Dealing with persisting abnormalities of mood. *International Review of Psychiatry*, **3**, 19–33.

Scott, J., Garland, A. & Moorhead, S. (2001) A pilot study of cognitive therapy in bipolar disorder. *Psychological Medicine*, **31**, 459–467.

Scott, J., Stanton, B., Garland, A., *et al* (2000) Cognitive vulnerability in bipolar disorders. *Psychological Medicine*, **30**, 467–472.

Scott, J. & Wright J. (1997) Cognitive therapy with severe and chronic mental disorders. In *Review of Psychiatry* Volume 16 (eds A. Frances & R. Hales), pp. 52–81. Washington: American Psychiatric Association Press.

Sensky, T., Turkington, D., Kingdon, D., *et al* (2000). A randomised controlled trial of cognitive behavioural therapy for persistent symptoms in schizophrenia resistant to medication. *Archives of General Psychiatry*, **57**, 165–172.

Skelton, P. & Croyle, D. (1991) *Mental Representation in Health and Illness*. New York: Springer Verlag.

Tarrier, N., Beckett, R., Harwood, S., *et al* (1993). A trial of two cognitive behavioural methods of treating drug resistant residual psychotic symptoms in schizophrenic patients: I: Outcome. *British Journal of Psychiatry*, **162**, 524–532.

Teasdale, J. (1988) Cognitive vulnerability to persistent depression. *Cognition and Emotion*, **2**, 247–274.

Thase, M. E., Greenhouse, J. B., Frank, E., *et al* (1997) Treatment of major depression with psychotherapy or psychotherapy–pharmacotherapy combinations. *Archives of General Psychiatry*, **54**, 1009–15.

CHAPTER 9

Group psychotherapy*

John Hook

The focus of this chapter is on work in small out-patient therapy groups using the group-analytic model, which is currently the most influential group model in the UK. Reference will be made also to other theoretical models applicable to larger groups or different settings. The work of Bion will be used to illustrate 'group-as-a-whole' phenomena. The aim is to structure the material in an experiential manner so that the reader who has participated in such a group (as member or conductor) will recognise it.

Historical background

Why therapy in groups? Ettin (1992) relates the legend of a friend of Socrates who asked the Oracle at Delphi if any man alive was wiser than Socrates. 'No one' was the reply. On being told this, Socrates tested people in argument to see if it were so, becoming disappointed to find no one was wiser than he. He had missed the point. Oracles should never be taken at face value: there was no one (i.e. single) person wiser than Socrates, but the collective wisdom of more than one, a group, could be.

Pratt (1922), an American chest physician, assembled a group of patients with tuberculosis in order to educate them about the illness. He noticed that it was not his expert input that proved therapeutic, but the 'fine spirit of camaraderie' between the group members that engendered hope. His contribution became relegated to an educational talk lasting only a few minutes. Although he had set out to see people in a group primarily to save time, he had the sagacity to recognise and duly publish his finding that relationships within the group itself provide a unique setting for therapy. Such knowledge continues to be rediscovered with the advent of the user movement and self-help groups.

Foulkes (1948) founded group-analysis on the premise that knowledge held by the whole group can benefit each individual member. Like Freud and Moreno (the founder of psychodrama) he was a Jewish exile from Vienna.

---

*A shorter version of this chapter appeared in Hook (2002), reproduced here by permission.

Personal experience led these men to question both the dark side of human nature, in individuals or groups, and the potential sources of healing. Foulkes described the group as being 'collectively the very norm from which individually they deviate'. Within the group the individual can test himself against the social standard which is held by the group-as-a-whole. In this context 'standard' refers to the highly complex system of values that governs human relations across the spectrum of intimate, social and organisational spheres of life. It is not that the group always knows best but that the 'common sense' of the group holds up a mirror to each member so he is seen as he is by others and therefore knows himself more truly.

Such processes occur naturally, not just in the somewhat artificial overt context of therapy groups. We learn who we are from how we are seen in groups within the family, school, work and social settings. These potentially conflicting views are matched against our growing personal sense of self, modifying and changing it throughout life. If the crucial early experience is not one of reciprocal nurturing, but is based on abuse, neglect or negative feedback, then we may develop mental illnesses, personality disorders or rigid character structures. Losing flexibility of interaction and the capacity to learn from experience, we respond in predetermined ways beyond our conscious control. The past gets repeated even when we desperately want to leave it behind.

The therapeutic leap which Foulkes made from the starting point of individual psychoanalysis was that if it is in groups that such psychopathology is formed, then it is in groups that the process can be reversed. Many people on being offered group therapy after assessment instinctively know this to be so. Yet it is a daunting thought to subject oneself to the scrutiny of the group process. To be at the receiving end of a group's disapproval is a painful and disturbing experience, however constructive ultimately. A group can become a frightening place. Powerful forces are activated which can be harnessed for good or ill. A group may quickly become a gang bent on violence, just as a crowd may turn into a rampaging mob sweeping all before it. In such instances the individual becomes submerged, impotent, his very survival at risk. It is perhaps not surprising that at first glance most individuals would prefer the private, intimate relationship with an individual therapist, who allegedly keeps his own affairs and agenda out of the room, concentrating solely on interpreting and analysing the productions of the individual/client. The fantasy of getting an ideal mother/father at last satisfies many narcissistic needs.

Formal therapeutic groups have been in existence for nearly 90 years, yet group therapy has not acquired the same status as individual therapy. This is changing. There is growing awareness of the potential for abuse in individual work, and the potential for fostering regression and dependency. The value of the genuine and spontaneous feedback that occurs in groups is being recognised. As service users fight to reduce the imbalance in power between psychiatrist and patient-group work becomes increasingly popular. The time is ripe for group work to be valued alongside individual therapy.

Classification of therapeutic groups

By size

A small group of 6 to 12 participants is the main therapeutic modality and will be discussed at length.

A median group of 25 to 30 members is often used on in-patient wards. This may be for administrative purposes or function directly as a therapy group. Unfortunately there is often little idea about what the aims are, and the groups are run because they are thought to be 'a good idea'. Given the range of severe disturbance coupled with often minimal staff training and experience, this can lead to reluctant and resentful participation. Patients are then deprived of the potential opportunity to create an environment of hope and optimism through the integrating function of the group.

A large group is the central feature of therapeutic communities where the 'milieu' is the driving force of therapy. A therapeutic community programme consists of a range of individual work, small and large groups, and other practical activities. The whole community and each individual within it take responsibility for the functioning of the community. The large group meetings serve as a focus for this, bringing together material from the different components of community life for observation and analysis. The authority of the whole community can be brought to bear on a problem, while providing a high level of containment and support for individuals, even if they need to be constructively challenged about behaviour.

By theoretical model

'Talking' groups

- group-analytic
- psychodynamic/object relations
- interpersonal
- gestalt.

Action groups

- psychodrama
- drama therapy
- art therapy
- music therapy
- dance therapy.

Learning groups

- cognitive–behavioural
- educational.

The group-analytic, small, out-patient group

Selection refers to choosing members who are assessed as suitable for psychotherapy in general and group therapy in particular (see also

Chapter 1). Composition refers to the rather more mysterious task of choosing people who will work well together in a group.

Selection

Many people will benefit from a variety of approaches. Group therapy is concerned with human relationships, difficulties with which lie behind many psychological problems. It might therefore be appropriate when carrying out a psychotherapy assessment to frame the question 'Why should this person not be offered a group?' To enable this to be a genuine option will require the ready availability of a group programme consisting of groups with different aims. If this is available, therapy can be provided for the majority of people referred for psychological treatment.

For optimum benefit patients must be able to view their psychopathology in a way that transcends diagnostic categories of mental illness (although such categorisation may be of use in defining exclusion criteria). While the presenting complaint is often couched in symptomatic terms, behind this usually lie relationship problems in intimate, social and work spheres. People either cannot form or sustain satisfying relationships, or they get stuck in unhealthy modes of relating, leading to a sense of failure and disappointment. They may feel lonely and isolated, put upon and criticised, with no self-esteem. Many have emotional and psychological problems, which leave them deeply scarred and disabled, often behind a deceptively normal façade.

Since such criteria apply in varying degrees to a large number of people, it is sometimes easier to describe exclusion criteria, not in the sense of 'rejecting' candidates, but minimising the risk that they will gain little from group therapy. This idea was introduced in Chapter 1, and will be elaborated here.

Exclusion criteria

People in acute crisis

Such people require a lot of individual attention. They are too preoccupied to make the necessary relationships within the group, and so have not earned their right to be heard. Once the crisis has subsided, it may however be relevant to offer group therapy to explore the antecedent factors, any repetitive features, and the traditional coping style which may have been inadequate in this instance.

People with poor impulse control

Those who misuse alcohol and drugs, or persistently harm themselves by overdose or self-cutting, or by gross eating disorders, deal with disturbing feelings by actions. Such behaviour may be too disruptive for a group focusing on refection and understanding. One of the cardinal characteristics of successful psychotherapy is the capacity to tolerate painful feelings long enough to talk them through without acting on them, and so understand the meaning of the experience.

As often, there is a 'yes but' addendum to such an exclusion clause. It is possible to treat such problems in homogeneous groups (people with the same difficulty or diagnosis) in special settings.

- alcohol and drug dependency within specialist units
- specialist groups for sexual deviance or perversions (e.g. the Portman Clinic)
- specialist groups for eating disorders.

The rationale for homogeneous groups is that maladaptive behavioural patterns and defences are not accessible to ordinary interaction but are able to be challenged by those who know best – people with the same *modus vivendi*.

People who have difficulty for largely organic reasons in forming reciprocal close relationships

- severe enduring mental illness (chronic psychosis)
- significant brain damage
- moderate to profound learning disability.

People with more severe personality disorders

- narcissistic personality disorder
- borderline personality disorder
- schizoid personality disorder.

Such people present special problems of management because of their faulty capacity for reality testing, which may verge on delusional. Generally a group can tolerate one member with this level of disturbance, as long as the therapist ensures that he does not become scapegoated. Such an individual may indeed become a useful facilitator to the group process, being particularly sensitive to more primitive levels of group functioning. For those whose disturbance leads to serious abuse or criminal behaviour then a specialist homogeneous group will be more appropriate, for example those in maximum security hospitals, in-patient psychotherapy units such as the Henderson Hospital or day services for personality disorders.

People who seek individual therapy only

A person who has experienced his family and other groups as alienating and frightening will have difficulty accepting that a group full of strangers, also with difficulties, can be a source of healing. Many people do need to have some individual therapy where they are the centre of attention, however brief, before they can cope with the public gaze of a group. This is balanced, of course, by those whose experience of individual authority figures is such that in no way will they trust their psyche to one psychiatrist/therapist in private, but who actively seek out peer support and solidarity within the group domain. The basic issue is that choice is important, and should be fuelled by adequate, non-biased information at the assessment stage.

Composition

How to compose a group that will gel together is scarcely a scientific endeavour and is often unduly influenced by who is seeking therapy at any one point in time. There are guiding principles (which will be described) but it is ultimately impossible to predict accurately how 8 or 9 people will turn into an effective work group. The guidelines are relatively basic and common sense. With a little thought one should be able to avoid a group consisting entirely of shy, retiring, unself-confident depressed people. Equally problematic would be a group only containing highly verbal histrionic characters.

Nowhere is it more true that variety is the spice of life than in a newly formed 'stranger' group. The aim is to select people heterogeneous along demographic variables such as age, gender, social class, marital status, having children or not, presenting complaint or (most importantly) style of interaction. It is essential to have some members who can get the group going, while the more reticent find their feet to contribute their reflective contribution.

If variety is one basic rule of thumb, the other is the constraining factor that no one should feel an outcast. Each person should have at least one other with whom there is a degree of identification. Nobody should be included who may be singled out for scapegoating, or be inclined to drop out, because of some outstanding feature that alienates them, such as being a perpetrator of a sexual crime. Such people will be better treated in a homogeneous group of peers. Less emotively the same principle applies to a lesser extent to the person widely divergent from the others in terms of age, gender or ethnic origin.

The role of the group conductor in group analysis

The aim of the conductor is to create a tolerable place where the individuals in the group can learn to be themselves in safety. People share details of intimate lives suffused with anxiety, conflict, guilt and shame in the hope of discovering new, more satisfying, ways of being with themselves and with others.

This kind of leadership differs from that in more educational or cognitive–behavioural groups, where the group leader is an expert delivering a relatively prescribed package. That style would be more didactic and active, with the therapist being the authority. Foulkes (1975: p. 3) described group analysis as 'therapy by the group, of the group, including the conductor'. The therapist is not the sole healer. In fact there is constant tension between his central role in organising the therapeutic process yet often being peripheral to its delivery. Therapy cannot proceed without him, yet the group mainly does the work. The therapist nevertheless continues to be viewed as the expert authority because of transference relationships involving parental and early authority relationships.

Foulkes' favoured term to describe the therapist or leader was 'conductor', which he likened to conducting an orchestra with the metaphors of modulating tempo, paying attention to individual instruments, sections and the whole orchestra, to harmonise the separate contributions.

The conductor has two interrelated tasks:

- dynamic administration (the group maintenance function)
- therapeutic activity (the task function).

Dynamic administration

The conductor has a responsibility to create and maintain the group. This involves establishing a boundary within which the therapeutic process can evolve unhindered within the psychological space which has been created.

Before the group begins it involves decisions about:

- what type of group: open (allowing entry of new members, especially when others leave) or closed (membership fixed from the start)
- duration: limited to a fixed time/number of sessions, or without a time limit. The latter situation is chosen more often for an open group
- time, place and frequency
- physical setting: size of room, type of chairs, waiting room arrangements, reception facilities etc.

Once the group begins there is continuing responsibility to provide a systematic approach to maintaining the boundary. This involves:

- no interruptions from outside
- time-keeping: punctuality in beginning and ending the group
- regularity of attendance: follow-up of those who do not attend, careful advance notification of annual leave breaks etc
- confidentiality: explicit rules about not discussing material from the group elsewhere.

Such activity is of paramount importance. First because the physical boundary becomes a metaphor for the psychological boundary. Freud said that for the individual 'the ego is first of all a body-ego'. For the group, the boundaries and rules constitute an equivalent of a psychic skin. Second, because much crucial therapeutic activity occurs around the group boundary, with patients often re-enacting conflicts about boundary issues elsewhere (boundaries about age, gender, family relationship, work role, authority etc). Third, because negotiating boundaries is a universal task in human relationships, how the conductor himself manages such issues can serve as a model for group members to learn from. Three examples follow to illustrate this.

Example 1

One evening my co-conductor and I arrived to find the group assembled in the corridor and the door locked. We had no key and were forced to find the security officer, who, among his vast array of keys, did not have the one we needed. I wanted to break the lock as the room contained nothing of value and no other room was obviously available. The security officer demurred. We eventually found an alternative venue and started half-an-hour late. The group sat for the next hour in furious silence refusing all attempts to engage them in discussion about what had happened. Clearly we were regarded as useless, beneath contempt and not to be trusted.

On a later occasion, we arrived to find the hospital management team encamped having been given a mistaken booking. This time I was successful in negotiating their departure. Whatever admiration the group may have felt for my intervention went unremarked.

The conductor therefore looks both inwards and outwards, providing a safe environment wherein the group can focus on the internal space. When the boundary is ruptured as in this example the group defends itself against the threat to its integrity. This group had an intensely dependent culture, hence the ferocity of its response of unspoken hatred at failure, and its taken-for-granted response to success.

The group is both intimate and private (yet paradoxically social) as opposed to public. There needs to be a flow of information across the boundary between the group and the outside world. The members need to talk about what is happening to them outside, as well as take back what they have learned in the group. This flow of material needs to be carefully monitored. An important explicit rule for a small analytic group is that members should not meet outside the group. People meeting regularly outside form a sub-group, which comes to have a secret agenda. Confidentiality is lost as group business is discussed without all participants being present. These formations are almost invariably defensive with members using the sub-group to avoid sharing something of import with the whole group. This denigrates the principles of openness and honesty which are the ground-rules of any group.

Example 2

A year into group, Jane revealed that she and Paula met each week after the group for a drink. It seemed that Paula's avowed intent in joining the group was to ensure that it would fail as far as she was concerned. Over a period of weeks Jane felt pressured by Paula to meet her separately. Paula told her information known to the conductors but not group members, and made it clear that she valued their discussions, which gave her a sense for once of being special. Jane however became increasingly uncomfortable as Paula avoided speaking about these issues in the group and the group in turn became incensed. The members and conductors failed to persuade them to stop meeting for some time.

When they did finally stop, Paula was able to tell the group her secret: she had a son by her estranged boyfriend but wanted nothing to do with the boyfriend. Her boyfriend was furious with her. Paula's venomous anger about the situation, which had echoed her ambivalence about her own mother, had been re-enacted in her treatment of the group. She split the group, choosing Jane as her ally and projecting the bad feelings into the rest of the group. This situation dominated the group for several weeks, although it was eventually worked through. In later groups Paula received considerable help, especially from Den who had himself been abandoned by a girlfriend in similar circumstances.

That example of extra-group activity caused considerable disruption, exemplifying the need for such rules. The conductor however has always to explore the underlying meaning and impact of such behaviour. No rule is hard and fast as is shown in the next example.

Example 3

A group was run for university students. Several of the members were characterised by marked social isolation, lack of support and serious suicide attempts. In such a small community it would have been impossible to avoid people bumping into one another outside the group. In addition some started meeting regularly after the group for coffee then visiting each other during the week. I reminded them of the rule and its rationale. There followed a healthy discussion where I realised the important social and supportive function the extra-group meetings were having. The group members also realised the importance of not having secrets from each other. Thereafter they reported the meetings to the group, especially when concerned that someone was feeling suicidal. The integrity of the group was maintained and its function in containing impulsive self-harm behaviour was enhanced through their taking shared responsibility.

Therapeutic activity

This has three components: leadership, analysis and interpretation.

Leadership

The conductor has to pay attention to two levels of activity simultaneously. There is manifest activity – what is actually being said and done by whom. There is also unconscious activity, giving meaning and significance to this activity for each individual and for the 'group-as-a-whole'. In non-analytic groups the leadership of the conductor is revealed in manifest behaviour such as setting the agenda, proposing tasks and goals, offering advice and fostering cooperation. The group-analyst does none of these things. His overt leadership in this way is simply to provide the setting as described under dynamic administration. This leads to a sense of frustration because it is expected that the 'expert' tells people what to do.

The group members unconsciously tend to endow the conductor with omnipotent, omniscient, magical qualities of leadership. His attitude to this is neither to foster it nor deny it. To encourage such a belief would actually be anti-analytic. Such a leader would require obedience, loyalty and dependency, which are qualities diametrically opposed to the empowering goals of analysis, where each individual learns to take responsibility for his actions and the impact they have on others. Instead the conductor allows the group to explore such projections and fantasies bit by bit in order to demythologise the power of the leader and allow the group to develop its own authority. Individuals then learn to derive the authority invested in the group for themselves.

This does not mean that the conductor abdicates all control. There are times when he has to exercise power and authority for the well-being of the group. This occurs at the manifest level, for example deciding that somebody should leave the group if they consistently defy the ground-rules, and at the unconscious level, for example challenging the group by interpreting a group resistance. The conductor must be strong enough to withstand the aggressive attacks of the group on himself and others in such situations.

His general attitude is to place the group-as-a-whole at the centre of his attention. By such free-floating attention to the latent content his counter-transference experience will be to the group rather than to individuals. An analytic attitude is fostered by the conductor bringing the unconscious to the attention of the group in his interventions. Of course a message is also given indirectly by what he chooses to comment on and what he ignores.

Analysis

People bring symptoms and problems to talk about in the group. This in itself is not sufficient for change although it can be therapeutic for those who have had little previous opportunity for open communication. For change to occur the problem must be felt in the group. This is exactly what happens as people begin to trust each other and work together. A dynamic 'matrix' is formed into which each person is drawn. 'Analysis' is the totality of work directed at making such unconscious processes conscious. Once the unconscious is understood and its effects evaluated, then there is the opportunity to choose healthier options. Foulkes understood this in terms of communication. The symptom is a closed communication with a predictable outcome. It serves to decrease anxiety or avoid something painful. Thus analysis is disturbing because it opens communication, making what happens next unpredictable. The analyst has to judge how much anxiety any individual and the group can tolerate at a point in time.

The tools of analysis are communication tools such as questioning, clarifying, pointing out and underlining. By watching how the therapist intervenes in this way and learning the impact on themselves and others, members of the group come to value this activity.

Interpretation

Linking current life experience with the past, including the here-and-now development of the relationship with the therapist, is valued in individual analysis as an instrument of insight and change. In the group context such interpretations are not solely the province of the conductor. They are arrived at spontaneously within the group. Each member can be the subject of another's projections as well as the observer of what takes place between group members and between one member and the group-as-a-whole. Each is therefore in the position to make interpretations. Pseudo-intellectual or defensive interpretations will quickly be spotted by fellow group members, but the experience of making an observation that lends emotional insight to a fellow member can be therapeutic on both sides. An interpretation can be about an individual or about the process going on in the group-as-a-whole. In practice the group members tend to make interpretations about each other, while the group-analyst comments on the process.

One of the most difficult aspects of such analytic work is deciding when and at which level to interpret, or whether to offer an interpretation spanning both the individual and the group. Theories which focus on group-as-a-whole phenomena such as focal conflict theory (Whitaker & Lieberman, 1964) or social systems theory (Skolnick, 1992) emphasise the need to interpret the group dynamic when the group is stuck. Otherwise the Foulkesian aphorism 'to let the group get on with it' holds true.

Example 4

The following excerpt took place in the last group before a summer break. The group, led by Jemma, were complaining about the long holidays taken by the therapists. Sam said he was not too worried because with the renewed communication with his mother he could always phone her if he felt bad. Jemma, whose own mother had died when she was 4 years old and whose father had been unable to support her emotionally from then on, attacked Sam for his dependency on his mother. I intervened on his behalf. He had only recently joined the group. I pointed out this was a good experience for him to be able to turn to his mother. Jemma then turned her attack fully on me, which was where her anger in the transference to me as father rightly belonged. In the ensuing heated debate about the needs of therapists to have a break despite the abandonment felt by the group members, Jim turned to Jemma and interpreted directly the absence of her mother throughout most of her life as behind her attack on Sam and me. I underlined this.

This example shows the therapeutic nature of the group in action at several different levels at once. The group had spent previous sessions strongly challenging two women members who had announced future absences. The atmosphere was charged with the feelings of imminent abandonment. The relationship of each member to the group-as-a-whole was to a persecuting mother. Jemma, whose personal experience had the best 'fit' expressed the anger felt by all. She identified particularly with Sam's need for his mother at a time of acute crisis for him and enviously attacked his good experience. The conductor chose to defend Sam because although his comments were judged to be in part defensive (later borne out by his returning to the group after the holiday a week early) his need at that moment was for an empathic response. This allowed the conductor to offer him the experience of parental concern, largely absent from his childhood, which could begin to stand against the previous abuse and neglect. The defensive aspect could be safely left until later.

This left the stage clear for Jemma to vent her hatred of the conductor as the father who never protected her from the loss of her mother. Jim, on behalf of the present live mother-group, offered her an analytic explanation of the infantile roots of her conflict. Either conductor could have interpreted this but often such an interpretation is more powerful when made by a member of the group. Furthermore, it gave Jim the experience of being potent in relation with a woman, something which he had failed singularly to be. Jemma however, hardened by years of keeping everybody at a safe distance through use of an aggressive, challenging interpersonal style, behind which lay a profound sense of emptiness and depression, could barely acknowledge this olive branch. At least she did not dismiss it and it clearly impacted on her as evidenced by subsequent events.

This exemplifies the complexity of interaction, all of which took place in a matter of minutes. Each member could be seen to be relating to one another through the process of projective identification, to the conductors as transference objects of particular (parental) significance and to the group--as-a-whole as a unitary object. It is this network which Foulkes named the dynamic matrix (see later).

In this example the traditional analytic interpretation forms one element of the therapeutic work. While it is an important element it is not the central therapeutic tool as it is in individual analytic psychotherapy. The context in the group process for all therapeutic activity is the here-and-now drama. This enactment of itself provides sufficient thrust so that a full analytic explanation of the infantile roots of a problem linked to the transference outworking is not always necessary.

Therapist transparency

An important question often asked is: 'how personally transparent should the conductor be?' In all analytically-derived therapies the emergence of the transference relationship in all its complexity is central to the task. The therapist must maintain a professional attitude that allows the patient to project freely onto him/her. The exposure of personal detail inevitably fills in the space available for this. Of course it can never be true that our patients know nothing about us, in fact such a pure culture would deprive the relationship of its necessary humanity. It is also true that we reveal a great deal, both consciously and unconsciously, about ourselves and our values. This can usefully encourage identification and modelling.

The pressure in a group to reveal oneself is often intense. The degree of exposure that any conductor allows will be a function of his capacity to contain his anxiety in this respect. The conductor must be guided by the overriding principle of what at any given moment is best for the group. Personal detail is almost always unhelpful but occasionally inevitable. What can be useful is sharing his experience in and of the group with the group.

Example 5
The scene is the same as in Example 4; the group after the summer holiday. There was a lively start with expression by Sam, Babs and Julie of different feelings related to the break. Sam was aware to a degree of the significance of his

turning up a week early but the other two told their stories oblivious to the link. I waited to see how the group would respond. Quite suddenly the atmosphere went flat and although the ensuing hour contained important communications there was no liveliness to the interaction. The style of communication was a familiar one for this group. Every time I was about to say something somebody else chimed in. The session was nearly at an end when I cut across the group and made a somewhat incoherent interpretation.

The next group was altogether different. Charles produced a dream which clearly related to what I felt had been my too-little-too-late intervention. In one scene Charles described a castle wall. He was peering round one side while I was peering round the other. I interpreted this as a dream for the whole group. The wall was the dividing line between conscious and unconscious.

I had been making a series of interpretations at the group-as-a-whole level in order to give the greater depth to the interactions, for which I judged the group ready. In relation to the previous week's material I went on to describe the group's dependency, their feeling of abandonment during the break and consequent anger; this was partially received. Later I enlarged on the theme to which Sam, a little irritatedly, wondered if it was not my need to be missed I was talking about. I had to reflect on this and acknowledge my lifelong wish to be needed. Although I considered saying this to the group I thought that Sam's question was a defence against his and the group's conflict and that to admit my need would most probably have been received as an admission of weakness rather than maturity. I turned instead to answering a previous question of Babs who wanted to know what it was that I could apparently see going on that they could not.

This last example further exemplifies the need for the conductor to interpret the group-as-a-whole level when the group becomes overwhelmed by anxiety and can no longer function effectively.

The healing process and underlying theoretical concepts

How does healing occur? This issue may be addressed by considering what happens when a symptom is produced. Individual analytic therapies are initially interested in how and why the symptom is produced. The group, in contrast, asks 'what is the result of producing a symptom?' It is not that a group is uninterested in analytic questions but it responds from the perspective of here-and-now relating in the group.

When an individual produces a neurotic symptom he produces a barrier to direct communication of emotions. His perception of self and other is distorted. He communicates in order to defend himself from further pain, which he believes the other will inflict upon him. Two particular emotions often contribute to this sense of isolation; shame and guilt. These emotions, experienced consciously and unconsciously, lead to the assumption that if the desired other were to know his dark secret he might again (because this has happened before) face rejection with all its attendant pain. The defence is thus reinforced.

The symptom is itself an attempt at communicating the nature of the problem but in a manner that hides as much as it reveals. What happens to the symptom in a group? Initially it is presented as 'the problem'. The group responds with each member identifying with different aspects of 'the problem'. This is one of Yalom's (1995) therapeutic factors; universality. The crucial process at this point is that the individual with 'the problem' feels less isolated. Until this moment he may have expressed his experience in such terms as: 'Nobody has ever been through what I have been through ... Nobody could ever understand.' This view cannot easily be maintained in the face of direct refutation by the other group members who may now feel more like allies than to be feared. Guilt and shame may thus be partially relieved by the recognition of the universality of the human condition, a recognition of what unites rather than what divides.

The individual who cannot enter into this process is likely to drop out. This may take the form of a protest that nothing in the group feels relevant. Precise examples of how others' comments were felt to be insufferable may be given. The group conductor finds himself thinking that this is, of course, just the point. The individual, instead of identifying with the shared experience projects his share of the problem onto the others and hence perceives it to be nothing to do with him.

Identification is only one aspect of the process. The problem has to be translated from a symptom to be talked about to distortions in relatedness to be felt in the group. Thus the unconscious dynamics driving the symptom come to be experienced in the group.

Group processes can be understood using object relations theory (see Chapter 3). By means of projective identification (Hinshelwood, 1989), in addition to the actual communication that all can observe, the individual repeats his past. Different members, including the conductor, come to take on the roles of the (internal) others. Since each is chosen for a particular role according to their characteristics the others will behave both according to the projection and yet differently from it. It is the difference that is vital.

Eventually the recipient of the projection will complain that he does not recognise the portrayal that is being painted through the projective process as himself. Thus he challenges the author of the projection to examine the distortion, own it as an aspect of his own character and modify his self-image accordingly. The group supports both participants in this dialogue but at the same time often intensifies the conflict. The end result is often to achieve change in both. Other members will also have an investment in the dynamic that draws them into the flame of the interaction whereby they too can profit. Those who remain silent are none the less participating and can learn through observation.

Foulkes (1964) described these interlocking processes as mirror, chain and condenser phenomena. Mirroring refers to the projective process; we all know from experience that it is easier to see in the other what one cannot see in oneself. Any single event in a group invites all members to share their associations forming a chain reaction. This has the effect of loosening resistance in the individual and group that in turn leads to an upsurge of repressed material; condenser phenomenon.

Example 6

(The same group as Examples 4 and 5. The fourth group after the break.) When we entered the room the whole group was, unusually, already assembled. The two remaining chairs were next to each other. This is also unusual as groups spend most of their time unconsciously trying to split the co-conductor pair. We were therefore put on our guard wondering about the meaning of this formation. We both, unknown to one another had the same fantasy of being king and queen on our thrones. Sam talked about the anger he had experienced the previous week towards his mother. Attention then shifted to Sol who had not attended for 2 weeks and had left the previous group angrily complaining that the group consistently ignored him. Suddenly Julie exploded angrily that she constantly had to look after everybody else. She left unsaid the obvious implication that nobody looked after her, which was Sol's complaint. Jemma, in obvious distress, talked of feeling depressed and suicidal and complained that the group was no use to her. She added that she had stopped her antidepressant medication during the break without consultation. It was now obvious to us that the reason the group had placed us together was to have a united parental couple who could contain the intense pain and anger no longer repressed. This enabled the group to work effectively with Jemma.

The matrix

The concept of the matrix is fundamental to the group-analytic model. It is the network of interaction which is described above and constantly evolves throughout the life of the group with each member as a nodal point. Foulkes (1964) described four levels:

- current reality
- transference (which connects each member's experience of the family group to the here-and-now of the group experience)
- part-object relations (at which level relatedness is governed by splitting and projection)
- transpersonal; equivalent to Jung's collective unconscious.

Foulkes drew a distinction between the foundation matrix and the dynamic matrix. The foundation matrix describes what each member brings with him to the group. This will include current and remembered past life experiences as well as unconscious material which has been repressed and that which is our human heritage, social and cultural. The dynamic matrix is the sum of all the interactions at every level, which is the life of the group. The preceding vignettes give a sense of the organisational complexity. They also make clear the impossibility of the conductor being able to track each level of development and predict the impact of any given intervention.

Phases in group development

In order to understand what is happening at any given moment an appreciation of the different phases of group development is necessary. This can be described from the perspective of any of the different theoretical models available.

Lacoursiere (1980) has described a useful overview. He postulates five stages:

1. Orientation; the group has to learn how to be a group. It is full of expectancy of magical change, dependent on the conductor and yet suffused with anxiety at the threat of loss of individuality. Nobody knows what to do. The purpose of their being there is expressed as wanting to be rid of unwanted symptoms. Drop-outs are common as individuals feel the group to be irrelevant to their problems.

2. Dissatisfaction; the idealisation of the leader crumbles in the face of his apparent inability to cure them. The group coheres around its frustration and disillusion. Aggression runs high and members jockey for position. On the surface it appears to be unproductive. Yet the scene is being set as past frustrations come to light. Drop-out is still common as the group is felt to be just a repeat of past bad experience.

3. Resolution; the group comes to a more realistic appraisal of the nature of the problem and of itself as a therapeutic vehicle. Their view of the leader as leader is less subject to splitting. He becomes more available for transference attributions. The general atmosphere is relatively benign and cooperative.

4. Production; the work group predominates. There is a strong feeling of everybody pulling together with common purpose. Accomplishments are acknowledged with a rise in self-esteem. Communication is open and challenging. Emotional expression is common.

5. Termination; the group becomes more conflicted as what has been achieved is measured against what has not been possible. Past losses resurface painfully. For some this is worked through to a satisfactory conclusion. For others defences are re-erected against the loss. Premature terminations occur.

These phases are not clear-cut and groups oscillate between them or may regress to earlier phases at times of crisis. They are more visible in training and dynamic therapy groups and in closed groups; less so in groups which are task-orientated.

The work of Bion

(See also Chapter 3.) The Second World War and in particular army psychiatry provided the impetus for major developments in group therapy. The army were faced with large numbers of psychological casualties requiring rehabilitation. Traditional medical model methods had proved ineffective. The Northfield Army Hospital became the unlikely setting for major developments in group therapy. Bion initiated what has come to be known as the first Northfield experiment. Although successful, his method, which was to allow the soldiers themselves to come to recognise the nature of the problem and then take responsibility for solving it, was too at variance with the army model of a strict hierarchy of discipline and he was transferred. None the less this brief experiment laid the foundations for his later work at the Tavistock Clinic. He was followed at Northfield by Foulkes and Main among others. They initiated the second Northfield experiment, which was more acceptable to the authorities. Out of this experience grew group-analysis (Foulkes) and the therapeutic community model pioneered by Main at the Cassel Hospital.

Bion (1961) went on to the Tavistock Clinic where he conducted small groups designed to explore how groups functioned. His observations focused on the functioning of the group-as-a-whole. In particular he drew attention to the dynamic between the group-as-a-whole and the conductor. He described and named two qualitatively different states of group mentality:

- work group
- basic assumption group.

The work group exists when a group is actively engaged in the task at hand, whatever that may be. The basic assumption group, alternatively, is beset by persecutory anxiety and is engaged in spurious forms of activity as a defence. This proceeds unconsciously and can be ascribed to Foulkes' projective level of the matrix. It is an ever-present phenomenon.

Bion enumerated three forms that basic assumption mentality could take:

- fight/flight
- dependency
- pairing.

He postulated that any one could be activated at any given time but, dependent upon the prevailing conditions, could be replaced by either of the other two. Each member has a valency which determines his propensity to join each of the three types. In basic assumption group fight/flight the group reacts to perceived threat either from inside or out by uniting behind a 'leader', not necessarily the conductor, who will focus attention critically on some outside agency or, as often occurs in the therapy group, choose a group member to 'treat'. In basic assumption group dependency the group shares a magical expectation that somebody will meet all their needs. This often prevails in the early stages of group life when the group expects the conductor to fill this role. In the pairing group there is a similar shared fantasy that a sexualised couple will produce a Messianic 'something'; a new member or idea, to save the group from its predicament.

In Example 1, where a predominantly dependent culture existed, that incident could be formulated in basic assumption terms as – the pair (group conductors) failed to open the door thus thwarting the dependency needs of the group who responded by taking flight into angry silence.

The import of Bion's formulation lies in the universality of the phenomena he describes. They can be observed in all group situations, therapeutic or otherwise. The relevance to therapy groups is that no matter what model of therapy is being used this formulation can be applied to understanding the reasons why a group has temporarily stopped functioning as a work group.

Looking again at the group material in Examples 4, 5 and 6 the question the conductor has to frame is, 'what is the nature of the anxiety felt by the group which is interfering with what has become its preferred mode of working?' The group was grappling with its dependency needs, which it had previously warded off by creating an illusion that it could look after itself – basic assumption flight. The forthcoming summer break that was imposed by the therapists fractured this cosy illusion and led to realisation of dependency on the therapists and concomitant rage at being abandoned. The conflict could not be expressed directly because as became clear an admission of dependency would lead to a breakthrough of painful early trauma. The holiday break aroused intense anxiety because of the perceived threat to the integrity of the group. As this process was interpreted the anxiety was replaced by another threat, this time from the volcanic irruption into the group of previously repressed feelings.

Bion derived his hypothesis from understanding how a group defends itself against persecutory anxiety. However, basic assumption formations can be useful and even at times desirable. A simple example would be of a class of students dependent on the teacher for information. After all the three types of basic assumption are basic human responses and needs.

Example 7

Unwittingly a group was selected that had a core common experience of absent fathering. The supervisor drew my attention to this and we wondered how the group might use me or the group-as-a-whole as father. I noticed a repeated pattern emerge. One member would speak, perhaps at length, about a matter which was clearly of import. I would respond, feeling myself to be interested and having ideas that seemed to make sense of what they were saying. A dialogue would ensue between the two of them. After a while I would notice that nobody else was joining in although they were obviously attentive. I would then withdraw from the dialogue and the others would become active. This process was repeated with each member taking a turn as it were.

This came to be understood as the group unconsciously promoting a situation whereby each member could have individual attention from me as a good father. A basic assumption pairing process was clearly in operation. While it was possible to understand this as defending against anxieties such as sibling rivalry its main purpose appeared to be therapeutic. Each individual had a personal experience while at the same time representing everybody else. In turn the group projected its painful longing for father into one member where it could be seen by all to be met in relation between that member and me. All could thereby identify with the one and introject a present, loved father to modify their earlier experiences of the absent, hated father.

Similarly in Example 6 the group unconsciously sat the therapists together in order to have a parental couple to enable them to contain and work with a high level of anxiety. If this had had a purely defensive function the group would have proceeded very differently. The emotional charge would have been muted and the group would not have been able to work with Jemma's suicidal feelings.

Is group therapy effective?

There is now a considerable research literature on group therapy. (For a helpful overview see Alonso & Swiller, chapter 24). Initially research focused on the question of effectiveness. The emphasis has now shifted to factors in the therapist, patient and group process that influence outcome.

The weight of evidence shows group therapy to be an effective treatment. It is at least as effective as individual therapy when the two are compared. It is cost-effective.

However, a serious problem exists in terms of current thinking about the hierarchy of the evidence base. Randomised controlled trial design is based upon having homogeneous patient samples. This is evidently not possible when dealing with mixed groups. It is difficult to conceive of an adequate control group. It may not therefore be possible to provide evidence about efficacy of this type of group treatment. However, many would argue against the applicability of this sort of evidence to a process as complex as psychotherapy, which is concerned with meaning and significance in emotional life.

Necessary qualities of group conductors

Foulkes (1975) drew attention to the twin necessities of adequate training and possession of certain personal attributes. The importance of regular, ongoing supervision has to be emphasised, especially for the relatively inexperienced group conductor.

Foulkes' list of personal attributes is daunting: ethical integrity with the capacity to take a high degree of emotional responsibility for oneself and the group; a genuine interest in the subject that is not too interfered with by a personal need to help others; a capacity for objectivity balanced with receptive listening; good intelligence, the ability to articulate problems creatively and succinctly allied with common sense; honesty and love of truth even when disturbing personally or to the group; mental and emotional balance, and able to lead a full and interesting life, relatively free from neurotic disturbance and serious character flaw. Above all the conductor must be able to handle group situations.

It might seem that the effective conductor has to be a paragon of virtue and have eyes in the back of his head. There is more than a grain of truth in this but fortunately it is not entirely so. A group that has been properly selected and which is conducted with respect to the principles outlined in this chapter will in large part learn to work to get on with it for itself. The overriding function of the conductor is to shape this process without getting in the way of it. The group endeavour is of itself a fascinating and exciting one.

References and further reading

Alonso, A. & Swiller, H. (eds) *Group Therapy in Clinical Practice*. Washington DC: American Psychiatric Press, 1993.

Aveline, M. & Dryden, W. (eds) 1988 *Group Therapy in Britain*. Milton Keynes: Open University Press.

Bion, W. R. (1961) *Experiences in Groups*. London: Tavistock Publications.

Ettin, M. F. (1992) *Foundations and Applications of Group Psychotherapy: A Sphere of Influence*. Boston: Allyn & Bacon.

Foulkes, S. H. (1948) *Introduction to Group Analytic Psychotherapy*. London: Maresfield Reprints.

Foulkes, S. H. (1964) *Therapeutic Group Analysis*. London: George Allen & Unwin.

Foulkes, S. H. (1975) *Group Analytic Psychotherapy: Methods and Principles*. London: Gordon & Breach.

Hinshelwood, R. D. (1989) *A Dictionary of Kleinian Thought*. London: Free Association Books.

Hook, J. (2002) Group therapy. *Psychiatry*, **1**, 52–55.

Lacoursiere, R. B. (1980) *The Life Cycle of Groups*. New York: Human Sciences Press.

Pratt, J. H. (1922) The principles of class treatment and their application to various chronic diseases. *Hospital Social Service Quarterly*, **6**, 401–411.

Skolnick, M. (1992) The role of the therapist from a social systems perspective. In *Handbook of Contemporary Psychotherapy* (eds R. H. Klein, H. S. Bernard & D. L. Singer). Madison: International Universities Press.

Whitaker, D. S. & Lieberman, M. A. (1964) *Psychotherapy Through the Group Process*. New York: Atherton Press.

Yalom, I. D. (1995) *The Theory and Practice of Group Psychotherapy*. New York: Basic Books.

CHAPTER 10

Child and adolescent individual psychoanalytical psychotherapy

Jean Robinson

This chapter aims first to describe the work of child and adolescent psychotherapists and their role in multidisciplinary child and adolescent mental health teams in the National Health Service, and second to describe the kind of individual child psychotherapeutic experience that psychiatrists in training might expect while on child and adolescent psychiatry placements. Other important models of psychotherapy with children and adolescents, for example cognitive and behavioural, are not discussed here (see Chapters 6 & 7).

Example: Alisdair; thinking the unthinkable, 'the lady who tries to understand'
Alisdair was re-referred, to child mental health services when he was 7-years-old. His first referral, at age 5 years, coincided with his expulsion from school because of soiling and wetting. In between referrals, sexual abuse by maternal grandfather was disclosed by a cousin, one of a network of cousins, including Alisdair, all abused by grandfather. Investigations revealed the high probability that Alisdair's mother and aunts had also been sexually abused by this man, although Alisdair's mother herself was unable to consciously think about this.

The second referral was made by the school psychologist because of Alisdair's hyperactivity and extreme violence towards other children in class. In addition, his obscene language and strange behaviour, which included crawling under desks and making animal noises, caused immense distress to his teachers and school. Although aware of his experiences of sexual abuse, the professionals then involved were unable to make links between this experience and his current difficulties.

Despite the high degree of concern expressed by the referrer, Alisdair's mother was relatively unperturbed about her son. Her greatest preoccupation was that his behaviour would threaten her recent marriage to a fourth partner (a man much older than herself whom she felt offered her good material security). Mother's first violent relationship of 12 years standing, produced three children now all in their late teens and living in social work hostels having for many years been in social work care. Mother's second relationship to Alisdair's father lasted 5 years ending when Alisdair was 4.5 years old. Their separation was blamed by mother on Alisdair. She perceived her partner as spoiling him and undermining her attempts to 'rule' him. Mother's principal recall of her pregnancy was of diarrhoea 'pouring out' and of a 'fall downstairs' which she worried would damage, if not kill, the baby. Following Alisdair's birth, mother thought he nearly died several times because of 'mucous'. Her account was spilled out, full of anxiety, 7 years after the event. Her thinking was jumbled with many gaps.

Alisdair had been in weekly psychotherapy for almost 3 years at the time of this account. Psychotherapy began after Alisdair secured a place in a day school for emotionally disturbed children. Early on in this period Alisdair's mother abandoned him with his biological father after she was admitted to hospital for major surgery. Initially his stay was intended to allow her to recuperate but once home she simply refused to have Alisdair back. It is likely that Alisdair received no explanation of this from his mother.

In his therapy, although his experience of sexual abuse has occupied much of the transference in the shape of rights of entry, feelings of humiliation, feeling small and confusion between good 'clean' fun and perverse twists of playfulness, a more fundamental and profound subtext coalesced round finding a safe space in his therapist's mind in which to feel he can locate his thoughts and feelings. This implies more than finding lost aspects of himself but rather finding the opportunity to conceive new aspects of his personality. After 1 year in therapy while debating his feelings about missing swimming because of his therapy, Alisdair argued in his therapist's favour 'but you're the lady who tries to understand things'.

In the past 3 years Alisdair has made gains. He has returned to mainstream schooling, is beginning to attain his academic potential and coping better in peer relationships. Much of this can be attributed to the containment of his anxiety in a specialised school setting and his settling down to live securely with his father. Alongside this he has been helped by the experience of his therapist's thoughtfulness and her attempts to seek to hold and reflect on his experience rather than pour it out in meaningless, 'diarrhoea like', jumping from one topic to another. It is likely that his mother's own mind was torn to shreds by her experience of maternal deprivation and paternal abuse. Alisdair's 'trying to understand' is a good starting place in which to think about the work of child and adolescent psychotherapy.

The above case description is a representative example of work with children who are severely deprived and traumatised. These children have internalised a severely damaged inner world, and are commonly referred for individual psychotherapy. Such children have had serious limitations placed on their emotional experience, often from birth, so that changing the external systems around them is insufficient in itself to significantly change their emotional view of themselves and relationships. However, there are many other kinds of less overtly harmful experiences and many of the children and youngsters seen, fall into a category of seeming to bring disasters down upon themselves. Before looking at some other clinical examples, a few of the major relevant psychoanalytical theories underlying child and adolescent psychotherapy will be described.

Relevant psychoanalytic theories in child and adolescent psychotherapy

Theories of psychoanalytic psychotherapy have been described elsewhere (Chapters 2 & 3) and all are applicable to work with children and teenagers. As in the adult field, there are several major schools of theory and these are reflected in the principal orientations of training schools. These include the traditional Freudian and post-Freudian; Kleinian and post-Kleinian; the Jungian and the 'independent' perspectives. However, in practice, experience suggests that child and adolescent psychotherapists have more in common with each other than not. Concepts from each orientation have found specific application when thinking about infant and childhood emotional development and the earliest organisations of primitive phantasy, thought and feeling states. For brevity these are listed as follows:

Anna Freud's enlargement of her father's work on the ego and instinctual development (A. Freud, 1936), particularly her work on developmental lines and their relationship to maternal and family constellations, provides a useful framework within which to think about developmental deviations from normality and pathological development. This diagnostic approach is increasingly finding application in research and audit initiatives in child and adolescent psychotherapy and has long formed the basis of the Hampstead Diagnostic Index (Sandler, 1962).

Melanie Klein's contribution to understanding the complexity of inner world functioning; the balance in emotional development between projective and introjective mechanisms; the richness of a state of mind built upon introjective identifications; the vulnerability of states of mind based on projective identifications; the resultant confusion when narcissistic identifications are the main tendency in relationships, have greatly enriched practice in many areas (Segal, 1964). Within child and adolescent psychotherapy this has particularly deepened appreciation of the complex interplay between the unconscious of mother and baby, even before birth and found verification in mother and baby observations, which are a fundamental component of all child psychotherapy training.

From different angles both Winnicott (Winnicott, 1971) and Bion (O'Shaughnessy, 1981) have approached the complexity, beauty and wonder of the earliest emotional interaction between mother, baby and father and the part this plays in the development of a sense of self, identity and the ability to give emotional experience words. Both Bion's concept of 'maternal reverie' and Winnicott's of 'mirroring' are useful as therapists reflect on the struggle to be therapeutic in the consulting room.

Jung's work on intuition as elaborated by Michael Fordham (Astor, 1991) finds resonance with Bion's work on transformation. Both take us into the realms of the links between the mother–baby relationship and its contribution to personality development and the therapeutic encounter.

Practice and technique

With this brief highlight of some of the principal theoretical orientations in child psychotherapy let us move to begin to consider what it is in practice and technique that distinguishes child and adolescent psychotherapy from adult psychotherapy.

While all of the fundamental principles of psychoanalytic psychotherapy, namely focusing on the unconscious as manifest in the total experience in the room, attention to setting and breaks, use of the transference and countertransference apply, self-evidently there is one striking difference – the patient is a child or adolescent. What are the differences that follow on from this?

Resistance

Struggling to engage in therapy is ubiquitous. However, usually in grown-ups, at least initially, there is some adult part of them that is aware of their distress and is prepared to get engaged in therapy. In children and perhaps especially adolescents, this mature response, is frequently located in another – the referrer. This may be parents, social worker, psychologist or others. Preliminary meetings and history taking will often therefore begin with a meeting with the adults concerned, alone or with the child. The fact, however, that children do not refer themselves (and some adolescents do), should not be taken as meaning that they do not experience psychic distress or cannot apprehend what therapy is about. Indeed perhaps because of their closeness to reality-based dependency needs, children often very quickly develop a sense of how therapy might help them. As with adults, a general comment about 'meeting a few times to see if coming to see me or somebody like me will help' is sufficient along with clarification of where and when, to explain the preliminary interviews. However, since it is normally (except in the instance of older and compliant adolescents) the case that children will be brought to therapy by parents or care staff, the viability of continued therapy partly rests on the carer's motivation and involvement in the process. Parents may be deeply concerned, or worryingly unconcerned about the emotional distress in their children and youngsters. For these reasons part of the overall assessment, in addition to the psychodynamic formulation reached with the child, will, of necessity, include an assessment of the parents, their understanding of the difficulties, their strengths and weaknesses and the role and participation of other child care agencies. In practice, unless it is clear from the referral letter or from consultation with the referrer that individual psychotherapy is the immediate treatment choice, a family meeting will usually precede further separate assessment of the child and parents. For this reason it is best to have two workers assigned to the case – a case manager who is often in addition the parent worker and a child worker. Experienced child psychotherapists may sometimes straddle both roles. This becomes increasingly difficult if a number of child care agencies are involved or the child is in care or attends a special educational placement. For those in training, seeking individual child psychotherapy experience, parent work and case management should be allocated to a separate worker, leaving them free to focus on the child.

The setting

Although aspects of the therapeutic setting may be taken as given in adult psychotherapy departments, these are often more difficult to establish in busy general purpose child and adolescent mental health clinics. However, a child or teenager is no different in his need for privacy, confidentiality and a sense of containment. This is communicated both by the attitude of the therapist and through physical characteristics of the room. It is insensitive and therefore unrewarding to interview a child where they can be seen or heard, especially by parents. Ideally the room should be neither too small nor too large, well ventilated and illuminated, with an engaged/free sign. Although the room should be comfortable and welcoming, too many interesting things readily provide distractions, so simplicity is an advantage. The therapist himself will be unable to maintain the necessary therapeutic stance if overwhelmed by concerns about the child's safety and possible damage to property and personal belongings.

For all these reasons most child and adolescent mental health clinics allocate or should allocate a child psychotherapy room in which all these features have been thought through and implemented, furnished with an appropriate range of nursery- to adult-sized chairs and tables, sometimes a couch and an assortment of play and drawing materials that can be taken into the room before each session and removed afterwards. Well organised departments will have a stock of children's toy boxes, often non-individualised for assessment interviews, with a personalised named box an option if the child proceeds to treatment. Under 5s have particular needs but it is unusual in basic training placements to see preschool children individually. Trained child psychotherapists may offer individual treatment to this age group.

More usual in a psychiatrist's training will be work with school-aged children or adolescents. For the school-age group an assortment of moving vehicles, family dolls, wild and tame families of animals, fences, building bricks, sellotape, glue, paper, children's scissors, pens and a soft ball are generally sufficient to give the child a range of choice and promote spontaneous play. Board games or mechanised toys are readily used defensively by children and sometimes therapists as a means of reassurance, diminishing anxiety, evading rather than exploring it. For this reason board games should not be introduced by the therapist. This, of course, will not prevent the well defended latency aged child coming 'armed' with a pocket computer game or a puzzle book but this then is his choice and is part of the process, open to thought and interpretation, rather similar to the adult who comes well prepared with a rehearsed story. It should be noted that these recommended toys, if they are to be sturdy and last, and not rapidly become meaningless bits and pieces, are often expensive and difficult to obtain. Departments and clinics offering psychoanalytic psychotherapy as a treatment option often have a procedure for replenishing stocks and a budget for this purpose. Junior staff are normally familiarised with these procedures as part of their initial induction course but if not, should find out what the routine is for play materials.

Many of the very disturbed children, for whom individual treatment is the necessary option, will however remain unable to play for many sessions if not months or years. An inability to play as we usually understand the word is a feature of their disturbance. This means the experience in the room is often inactivity and silence or chaotic movement and sound and above all, intense anxiety and fear in the child and therapist. These difficulties are encountered by everyone seeing a new case. Indeed part of the work is the experience of these early primitive anxieties. However, since meeting with a child often evokes particular feelings of vulnerability, it is especially necessary for beginners to have available supervision from a child psychotherapist, ideally even before seeing the child. In addition it is recommended that junior psychiatrists in training see children who are relatively well, whose difficulties are focused and of recent onset, perhaps related to a life event and who are functioning well in other aspects of their life and cared for in a reasonably functioning family. This will not remove the anxieties inherent in the beginning but offer greater likelihood that after the initial tackling of anxieties, the child will be able to settle down to use symbolic play to demonstrate their area of particular concern. Adolescents vary widely in their proclivity to play or talk. As a general rule, early adolescents often benefit from the opportunity to fall back on drawing or doodling when anxiety is high although they may initially show disdain for such childish trifles.

Communication style

Children and adolescents like adults may communicate their unconscious phantasies and inner world of good and bad experiences, sensations, feelings and thoughts via verbal communications, reports of dreams and day dreams. As with adults, these apparent communications may actually turn out to be miscommunications or attempts to prevent emotionally meaningful relatedness. However, children frequently use other means of communication. These are now listed with some examples.

Symbolic play

Example
Brodie; this, almost 3-year-old boy, had a history of repeated and unsuccessful surgical intervention for hypospadias (urethra opening onto the shaft of the penis, rather than the tip) following a complicated circumcision. He was seen with his mother twice for assessment and on both occasions used the hospital scene toys to reveal something of his preoccupations; the boy in the hospital bed

was pushed by the nurse with 'hands sticking out' towards the stairs, but the nurse did not hold the boy properly, he fell out and 'got hurt'. Brodie became anxious when introducing the doctor figure who went for a walk 'with boots on'. Brodie was now unable to finish this piece of play, brushed the toys from the table and turned to drawing a safe picture of a puppy dog with his parents. In addition to the content of this piece of play what was of interest was the form that it took and Brodie's associated affect; the story was repeated many, many times, but without a clear beginning, middle or end. There was no satisfactory resolution and his handling of the toys was very controlled and obsessional. Each piece had to be in exactly its right place.

Thus, this little boy conveyed a sense of an experience, which he had been unable to put into place and forget about, which continued to alarm him, and to which he responded with obsessional omnipotent defences.

Example
Calum; an 8-year-old boy was referred for assessment because of his lying, tall stories and lack of emotional depth. Calum, when a few years old was abandoned by his mother and raised by his father who sexually abused him over a long period. Since coming into social work care he had been in a number of foster placements that broke down because of his subtle but corrosive undermining of the goodness available to him from his foster families.

In his second assessment session Calum added to the plasticine house he had built in the first session, a path, flowers, trees laden with fruit, a long windy road with a lay-by in case cars 'broke down' and a church with a ramp for people who 'break down'. Calum then turned briefly to drawing a clown face with an enormous nose. The impression of the drawing was intrusive and frightening. Now Calum became rather lost with 'no ideas'. Rain outside became linked in his mind with the possibility of lightning, 'like a light gun which makes holes through teddy bears'.

This sequence suggested many possibilities of interrelated communications. In the symbolic representation of the idyllic cottage and orchard, Calum communicated his search for a perfect, ideal existence and parental object. This wish too was communicated in his attitude towards the therapist who at times felt very warm and compassionate towards this boy. However, the cosy scene was interrupted by thoughts of 'breakdown'; his own psychic breakdown and breakdown of his foster placements. More hopefully support and help were available in the lay-by and ramp. More anxiously there was a link with an intrusive false experience (the clown meant to be funny is actually frightening) and a shift to a highly persecuting attack. This movement was experienced by the therapist as a communication both about Calum's view of her, quickly shifting from a bounteous, idealised mother to a highly alarming, intrusive father figure and a statement about Calum's own internalised capacity to spoil and destroy via intrusive entry into his objects.

Drawing

Example
Douglas, 8-years-old at the time of the referral, one of non-identical twins, was born prematurely with a lengthy and very ill period in a special care baby unit. He was subsequently discovered to suffer from moderate cerebral palsy, and was

referred to child psychiatry because of extreme temper tantrums at home, over-activity and difficulty in school. In his first assessment session, Douglas drew a house; this was light and spacious but was subsequently darkly and heavily filled in as Douglas went through each felt tip pen in order to ascertain whether they 'worked well'. Then he moved to tracing an outline around the small plastic truck, taking care that all four wheels were in place on the paper.

Over a few minutes these rather carefully executed drawings moved on to a series of 10–15 frantically rushed drawings, each moving further away from what first looked like a segmented clock through to loose, wobbly, squiggly shapes resembling spider's webs, flowing over the edge of the paper onto the table. These were finished at a rate of about two per minute. In between each drawing Douglas wobbled unsteadily on his broad-based gait to the corner to collect the separate sheets of paper.

In these drawings form is as interesting as content. What begins as a potentially symbolic drawing of a containing house and himself is filled up with solid weight, via the question of whether the pens work or not, which is echoed in the care taken over the truck's wheels/limbs with the drawings finally breaking down in uncontained spilling out of wisps of disconnected experience.

This boy's and his parent's subsequent treatment revealed how Douglas's psychic steadiness was repeatedly threatened by his parents' depression around his disability and his own fury and resentment that he unlike his twin had not been 'finished off' properly.

Constructions

Example: Douglas (continued)
Later in Douglas's treatment and over a period of many months he moved through a series of paper constructions. Again these were of interest not simply in content but in how they were made, what position in space they occupied etc. The first of these paper sculptures involved endlessly and laboriously (given his severe coordination difficulties) sellotaping tiny scraps of paper to a growing expanse of paper over the couch. Additionally this play worked on his relationship with his therapist, sometimes adding to it, sometimes tearing it up. After perhaps 6 sessions of flat growth, the sculpture moved on to become a crocodile/boy with a formidable array of teeth, two layers deep and badly misshapen fingers and toes.

This was a 2-D life-size image imbued with great anger, pain and sadness. Towards the end of 3 years of treatment, Douglas attempted a very complicated 3-D construction of a beautiful bird singing in a cage. These and many more miscreations and creations provided the medium through which he and his therapist worked together.

Enactment and projective identification

While adults will often reveal split-off parts of themselves through their narrative and the emotional fluctuations in the therapeutic encounter, children and younger teenagers are as likely to do this through physical role play and enactment.

Example

Elsie; an 8-year-old girl, had presented with problems since birth. She was described as an irritable baby who would not eat or sleep. Mother was very depressed at the time of her birth and the marriage unhappy. Mother later revealed that she entertained thoughts of suicide and infanticide at this time. A thin and largely negative relationship was described between mother and daughter.

In this session Elsie was busy, lovingly tending her 'perfect' baby doll. Her therapist was left with the ugly doll and told to leave her face down on the ground. Elsie continued as a competent, 'in control' mother, while the therapist increasingly felt forlorn, abandoned and vulnerable. This became so unbearable that despite her instructions from Elsie, she did pick up the ugly doll and tend to it. What she powerfully experienced were bad, neglected baby experiences and Elsie's defence against this in her identification with an idealised loving mother.

Example

Fergus; a 13-year-old boy was severely and perversely abused in his family of origin. Complicated by his adolescent psychosexual development, much of his sessions were taken up in bullying and terrorising his therapist, with the re-enactment of the victim/abuser scenario. His therapist at times experienced deep humiliation, fear and dread. At a period when these aspects of the relationship were becoming easier to talk about, Fergus verbally tyrannised his therapist, 'take your clothes off, go on, go and lie face down on the couch' and when this met with no movement, tried to bribe her, 'look how much money I have' then tried to catch his therapist out 'quick, look over there, a spider in the corner'. Struggling through these very difficult experiences allowed Fergus's therapist a sense of his inner world of tyranny and brutality.

Assessment sessions and beginnings

Most training psychiatrists' experience of individual child psychotherapeutic work will be limited to a number of individual assessments, and perhaps a piece of brief, focused work, rather than a long-term treatment case. Trainee staff often find themselves instructed 'to simply be with the child' or to do nothing (making the experience potentially as frightening to the therapist as to the child). For this reason emphasis is now given on how to begin. However, it must be emphasised that what follows is not prescriptive, each therapist/child dyad is unique and without question the most helpful way to think about this is not by reading, but through having an experience with a child in the room and then having the opportunity to reflect on this in supervision. Just as the child may be paralysed with fear, frozen into immobility, want to flee the room, so may these feelings be experienced by the therapist. Other beginnings are coloured by driven activity, forced cheerfulness and jokiness, which again the therapist may find himself colluding with. All these countertransference experiences constitute the real work of beginnings. However, there are some physical preparations that require consideration.

If the assessment of the child requires more than one session, as is often the case, effort should be made to keep the setting constant. Subsequent appointments should not be made until the room is known to be available. Many children will have used the room in the intervening time, so a few minutes should be spent, preparatory to the session, returning it to its quiescent, steady state, especially if the room is used for many different purposes. In a multi-purpose room, all sorts of varied articles may be left behind by previous occupants, for example cigarette ends, keys and even used nappies.

In most departments, therefore, there is an expectation that therapists return the room to the state in which it was found and for this reason more than usual time should be left between sessions.

Choice of toys has already been discussed. There are some special situations that require more thought regarding range of toys. These include work with children with autism, disabilities, sensory impairments, those in preschool and those who have been sexually abused. However, these would seldom be seen for individual psychotherapy by other than trained child psychotherapists. If the assessment extends beyond one session, then the toys should be kept safely locked up. A special container for the toys, i.e. a plastic stackable box, ideally with a lid, symbolically highlights the privacy and containment of the sessions. The manner in which the box is used or perceived will provide considerable information about how the child views the therapist and hence his basic object relationships. Boxes may be trampled into the ground, ignored or adorned with every variety of graffiti or self-identification. The continuity of the box of toys is an external representation of the continuity of the therapist's attention. Some children will remain totally unconvinced that the box/session time is just for them, or will be adamant that something has been removed or put in during their absence. The therapist needs to be able in his or her own mind to know this is untrue in order to withstand this attack on reality and work with the fantasy. What is required is a setting that allows the therapist as well as the child freedom for thought.

Drawings should be retained and returned to subsequent sessions as an indication that communication between individuals does not just vaporise but can be built up into memory and personal history. Some children will very persistently attempt to leave their mark on a room, for example leaving paintings on walls. This is best taken up with the child so that the therapist is not left after a session wondering whether to detach a very intricate piece of work from the wall. Before the session ends, if the child has not brought it up themselves, they can be asked 'what are we going to do with your drawings?'

The therapist's first contact with the child, for the purpose of the assessment session is in the waiting room. In the ideal situation the child will come willingly to the therapy room with a minimum of fuss and the maximum amount of cooperation from child and parent. Needless to say, this is not often the case and the therapist may need to anticipate considerable emotional and perhaps physical struggle. The child may be reluctant to leave his mother, fearing what the therapist might do to him in the room. Mother may be reluctant to leave her child on his own with the therapist, not having fully anticipated her absence from this part of the assessment.

Sloppy introductions or diffidence by the therapist can only serve to heighten such a dilemma, and it is, therefore, essential to be prepared, to have the child firmly in mind, to remember, whatever anxieties are transmitted by the child, that his mother will still be there at the end, provided she has already been asked to do so and that the therapist will return him to her after 50 minutes. In most cases this reality reminder is sufficient to get the child into the room and thereafter emergent separation and persecutory anxieties can be dealt with as they arise. In some rare cases, however, often indicative of severe psychotic pathology between mother and child, it may be absolutely impossible to separate them. In these very unusual circumstances it may be necessary to have mother present initially. In this circumstance she will require some guidance about her role in the session, for example 'mummy's going to sit in the corner and just watch, so as to help you spend some time with me'.

In the initial greeting the therapist wishes to convey friendliness without appearing overly solicitous or indulgent. The latter is as likely to lead to mistrust and suspiciousness as is a cold aloof manner. Every effort must be made to be punctual. This is not easy in the life of general child and adolescent psychiatry clients, but unless rigorously pursued, the predictability and dependability of the therapeutic space is readily eroded and may be misconstrued by the child and parents as an indication that this part of the assessment is unimportant. The parents' attitude to therapy will frequently be modelled on what they perceive is the therapist's attitude, so that irrespective of what is happening with the child, if the parents get the message through lateness or badly managed cancellations that the work is unimportant, their commitment will falter and failure to engage will be the outcome. Lateness also can only increase the child's anxiety and may make separation more difficult.

Once in the room, the therapist should provide some brief simple orientation, for example, 'we are going to be here for 50 minutes and then I will take you back to the waiting room. There are some things in this box that you might want to use'. Thereafter the amount of talking done by the therapist will depend on the degree of the child's anxiety. Ideally, one hopes that the child will proceed to play or otherwise communicate spontaneously. If the child is immediately suffused with anxiety, to the extent that he is inhibited in proceeding, then he is going to need some help. Reassurance is a natural response but not one that sheds much light on what it is that is blocking the child. Immediately the therapist needs to be in touch with any slight clue internal or external that might help to understand the child's difficulty. Unfortunately this is the very time when the therapist is most likely to be filled with his or her own anxiety about beginning. In this situation there is a very understandable, but not very helpful tendency to resort to action or make leading statements, for example 'why don't you paint?' or 'what did you do at school today?' or in sheer desperation 'I'm not going to hurt you'. However, there is every chance that this will not address what is worrying the child. If the therapist can hold onto and reflect on her own anxiety for a bit and wait for a response from the child, this may become clearer. However, the therapist may need to directly acknowledge some general causes of anxiety, for example 'it's difficult for you to leave mummy and be with me at the moment', or 'some boys who come to spend time with me might be worried that I won't take them back to mummy at the end', and see what fits for this child.

Throughout the session the therapist is trying to remain in tune with the child's anxiety and needs and responds accordingly. This may mean that the child will require frequent interpretation of his negative transference fears or he may require some practical help, for example, to undo the glue top or find the toilet. There is often a mistaken view that children require no limits in a session, leading trainees to confidently announce at the beginning of a session, 'you can do whatever you want here' in the hope that this will lead to spontaneity. Children are dependent on adults for their ultimate physical safety, and this equally applies within the psychotherapeutic setting.

The required attitude of the therapist is that of an attentive, detailed observer, taking in the totality of the child's presence in the room in concert with reflection of his own countertransference.

For this reason it is considered a definite advantage for senior house officers, and specialist registrars in training to have the opportunity to conduct supervised baby or child observations (MacFadyen, 1991) as this enormously increases skill in observation, the prerequisite step in all hypothesis making. These observations begin to make links in the therapist's mind with what is already known about the child, his background and current family constellation and thus begins to form the matrix from which therapeutic interpretations can be made or a psychodynamic formulation derived.

The role of child and adolescent psychotherapists in the multidisciplinary team

Many child and adolescent mental health teams in the UK have no access to child and adolescent psychotherapy services. However, it is to be hoped that this situation will be steadily remedied over the next decade. In an ideal situation child psychotherapists, alongside psychiatrists, child psychologists, social worker, nurse therapists and all other disciplines working with children and teenagers, would contribute to assessment and treatment options. The work of these is not only limited to long-term weekly or intensive psychotherapy. In addition to consultation, teaching, supervision, research and audit, there exist many less intensive therapeutic modalities applying the expertise of this training through a range of techniques. Some examples are given:

- under-5 counselling services; these normally offer up to 5 sessions working with preschool children and their parents, frequently addressing feeding, sleeping, toileting and overactivity difficulties
- young people's counselling service; again this normally offers up to 5 sessions with teenagers and young people providing as well as treatment an opportunity to think further about longer-term treatment for youngsters who need and want it
- group work; this may take the traditional form of work with a selected group or a family group of siblings, for example, those who have witnessed or experienced similar trauma (e.g. murder of a parent, abuse, etc.)
- paediatric liaison work; this may take many forms, for example, contribution to psychosocial ward rounds, often with those who are chronically sick or with disabilities, liaison to special care baby units etc.
- brief assessment work; again this may take many forms but is frequently requested for court and social services
- general practice liaison work; for example, consultation to health visitors and baby clinics.

In addition to these particular models of treatment the past 10–15 years have seen the flourishing of psychotherapeutic work with complex and specialised areas. These include children who have autism, borderline personality disorder or psychosis, those with mental or physical disorders, those who have been severely abused and/or deprived, refugee children and those children or adolescents who are adopted, fostered or accommodated.

Training opportunities

It has already been stressed that the best way to begin to develop skills in this realm is to seek some relatively uncomplicated assessments and to have these supervised, ideally by a child psychotherapist. If there is a desire to take this experience further, many centres throughout the UK offer a range of courses and training in working therapeutically with children and adolescents (contact the Association of Child Psychotherapists). Particularly valuable for senior house officers and specialist registrars are work discussion and infant observation seminars. The former allows exploration of individual case material within the context of a variety of professional settings, the latter the opportunity to observe in depth the emergence of an infant's personality in the context of his own temperament and family, thus reflecting on basic processes of human interaction. Full professional training in child psychotherapy, recognised by the Association of Child Psychotherapists, is now available in 6 centres in the UK, 3 in London, 1 in Birmingham, 1 in Scotland and 1 in the north-east of England (see Box 1).

Box 10.1 Training resources

Association of Child Psychotherapists
120 West Heath Road, London NW3 7TU, Tel: 020 8458 1609

Training institutions
There are 6 training institutions recognised by the Association of Child Psychotherapists

The Anna Freud Centre for the Psychoanalytic Study and Treatment of Children
21 Maresfield Gardens, London NW3 5SD, Tel: 020 7794 2313 (Details from the course tutor)

Birmingham Trust for Psychoanalytic Psychotherapy
Flat 1, Queen's College, Somerset Road, Edgbaston, Birmingham B15 2QH, Tel: 0121 455 9393 (Details from Mrs Shirley Truckle)

British Association of Psychotherapists
37 Mapesbury Road, London NW2 4HJ, Tel: 020 8452 9823 (Details from the secretary)

Scottish Institute of Human Relations
18 Young Street, Edinburgh EH2 4JB, Tel: 0131 226 9610 (Details from the course organising tutor)

Tavistock and Portman NHS Trust
Tavistock Centre, 120 Belsize Lane, London NW3 5BA, Tel: 020 7435 7111 (Details from the training administrator)

Northern School of Child and Adolescent Psychotherapy
Fairbairn House, 72–75 Clarendon Road, Leeds LS2 9PL, Tel: 0113 343 4868

References and further reading

Astor, J. (1991) The emergence of Michael Fordham's model of development: a new integration in analytical psychology. In *Extending Horizons, Psychoanalytic Psychotherapy with Children, Adolescents and Families* (eds R. Szur & S. Miller), pp. 405–421. London: Karnac (Books) Ltd.

Boston, M. & Szur, R. (eds) (1983) *Psychotherapy with Severely Deprived Children*. London: Routledge and Kegan Paul.

Freud, A. (1936) *The Ego and Mechanisms of Defence*. London: Hogarth Press.

Hunter, M. (2001) *Psychotherapy with Young People in Care. Lost and Found*. London: Brunner-Routledge.

Lanyado, M. & Horne, A. (eds) (1999) *The Handbook of Child and Adolescent Psychotherapy. Psychoanalytic Approaches*. Routledge.

MacFadyen, A. (1991) Some thoughts on infant observation and its possible role in child psychiatry training. *Association of Child Psychiatry and Psychology Newsletter*, **13**, 10–14.

O'Shaughnessy, E. (1981) A commemorative essay of W. R. Bion's theory of thinking. *Journal of Child Psychotherapy*, **7**, 181–192.

Sandler, J. (1962) Research in psycho-analysis. The Hampstead Index as an instrument of psycho-analytic research. *International Journal of Psychoanalysis*, **43**, 287–291.

Segal, H. (1964) *An Introduction to the Work of Melanie Klein*. London: Heinemann.

Waddell, M. (1999) *Inside Lives. Psychoanalysis and the Growth of Personality*. London: Gerald Duckworth & Co Ltd.

Winnicott, D. W. (1971) *Playing and Reality*. London: Penguin.

CHAPTER 11

Family therapy and systemic practice

Graham Bryce

Systemic theory is useful in a variety of ways. Translated into practice, it provides the main theoretical framework for family therapy but also helps in the area of family-sensitive practice, a core issue in delivering contemporary mental health services. Also, as a way of considering how systems (whether groups of people or sets of ideas) get along together, systemic theory has a contribution to make to the important issues of working in teams, interdisciplinary and inter-agency work.

This chapter illustrates how systemic theory can inform the work of practitioners on a day-to-day basis. Following an introductory description of systemic theory, some key concepts in family therapy are set out. After a brief review of evidence, the application of family therapy and the wider application of systemic ideas are considered, and the chapter concludes with a brief discussion about learning processes. The account is illustrated and supported throughout by references to research and practice.

Systemic theory

Systemic theory is a set of propositions about how people's lives are informed and influenced by the contexts in which they lead those lives. Work with members of a family group to consider events and dilemmas in the context of important relationships between family members and in the light of experiences and beliefs that have shaped those relationships (that is, the practical definition of family therapy in this chapter) is a particular application of this widely useful theory.

Informed by systemic theory, practitioners consider the way in which patterns, themes and beliefs develop, become established and transform within people's lives over time. In therapeutic work with families, practitioners aim to engage with family members, draw on their understanding of relationships, investigate ways of teasing these matters out and so support change.

In this continuously developing field, ideas that have gained prominence in recent years, such as the importance of the personal and the shared narratives of family members, have added further richness and depth to earlier ideas about family process, which were typically expressed in terms of the structure and patterning of relationships. This development has occurred in parallel with a number of important social trends:

- the increasing diversity of family structure
- changing attitudes towards social roles, especially gender roles
- the growing acknowledgement of cultural diversity.

At the same time, social constructionism has gained currency as a theory of knowledge, not least within the field of family therapy and systemic practice. By inviting attention to the social and cultural contexts in which theoretical frameworks have been developed, a social constructionist perspective ushers in a series of new questions about these notions. This is reflected in heightened attention (in theorising, in research and in practice) to issues of gender, race, culture, power and class.

This continual revisiting and revising of the adequacy of the concepts that shape practice, or reflexivity, has become an integral part of systemic thinking and will weave its way through the account that follows.

Key concepts in family therapy and systemic practice

There are many ways to describe and discuss people's lives and the dilemmas that arise within them. That diversity holds the potential for both conceptual richness and complete confusion, as any serious student of family therapy quickly realises. There are a number of ways of addressing that challenge and this section begins by considering this.

For the purposes of this chapter, the story of family therapy will be recounted as a tale of two metaphors: process and narrative. Each of these themes is important in contemporary practice and this way of telling the story has been chosen to allow each to be considered in its own right and also to allow the opportunity to consider the relationship between the two.

The process metaphor

Many of the earliest accounts of family therapy were based on the idea that particular patterns in the interaction between family members (i.e. family processes) were critical factors in understanding and assisting with the difficulties that were being experienced within those families. A good example can be found in the structural model developed by Salvador Minuchin (1974), where the pattern of relationships was considered in terms of boundaries and hierarchy. On the strength of hypotheses about a causal link between problems in these areas and the presenting difficulty, an intervention designed to improve upon these aspects of family relationships was introduced.

The process paradigm was, for a long time, the dominant theme in family therapy theory and practice, and remains important. One of the strengths of process-based approaches is that many were based on models of family relationships that had their roots in research in non-clinical families.

Reviewing this family relationship research, Froma Walsh (1993) warns of the pitfall of deriving concepts of 'healthy family functioning' from what is regarded as 'typical', 'average' or even 'optimal' family life. She reserves particular attention for the conceptualisation of normal families as asymptomatic. According to Walsh, the related assumption, that families with a symptomatic member are dysfunctional, is commonplace among clinicians: 'a family is regarded as normal (and healthy) if there are no symptoms of disorder in any family member' (Walsh, 1993, p. 5).

Walsh (1993) points out two particular problems with this perspective. The first is that practitioners are less likely to pay attention to strengths within families where a member has a problem. The second is that responsibility for individual difficulties is attributed to 'family dysfunction', although, as she points out, the evidence for this is not clear.

From these empirical studies of non-clinical families (all of them carried out in North America), Walsh (1993) derives three key notions:

- that normal family processes 'involve the integration and maintenance of the family unit and its ability to carry out the essential tasks for the growth and well-being of its members' (p.7)
- that these processes have to be considered in a developmental context; they may be different within the same family at different points in the life cycle
- the importance of considering these processes in a sociocultural context. In other words, they may well be different between families from different cultures at the same point in the life cycle.

Resilience

In further development of this work, Walsh (2003) among others has addressed herself to the question suggested by any process dominated account, namely how do you know which processes produce good outcomes for family members. This has seen systemic writers exploring the overlap between the research on family relationships and the research on resilience (Hawley & de Haan, 1996). Walsh has gone on to distil this work into a 'family resilience framework' which combines findings from many studies. She 'identifies and synthesises key processes within three domains of family functioning' (Walsh, 2003, p.6):

- communication processes, with a particular emphasis on clarity, openness and collaboration in problem solving
- organisational patterns, for example, the balance between flexible adaptation to changing circumstances and the maintenance of stability and continuity
- family belief systems, including the sense family members make of adverse experiences.

These ideas translate readily to a framework for practice which considers:

- communication and organisation
- the 'fit' between these processes and

- the various needs of family members
- the individual and shared histories of family members
- the family's cultural context(s)
- the beliefs which shape these processes.

Example

Alice has looked after her teenage nephews, Tommy and Jackie, since her sister died 4 years ago, after years of struggling with drug and alcohol problems. The boys live with Alice and her four children, three girls in their teens and a boy in his early 20s.

Tommy, the younger boy, who has significant learning and concentration problems, is in contact with psychiatric services. Family members speak warmly of him as a friendly, restless boy who loves winding everyone up. Jackie has always coped well in school but has lately been missing classes and reported as being in fights. At home, Alice gets frustrated when he quietly resists her attempts to talk to him about these things and when he defies the rules which work well for the rest of the household.

In a family meeting there is palpable frustration between Jackie and Alice, but the affection between the members is clear, as is the strong sense of organisation and working together that Alice and her birth children share.

After a lengthy discussion of household routines and the expectations attached, Jackie mentions quietly that the care which Alice shows is great but he cannot help but think that, if his mum were alive, he and Tommy would be free to come and go as they please.

The explanations of this dilemma that family members were offering to one another had been in terms of organisation, roles and communication. But here we see how the beliefs that Jackie (and his brother) hold about family life were shaping their way of relating in their 'new' family experience.

The arc of Walsh's work echoes an important development within family therapy: the early attention to family functioning adapted, in light of growing appreciation of diversity of family form and culture, in this case, into an eclectic and pragmatic resilience-orientated framework. It is noteworthy that, as that adaptation takes place, beliefs gain increasing prominence as a theme.

The Milan model

The Milan group, who have been very influential in the development of the field within the UK, took a different course, with their commitment to studying how family difficulties were encoded in their communication patterns.

Mara Selvini Palazzoli and her colleagues in Milan were experienced mental health practitioners interested in developing 'precise methodologies' as a 'detailed guide to the therapist who ventures into the labyrinth of the family session', as they say in the introduction to their 1980 landmark paper 'Hypothesising, circularity, neutrality: three guidelines for the conductor of the session' (Selvini *et al*, 1980). Their theoretical framework was built around Gregory Bateson's (1972) work on how information is communicated in complex systems and, in particular, on the important function of difference.

The method saw the team develop hypotheses about what was happening in the family, with a particular interest in the logic of existing patterns. Circularity referred to the interview style, which sought information about relationships, evolved in response to feedback from the family, and led to increasingly refined, increasingly systemic hypotheses. They proposed that the practitioner would be experienced by family members as neutral, that is 'allied with everyone and no one at the same time'. Their interventions commonly involved positive connotation of the problem behaviours in the family, as a way of highlighting the dilemmas associated with change.

During the 1980s, the Milan model was at the heart of a debate about its systemic epistemology meaning that 'the therapist was more interested in provoking feedback and less apt to make moral judgements of any kind'. A particularly robust critique came from those working in the field of domestic and sexual violence, who argued that a therapeutic stance of neutrality was unsustainable in family relations work; this against the increasingly accepted reading, during this time, of domestic and sexual violence as abuses of power.

During this period the original Milan group divided. Cecchin and Boscolo were involved in what might be regarded as a move into a more explicit human relations theory, with Cecchin (1987) revisiting the concept of neutrality and proposing instead the idea of curiosity. In the post-Milan development family dilemmas were increasingly considered in terms of their sociocultural significance, with gender and, later, culture and ethnicity taking a place, alongside the more local and unique circumstances of families and family members, as important contexts.

The narrative metaphor

The narrative theme indicates the interest within the field of family therapy and systemic practice in how families and family members make sense of their lives. This interest in narrative is by no means limited to family therapy, nor was it a new concept in this field when it began to gain prominence in the early 1990s.

Charlotte Burck talks about narrative in this way: 'the central tenet of narrative theory is that the self is constructed – is storied through interaction with others, and that in this process language produces meaning and does not just reflect experience' (Burck, 1997, p.64).

In other words, while the process metaphor regards families as systems and discusses their dilemmas in terms of patterns and the processes which organise them, the narrative metaphor takes a different approach, casting families as meaning-generating systems, with family members shaping their lives through the meanings they give to their experience.

In terms of a theory of change, the process metaphor suggests therapy as a context in which language is used as a tool to investigate and reveal the ways that family dilemmas are coded, in terms of their relationships and beliefs. According to the particular model, interventions of various kinds are offered, again with language as the medium or vehicle.

The narrative metaphor takes a different view, as Anderson & Goolishian (1988: p. 377) put it 'this emphasis creates an alternative to thinking of social role and structure as existing in some kind of reified and empirical social reality. It construes language and communication as basic to social conduct. Thus, social organization is the product of social communication, rather than communication being a product of organization'.

So the narrative metaphor considers meaning as being coded in language, and therapy, therefore, involves working with language. The language used to describe problems, the terms used to describe the meanings attributed to important experiences, the words used to denote identities, as well as the meaning themselves, therefore constitute 'the stuff' of narrative work.

The work of Michael White & David Epston (1990) is a particular expression of the narrative metaphor. Narrative therapy, as it is known, is an elaborated method for working with narratives, central to which is the idea that identities are shaped by the narratives that hold sway in people's lives. These may be local narratives, for example, a view within a family of a member as a problem; these may be societal narratives, for example beliefs about gender roles. The critical issue for the narrative therapist is that the person in question has the opportunity to review these ways of interpreting their life and is able to call on alternative stories (additional sources of information or knowledge about their lives) that contribute to the development of a more affirming identity.

Thinking systemically

This admittedly brief account is set out as a tale of two metaphors to illustrate that, as an evolving body of knowledge, systemic theory comprises different sets of ideas, of rather different orders. One can describe the various process models as modernist projects, interested in developing adequate representations of the world. By contrast the narrative ideas have developed in the light of postmodern notions of the problems inherent in regarding the observer and the observed as separable.

One of the contemporary dilemmas for systemic theory is how to construe the relationship between these sets of ideas. Some take the view that the narrative developments render the insights and practices derived from the process paradigm redundant, or worse.

Glenn Larner (1995) proposes an (ironic) position of paramodern, within which the division into modern or postmodern can be resisted since 'the various perspectives in family therapy mark a difference and plurality rather than an opposition. All enrich our understanding and practice of "therapy" as a setting in life' (p.211). He later identifies this 'bring(ing) contradictory and opposing voices and perspectives into conversation' as part and parcel of systemic practice.

David Pocock offers a useful way of dealing with this dilemma with his 'better story position' which suggests regarding the explanations we develop, theoretical or clinical, as 'the best efforts, from different standpoints, at making sense of a real but never certain world' (Pocock, 1995: p. 160).

Evidence and systemic practice

In a recent article on evidence and family therapy, Glenn Larner wrote:

'While there is a wealth of outcome research showing that family therapy works, it remains on the margin of mainstream therapy and mental health practice. Until recently it has been difficult to satisfy 'gold standards' of randomised control research which require manualisation and controlled replication by independent investigators. This is because systemic family therapy is language-based, client-directed and focused on relational process rather than step-by-step operational techniques.' (Larner, 2004, p. 17)

Before going on to look at systemic theory in practice, the evidence that has a bearing on family therapy and systemic practice is considered. This brief discussion is not confined to family therapy research, since there is much of relevance to family therapy emerging from other fields. Nor is it confined to outcome research, important as that is, since there is much of value emerging from other kinds of research.

Outcome research

Larner was, effectively, replying to David Sackett, who wrote of evidence-based practice, that:

'It is when asking questions about therapy that we should try to avoid the non-experimental approaches, since these routinely lead to false positive conclusions about efficacy. Because the randomised trial, and especially the systematic review of several randomised trials, is so much more likely to inform us and so much less likely to mislead us, it has become the "gold standard" for judging whether a treatment does more good than harm.' (Sackett, *et al* 1996, p.72)

Sackett's proposition distils an interesting dilemma for systemic therapy and, perhaps, psychotherapy in general (see also Chapter 12). There are, at least, two strands in this, as Larner indicates. One is practical; that is the extent to which systemic therapy is amenable to the kinds of investigations that are central to outcome research. The second is of a different order, reflecting the lack of academic tradition and, even now, the lack of academic infrastructure and capacity within family therapy.

Projects such as the London Depression Intervention Trial (Leff *et al*, 2000), where systemic couple therapy proved as effective and more acceptable than antidepressants, in a randomised study (conspicuous as much for its rarity as its success), indicate that these issues can be addressed. So the demanding work of manualising systemic therapy, undertaken by Jones & Asen (2000) for that study, seems to beckon as one direction for systemic researchers who would develop the evidence base.

Addressing another of the traditionally confounding issues in a recent review, Alan Carr (2004) noted the emergence of meta-analytically supported treatments as a way of gathering sufficiently large numbers of subjects to demonstrate effect size.

Ivan Eisler (2003), who has consistently argued for systemic practitioners' engagement with all forms of research, recently reflected on whether the value of such studies might lie in helping to tease out the necessary components of effective interventions and the circumstances in which they have that effect. So while Carr (2004) was able to conclude from his review that 'there is good evidence for the efficacy of marital and family therapy with common child- and adult- focused problems' (p. 434), further research should allow that efficacy to be described increasingly specifically.

At present there is evidence for the role of family therapy as a treatment of choice in some circumstances, for example, for some adults with depression who are in couple relationships (Leff *et al*, 2003), or for young people with anorexia nervosa (Eisler *et al*, 2000). There is also evidence to support the role of family therapy as part of a coordinated multi-dimensional intervention, particularly in relation to young people with antisocial behaviour problems (Henggeler *et al*, 2003) and in relation to problem use of drugs and alcohol (Rowe & Liddle, 2003).

There are a number of other interventions of proven effectiveness which focus on changing interactions within close relationships, for example parent-training work (Webster-Stratton & Hammond, 1997) or family intervention in psychosis (Kuipers *et al*, 2002). These, and other interventions that derive from behavioural analyses of problems in relationships and behaviour, are important sources of information for all practitioners working with families.

Other research

The field of family therapy has long been crossed by research paths, stretching back to the work of Bateson and his colleagues at Palo Alto in California in the 1950s into communication patterns. It is beyond the scope of this discussion to consider this in any detail, but Dallos & Draper (2000) provide a good account. Rather, this is an opportunity to describe some current research as a way of illustrating the activity and breadth of the field. Three recent examples have been chosen which deal with language, processes of therapy and gender.

Charlotte Burck's work considers how 'living in several languages' influences the way that people experience themselves, their relationships and therapy. In her qualitative study of 24 adults living in Britain, none of whom had come to English as a first language, Burck noted that 'reflections on the difference their languages encoded provided a recontextualisation which generated new ideas and moved a story from blame towards curiosity' (Burck, 2004, p.333). This interesting work raises a number of implications for practice. For example, in therapeutic work with bilingual individuals and families it is possible that the particular meanings that come to the fore in therapy will be influenced by the language used. Burck (2004) concludes that 'if an individual and family can use all their languages within a therapeutic session, a context may be created in which their multiplicities, contradictions and loyalties will be helpfully explored' (p.335).

As indicated in earlier discussion, there is a long history in the systemic field of interest in matters of process. The discussion to date has illustrated this in relation to family functioning. But the issue of process of therapy is another rich area for study. Among recent projects that have looked at this are efforts to examine the exchanges within therapy in light of other well-researched models of relationships. So, for example, there is a considerable amount of research applying the precepts of attachment theory to such exchanges (for example, see, Fiese & Wamboldt, 2003; Dallos, 2004).

Another example is the study of processes of blaming using attribution theory. In his work, Peter Stratton describes a method for coding attributions in family sessions that provided 'an effective way of gaining insight into the habitual but sometimes unproductive explanations used by some families' (Stratton, 2003: p. 156). From this qualitative study he suggests 'it was possible to see how limited changes in these forms of attributions could convert them into more benign and productive contributions to the family discussion'.

The third illustration comes from a study that set out to examine the relationship between depression and power in partner relationships. Michael Byrne and his colleagues studied 20 couples where the female partner was depressed, comparing them with 20 couples where the female partner had a different, significant mental health problem (panic disorder), with a further 20 couples acting as a control group (Byrne *et al*, 2004). Using a number of pre-existing measures, this quantitative study considered how aspects of relationship power (expressed in terms of economic factors, gender roles, interpersonal violence and communication, among others) varied across the three groups. They reported that the results of the study 'underline the unique association between depression (as distinct from other psychological problems) within the long-term relationships and a sense of economic powerlessness on the part of depressed females and domestic violence within their relationships' (p.426).

Future research

As interest in research grows, as methodologies develop and discussion about the nature and uses of evidence moves on, the questions for family therapy are already moving away from narrow debates on 'does it work?'.

We can anticipate that further research will allow more clarity about the range of contributions that systemic therapy, alone and in combination, can make to the range of frequently complex dilemmas facing those who consult services. We should also anticipate further research that allows examination of the ways that dilemmas are embedded, not just in patterns of relationships, but also in the language used to voice and to address those dilemmas.

243

Finally, systemic therapy is one of a number of strands of practice where there is now a sustained effort to engage and involve those who consult services in commenting on their experience. David Campbell's description of the client's experience of therapy signals the potential for research becoming increasingly collaborative, with clients making a growing contribution to the learning process (Campbell, 1997).

Using systemic ideas in practice

Before going on to look at working with families, there are the wider applications of systemic theory to consider. As is already plain, this approach to practice proposes that the dilemmas our clients bring, the initiatives we develop and the arrangements we make to offer help are always part of a bigger picture. Even when our client's dilemmas can be described as 'schizophrenia' or 'depression' or 'chronic pain', relationship and other contextual issues continue to have a major bearing.

What does this mean in practice? No apology is made for proposing that such an approach should become more widely available, but this is not a plea for family therapy for everyone. It simply means that we should regard our client's problems in context and seek to work with them in that light. The following are examples.

Partners

When a woman who is in a partnership reports depression lasting for a period of time, it is important to consider her life circumstances, ask about her partnership and discuss with her whether joint work with her partner may be useful.

Parents

In those situations where there may not be a case for family therapy, it remains important to consider relationships. For example, advice and support for family members of a young man with schizophrenia is likely both to be helpful to them and to promote and sustain the best outcomes for him.

Children

We know that a substantial proportion of people who develop a significant mental health problem have dependent children, while a substantial proportion of children who develop mental health problems have parents who have mental health problems. This should prompt us to develop services that consider the needs of children of parents with mental illness as a matter of routine.

Teams

Mental health teams, even small ones, are typically complex groups. They have practitioners from different professional backgrounds, trained in different ways, who offer different skills. There are usually formal hierarchies as well as beliefs and assumptions about hierarchy to be found within them. They often have networks, rather than lines, of accountability.

They often work in demanding circumstances. Yet these groups are also the main professional context for developing and sustaining coherent identities, relevant skills and resilient processes.

Example: a dilemma of the kind that teams commonly encounter

Chris is a woman of 28 who has had several episodes of depression, including one that required compulsory admission to hospital. She has been living at home, supported by mental health services, and looking after her children, aged 6 and 7, on her own. The children had been looked after in foster care when Chris was in hospital.

Joan, a community psychiatric nurse who visits regularly, has noticed that Chris seems to have been tearful and increasingly short-tempered with the children when they come in from school. She arranges to visit Chris when the children are at school and asks if they might talk about what she has noticed. Chris tells Joan that she is feeling particularly depressed. She has not wanted to discuss it for fear that her children will be taken away from her.

When Joan raises this at the team meeting, there is disagreement about what to do. The social worker in the team says that he would like to visit to establish that the children are being well cared for. The psychiatrist argues that addressing the depression was the priority and that focusing on her parenting at this point may make Chris more depressed and increase the chances that she will become unable to care for her children.

In their attempts to be helpful to Chris, team members find themselves in conflict. Each response is understandable, but together present something of a dilemma for Joan. Rather than choosing between two conflicting options, Joan meets separately with each colleague to discuss the concerns and ideas that each had in mind. She then meets with Chris to discuss these ideas. In the event, both colleagues' suggestions have something to offer; thinking about how to support Chris and her children as a family would contribute to helping her to deal with her depression; addressing her depression would help her and her children.

One of the strengths of multidisciplinary and inter-agency working is the potential for building fuller and more useful descriptions of the dilemmas with which clients are struggling. Valuing difference and looking for ways to promote constructive coexistence of different perspectives is a foundational issue for teams. Beliefs about difference of view and how these are to be understood are a core element in systemic theory, while the capacity to engage in 'both/and' thinking, as well as 'either/or' approaches to problem solving, are a core feature of systemic practice.

In other words, as well as those occasions when direct family work is appropriate, there are many situations where systemic theory can offer useful perspectives for those using services and those providing services.

Meeting with families: things to do and say

Family therapy involves meeting with people as they look for more useful ways of managing the dilemmas in their lives. The work involved in that process requires a capacity to think systemically and the skills to translate that into practice. This section looks particularly at those skills, which range from very practical considerations to more particular matters of technique and application.

We begin by looking at basic steps for setting up and conducting a family meeting. Then we consider a wide range of skills associated with systemic therapy that are designed to support the development of curiosity and new ideas about the dilemmas facing family members.

Basic steps
Before the meeting

When meeting a family, some preparation is necessary. When considering who should be involved in the meeting, it is important to bear in mind the notion of families generating meanings in the context of their relationships: this suggests that the outcomes will be significantly influenced by who is involved in the process.

Whatever the decision, it should be clear from correspondence who is invited to attend. Where there are children in the family, some advanced discussion about whether they will join the meeting can be helpful.

If children will be there, the availability of developmentally appropriate play materials is important. A supply of large sheets of paper and marker pens helps when drawing up a genogram. If a one-way screen is to be used, it is worth checking that all the necessary equipment is available and working.

Start of the meeting

When family members arrive for a meeting, the usual concerns associated with attending a clinical setting are often compounded. There can be uncertainty about what happens in a family meeting and what will be expected of family members. Some family members may be experiencing difficult emotions, reflecting what is happening in the family; guilt, anger, anxiety and even apprehension about how family members will behave are common.

It is therefore important to offer a warm welcome to all of the members of the family group and, in the early part of the meeting, take the lead in negotiating the purpose of the meeting. This should be done in consultation with family members, including children, as far as they are able to contribute. It is also helpful to ask what members think about attending.

This is not an exhaustive account but is set out here to emphasise that while a well-crafted systemic formulation is important, some basic steps are necessary to set up a useful family meeting.

Systemic skills
Promoting communication

The practitioner wants to ensure that the developing discussion is informed by the views of all family members. It is important therefore that each has the opportunity to contribute. This means that the practitioner has to note how discussion proceeds, as well as what is said and, where family members are excluded or ignored, to act to include them in the discussion.

Example

When two members of a family become engaged in an intense exchange, it is often useful to invite other members present to talk to one another about their relationship with this discussion.

Similarly it can be helpful, when a family member has not come to a meeting, to ask, 'if he were here, what might he say about this?'

Family members communicating with one another is an important part of family therapy. As well as encouraging this interaction, the practitioner is interested in noting how family members go about this and, in particular, the extent to which communications are recognised and validated. This extends beyond the realm of what is said, to include non-verbal communication.

The beliefs which shape communication arise both in response to the unique experience of the particular family and also as a reflection of wider social and cultural attitudes. For example, drawing on the notion of voice, Lynn Hoffmann illustrates how beliefs about gender roles shape the communication, among family members and with the practitioner (Hoffmann, 1990).

Pace

It is important to pace the meeting in light of feedback from family members. As this example indicates, consulting family members about these judgements can be very helpful:

Example

Concern about 8-year-old John's behaviour had lead to him attending the local child and family psychiatric clinic, with his mother and sisters. As the members of the family began to talk about their concerns, the practitioner noted there were repeated references to the children's father having left the family home 9 months before.

When John's sister began to look particularly upset, the practitioner asked, 'I notice eyes filling with tears…is this a discussion you wish to continue?'

Family members looked at one another. John began nodding and others soon said that they did want to talk about this. Over the following period, they talked together, at times tearfully, of the different ways in which his departure had affected each of them.

Talking about problems

A meeting can take a systemic turn when the subject of the problem is raised. One member of the family might venture a view that the behaviour of another member of the family is 'the problem'. There are, of course, many ways to conduct a discussion in a clinical setting, but in contrast to a line of enquiry that seeks to elicit patterns of symptoms or behaviours, a systemic enquiry traces sequences and the perceptions and beliefs that inform them.

Example

A father points at each of his daughters in turn and says, 'her behaviour is not a problem, but hers is'. The systemic practitioner would usually decline any implicit invitation to construct an enquiry around the 'nominated' child's behaviours. Instead attention turns to how, within this family group, this picture has been developed, how it has been validated, challenged, transformed, and so on, in the course of that process. To do this, the practitioner involves others, at an early stage, inviting their descriptions and their views of each other's descriptions.

This process will, often, lead to a revision or unpicking or qualification of the initial account of the problem. With time and perseverance this can pave the way for the development of new, more fully negotiated, shared accounts of the dilemmas confronting family members.

This is an example of circularity, with the practitioner proceeding 'on the basis of feedback from the family in response to the information he solicits about relationships and, therefore, about difference and change'.

In other words, rather than following a prescribed menu of items, the themes emerge and evolve in light of the developing relationship between the practitioner and the family members.

Solutions, strengths and exceptions

Attention to the concerns of family members is important, as is developing systemic accounts of problems. But other issues are also important.

Identifying strengths such as generosity, compassion and patience, and acknowledging these is an important activity. It is very helpful for family members involved in reviewing and revising their accounts of their lives and experiences that they are able to recall, and call on, the strengths in their relationships.

Solution-focused ideas (deShazer, 1994) with their interest in identifying what is working well, and narrative therapy interest in exceptions, when the expected sequence or consequence did not materialise, help to draw attention to strengths and successes.

Externalising conversations

Michael White is particularly interested in the construction of identities that are dominated by problems (White & Epston, 1990). Narrative therapy makes use of externalising conversations to address this. The externalising conversation challenges the way that people's identities become subsumed by the problems they experience.

For example, embarking on an externalising conversation with a member of a family who is responding angrily to being referred to by others as a problem, might involve drawing attention to the difference between having a problem and being a problem, and then inviting discussion about those situations where the problem has more influence and those where it has less.

As well as being a useful technique, the externalising conversation also brings the underpinning values of narrative therapy into the process, in that it makes explicit the ways in which preferred identities have been marginalised by the effects of the problem, and offers the opportunity to construct these preferred identities.

Language

There is the matter of choosing language and forms of communication that are developmentally appropriate, particularly when young children are involved in the meeting. This can present difficulties, particularly for those practitioners with limited involvement with children. Asking other family members to act as consultants in tuning the meeting to a 'frequency' on which the children can contribute can be a very useful step.

It is important, particularly when meeting multi-lingual families, to work out how the discussion can be conducted so as to promote the inclusion of all family members present. At the very least, this acknowledges the risk of creating or perpetuating a hierarchy between languages. But, as Burck (2004) suggested, this can also open rich seams of experience, which are left out when the focus is on a single language.

In terms of the process metaphor, such attention to language is important, aside from courtesy and respect, because it promotes access to the family processes where the difficulties are encoded. But the narrative metaphor invites a different reading in which such steps are part of the fabric of a therapy where new narratives are storied through interaction with others.

This means that the way that issues are talked about is important. So, for example, suggesting that a practitioner takes care to use terms that are understood by other participants becomes an important indicator of what the practitioner proposes as the 'terms' of the therapeutic exchange.

For practitioners, and perhaps psychiatrists in particular, this raises interesting questions about the way that a diagnosis is incorporated into personal and family narratives. It is important, therefore, to track a diagnosis, that is, investigate its orientating powers. So, for example, consider how family members (and practitioners) use this idea to explain aspects of behaviour and relationships and shape expectations. Similarly, it can be useful to ask whether there are ways in which this diagnosis invites family members to make unhelpful use of its powers.

Reflecting processes

So far we have looked at how the practitioner, prompted by curiosity about alternative explanations, draws on a range of skills to enable family members to set out accounts of their lives and experiences. Family therapy also seeks to work with family members as they review and revise these into narratives that constitute a 'better story'. A development called the reflecting team illustrates one way of supporting this process. The first account of a reflecting team came from the work of Tom Andersen and his colleagues in Norway (Andersen, 1987).

In the context of live supervision, a standard practice within family therapy, Andersen noticed that their observations and suggestions were not being passed on to families by the trainee therapist. He therefore arranged that the family members and the therapist take a break and listen in together as the observing members of the team discuss their thoughts about the interview. Once this was finished, the family and their interviewer then discussed what they had heard (Andersen, 1987).

This was conceived of as a strategy to communicate to the family; family members reported that the approach was both acceptable and helpful. But Andersen records that they soon found some unintended effects. The usual aim of live supervision was to get a single, often layered, message across to family members; and this was Andersen's aim here too. But family members reported that what they found particularly useful was listening to the different views of team members as they reflected on the family's dilemmas.

In a sense this, almost accidental, development crystallises something about the shifts in systemic therapy. Not only were members of the therapy team 'showing their working', family members were explicitly free to choose the elements in the reflection that they found most useful for their particular situation.

We return to Anderson & Goolishian (1988: p. 383) who referred to the practitioner in this collaborative language-based approach as 'an architect of dialogue whose expertise is in creating a space for and facilitating a dialogical conversation'.

The practitioner interested in developing the capacity to support and promote the sense of space for reflection has to find ways of managing the sense, the urgency and impatience that family members at times bring into the therapeutic process. Throughout this account we refer to conceptual and practical steps that can help in this process.

Example

Claire, who is 8, and her sister Stephanie, who is 10, have lived with their foster carers, Anne and Bob, for 2 years. They came along to the clinic initially because Bob and Anne were concerned about the behaviour of Claire, who had been prescribed methylphenidate some months before.

Over the course of some weeks, discussion had focused on exploring the usefulness and the limits of the usefulness of the notion as Claire 'having attention-deficit hyperactivity disorder (ADHD)' and the concern about Claire's situation was now much reduced.

But in the course of these discussions, concern had increasingly focused on Stephanie. So much so that the practitioner had introduced the 'remote control' technique; that is offering Stephanie the facility to 'pause' the conversation when others have missed how it was affecting her.

Claire, who had participated in an externalising conversation about ADHD some weeks before, suggested doing 'that thing where you give the problem a name and then build a wall so that it can't get at you'. Stephanie clearly appreciated her sister's support but did not want to do that.

Bob confessed that he was unable to understand that, even after 2 years, Stephanie seemed unable to trust them. Anne turned to Stephanie and said 'it's as if you've never unpacked your bags since you came'. Stephanie was unsure how to respond to this but, noting them all puzzling to find a different meaning for their dilemma, the practitioner asked if he might have a conversation with his reflecting team.

The reflecting team format is particularly useful as a way of offering family members an opportunity to listen to a discussion about themselves without having to participate directly in it. On this occasion there were no available colleagues and so, with permission, the practitioner involved a team of puppets. Family members, already comfortable with playfulness, listened to the 'discussion'.

The 'team' spoke positively about the strengths the family members shared and offered to one another. A range of comments followed, touching on the position of each of the members of the household, exploring Stephanie's 'backpack' as a metaphor for their dilemma; how to create a narrative which accommodated all of their stories. In particular how could the girls' experiences, in an inner city area, exposed to drug problems and serious violence, become fully reflected in their story of their lives together in this very different social and cultural setting.

Prompted by the reflecting team comments, the girls began to talk about their previous life. Many of the 'facts' had been shared before but the position of other members had changed and Stephanie's 'backpack' now offered a new way of storying their evolving relationships.

This illustrates that new narratives evolve and emerge often via the development of provisional and transitional ideas, and that reflecting processes can provide space for investigating and developing these.

Reflection on things to do and say

The practitioner has travelled a long way in this section, from the modest beginnings, so to speak, figuring out the number of chairs needed, to Anderson & Goolishian's notion of 'architect of dialogue'.

The journey between these two positions necessarily involves identifying and practising these and other skills. The path sketched here takes in skills from process-based approaches, from narrative approaches and beyond, reflecting a view that 'family therapists remain open to and interested in all metaphors for change, while cognizant of their limitations, excesses and risks' (Lamer, 1995, p. 213).

Working with families: building therapeutic relationships

The relationship between family members and systemic therapists was not much discussed before the mid-1990s (Flaskas & Perlesz, 1996).

Speed (1996) suggests that preoccupation with complex technique and the emphasis on teamworking may have contributed to this being the case among Milan model practitioners. She reports that 'on the whole, as evidenced by their writings at least, many family therapists were not relating to clients…on a basis of intimacy and engagement of feelings' (p. 111). And it is true that many of the early accounts of family therapy emphasised what the therapist was doing, from the inventive manoeuvring of the structural therapist (Minuchin, 1974) to the creative ideas of the strategic therapist (Haley, 1976).

Collaboration

In their discussion of an ethical basis for systemic practice, Inger & Inger (1994: p. 18) argued that a commitment to introducing change, which they reported as the dominant culture in early family therapy, led to therapists being wedded to change at the expense of 'respect for the lifelong struggles of individuals'.

In parallel with other shifts described in this account, there has been a move towards working in ways that are more explicitly collaborative. Collaboration is a property of relationships and the term denotes the approach that the practitioner brings to the relationships she/he seeks to develop as a basis for therapeutic work.

It does not mean that the people consulted have to be willing to work or ready to agree with the practitioner in the first instance. It does mean that if someone is uncertain, or perhaps even hostile to the idea of meeting, the practitioner will look for ways of discussing those concerns in the hope of finding some agreed way to proceed.

Indeed, useful therapeutic work can sometimes proceed in circumstances that might at first appear unpromising, given careful attention to getting the context right. Arlene Vetere & Jan Cooper (2003) offer a good example of this approach in their work on domestic violence. Here they offer therapeutic work that is legally sanctioned but also negotiated with the participants to ensure the appropriate supports and safeguards are in place.

In practice, the practitioner takes steps towards a collaborative relationship by being willing to negotiate the purpose of meeting, the structure of work together, the handling of information and so on. Problems in maintaining a collaborative relationship then become a matter for discussion, since this is part of the fabric of therapy.

Limits to collaboration

There are occasions, however, when the practitioner needs to step out of collaborative mode. One is where the risk of violence emerges in a session. Another is where it becomes apparent that one member of the household is abusing another, for example, where one partner is being violent towards another or an adult is sexually abusing a child in the family.

While a detailed discussion of these difficult situations is beyond the scope of this chapter, there are some important principles to bear in mind. The first is that it is neither feasible nor appropriate to try to work therapeutically with a person who is in danger from a member of their family. The second is that practitioners have a responsibility to take action when children are at risk.

Challenging these issues will usually create conflict. Some, occasionally most, members of a family might argue that the victim is telling lies, that the practitioner is misinterpreting innocent activities, or perhaps, that therapy can sort this problem out. There may also be disagreement among colleagues about how to respect the principle of confidentiality.

While guidance is now completely unambiguous about the child's right to protection, the situation presents one of the most testing moments for any professional. Contact with the local child protection service is mandatory in such circumstances, while early consultation with an experienced colleague is strongly advised.

Authority, safety and certainty

The earlier description of collaborative practice refers to practitioners using their authority in ways that are qualitatively different from that which is evident in the early accounts of family therapy. In this account, a practitioner who is willing to negotiate the therapeutic 'contract' is effectively taking a stance in relation to her/his own authority, choosing not to assert that the professional view is pre-eminent in all matters.

Researchers Carolyn Taylor & Susan White (2000) provide an interesting discussion of professional authority in health and welfare services generally, based on their study of transcriptions of exchanges between clients and professionals. They reported that the aims of these client–professional exchanges were seldom made explicit and that the process was seldom negotiated. This, in their view, shaped the roles available to the participants.

In narrative terms, we construct our roles by the language we use, an important perspective, if we are interested in family members acting as creative participants in the therapeutic process. This timely research suggests that professional training might usefully involve both the accumulation of knowledge and learning how to negotiate its appropriate use within the client–professional relationship.

Such a stance is, of course, not without its challenges, and so versions of the client–professional relationship that afford practitioners some comfortable certainty have their appeal. Barry Mason calls this 'unsafe certainty' and suggests that it is of limited value in therapeutic work. He describes the more open collaborative stance, 'safe uncertainty', where the practitioner acknowledges and takes responsibility for the extent of, but also the limits of her/his own knowledge (Mason, 1993).

In this scenario, the practitioner's knowledge and experience is a resource for the therapeutic endeavour. But there are other resources, in the form of knowledge and experience that family members bring.

In practice, then, a practitioner might call on a robust knowledge base that confirms that loud arguments between parents in front of children are very likely to create significant difficulties for the children or that a harsh or critical family atmosphere greatly increases the risk of a person with a schizophrenic illness becoming unwell. Such knowledge is a useful resource for family members and should be shared with them. However, in many instances the practitioner does well to encourage curiosity among family members and invite them to consider how they might bring their own knowledge and experience to bear on the dilemmas they face. Mason suggests that such a position helps to foster curiosity in therapeutic work.

There is some resonance between Mason's ideas and John Byng-Hall's application of concepts from attachment theory to work with families. Byng-Hall (1995) conceptualised the therapeutic context as a secure base: the metaphor that Mary Ainsworth (1967) used for the kind of care-giving relationship that fosters a child's creative and confident exploration of the environment. Byng-Hall concluded that 'the overall aim of therapy is to establish a secure family base from which the family can explore new solutions to family problems both during and after therapy' (p. 45).

The contribution of the problem

So far we have considered the part played by practitioners' preferred ways of working on the shape of the therapeutic relationship. We turn now to consider how the issues with which clients are dealing influence matters.

Considering the client–practitioner relationship in his tellingly titled *Terrors and Experts*, contemporary psychoanalytic writer Adam Phillips suggests that certain dilemmas, for example anxiety, tend to cast the helping relationship in terms of client and expert. He proposes the importance of recognising that process and suggests that the work of resisting that 'invitation' is a core part of the therapeutic process (Phillips, 1997).

In trauma organised systems, Arnon Bentovim (1992) talks about sexual abuse having long-term organising effects on the functioning of individuals and their relationships. In practice this means that it is useful, when reflecting on the way that the relationship systems are working for a particular client or family, to consider how the dilemmas that led them to seek consultation might be contributing to the shape that those relationships are taking.

Creativity in the therapeutic relationship

Throughout the history of family therapy, there has been evidence of much creativity. In common with our earlier observations in this section, the accounts have been particularly focused on the therapist and the therapeutic team as the source of creativity.

The practitioner's capacity for creative thinking is important. This seems much in keeping with what Gianfranco Cecchin (1987: p. 405) had in mind when he proposed that, in approaching the family's stories, the practitioner adopt a state of curiosity that 'leads to exploration and invention of alternative views and moves, and different moves and views breed curiosity'.

In this account we have described an approach to therapeutic work that invites family members to become curious about their situation. One of Cecchin's later ideas (1992), reminding us that the Milan model explored the logic of current patterns, was that practitioners consider a stance of irreverence towards the explanations and beliefs family members hold about their situation, as a step towards considering alternative explanations.

The value of this sense of playfulness is something which Jim Wilson (1998: p. 7) takes further, 'this (state of play) is a domain in which alternative ideas may be explored and experienced. Without playfulness in this sense, no change is likely to occur'.

This playfulness is not to be confused with a lack of seriousness of purpose, just as irreverence is not to be confused with a lack of respect for the dilemmas and the clients who bring them. The purpose here is to create a context that will allow consideration of alternative explanations, as part of the process of developing a 'better story'.

Example

Joyce is 39 and has been attending therapy for 4 weeks, having been referred because of persisting feelings of depression. She has spoken several times about arguments at home, both with her husband, Joe, and teenage daughter, Lisa.

Having noticed these names coming up repeatedly, the practitioner asked whether she might like to invite others to attend. Joyce was initially apprehensive about this, saying that 'Joe doesn't like to talk about things'. However in the conversation so far, she has become more interested in the connection between her depressed mood and her relationships and decides that she would like to invite Joe, in the first instance.

In the first meeting with both, Joe says that he is not sure that this contact is helping Joyce, adding, 'talking only makes her worse'. Joyce has become quieter as the meeting progresses.

The practitioner has a dilemma; wishing to treat Joe's views seriously but wondering about the coincidence of Joyce falling quiet. He considers pointing out the research evidence about the effectiveness of couple work in depression, but judges this offers unsafe certainty.

While he is considering asking Joe to talk about a time when he has found talk between them useful, Joyce says that she thinks Joe is trying to protect her. They go on to talk about Joe's role in the months after their first child was born when Joyce had become depressed.

That narrative of care and protection reflected Joe's experience in his own family, where his mother experienced violence at his father's hands. Joyce's dilemma was that as she now began to review her own life story (less child-care demands meaning a better job opportunity) the gender roles which may have fitted their relationship in earlier years were no longer working well for her.

Themes for practitioners

This discussion of family therapy and systemic practice has referred to several routes by which professional practice develops. As well as engagement with the continuously evolving professional literature, the process of reflexivity provides continuous feedback about one's theories and practices. But in this section we briefly review some specific activities that promote learning and facilitate professional development within systemic practice.

Formulation

It is important that the practitioner has a way of managing the information which emerges from meeting with a family. The use of formulation within systemic practice might appear to be at odds with a therapeutic process designed to encourage family members to review and develop their own explanations of their experiences. But by distilling her or his ideas into a systemic formulation, the practitioner is essentially developing a summary of what she or he understands as the best explanation so far available of the presenting dilemmas. This is an important process, given the amount and range of information that emerges in the course of a family session. Practising formulation is a step towards familiarity and confidence with the key concepts of systemic theory.

Froma Walsh (2002) suggests that 'a family time line and a genogram are essential tools' (p.131) in developing a formulation. A family time line, as the name suggests, is simply a graphical representation of historical events in chronological order. A genogram (McGoldrick *et al*, 1999) is a systematic method for drawing a family tree which graphically represents issues of life cycle and family history. Many practitioners invite families to construct a genogram as part of their clinical work, finding that the process of doing this often allows richer accounts of family heritage, traditions, losses and affiliations to emerge and contribute to the process of reviewing and revising current family narratives. A genogram can also serve as an aide to curiosity, prompting ideas and suggesting new questions.

There are a number of ways of constructing a formulation. Alan Carr (2000) has developed a particularly comprehensive model that incorporates:

- a description of the dilemmas set within the current pattern of relationships
- a description of processes and narratives that inform these patterns
- an account of the contexts that have shaped these processes and narratives.

Carr's (2000) model facilitates the use of multiple modes of explanation and, as such, is particularly for use in training.

The practitioner's own stories

A further important development within the past 10 years has been attention to the ways in which the personal and professional development of the practitioner interacts with the course of therapy. Family therapy involves the deployment of a range of therapeutic skills, but important as those are, it is also important to appreciate that working systemically goes beyond developing an account of the dilemmas presented by a family and matching up a set of interventions. In this respect, family therapy is a psychotherapy, that is an endeavour grounded in human relations and depending, for its usefulness, on the willingness of those participating to identify ways to engage that are personally meaningful.

This recent interest has some resonance with the psychoanalytic themes of transference and countertransference (see earlier Chapters 2, 3 & 4), and indeed there have been numerous papers over this time discussing this (for example, see Donovan, 2003). Furthermore, there are practices in family therapy training, such as constructing a personal genogram or identifying 'trigger' families whose histories present particular challenges, which bear scrutiny as analogous developments.

However, the systemic approach to this issue, again reflecting the impact of social constructionist ideas, has been to consider the practitioner's preferred theories, and the related practices, in a systemic light (Hedges & Lang, 1993). The term self-reflexivity is a shorthand way of describing this work that involves looking at how these matters have been informed and shaped. How best to enable this process is a leading question in systemic training in the UK at present. Most courses currently provide opportunities to reflect on personal and family experiences, local and wider cultural beliefs and traditions, professional history and professional traditions, among others. But generally speaking, in contrast with analytical psychotherapy, personal therapy is not part of that training process.

A further useful development of the application of genograms came when Hardy & Laszloffy (1995) published their account of the cultural genogram. By illustrating cultural backgrounds in the genogram, additional stories, in particular, of migration and acculturation become more explicit.

The cultural genogram is a useful addition to the process of training culturally sensitive practitioners. Systemic therapy is explicitly committed to anti-oppressive practice and all professionally approved family therapy training in the UK involves engaging with this agenda.

Supervision

Case discussion

As with other forms of psychotherapy, case discussion is widely used in family therapy. Case discussion is a particularly useful forum for considering conceptual aspects of working with families, for example developing hypotheses, reviewing formulation, discussing family process, identifying individual and family narratives.

Video review

Regular review of video recordings of family meetings acts as a very useful learning device. Watching with the remote control in hand, the practitioner pauses the tape regularly to ask, 'what is happening now?' and 'what else might have been said or done at this point?'.

This is a useful process done alone, with a supervisor or with a group, with each arrangement offering different advantages. In all cases, this is a particularly useful medium for reviewing practical skills and the choice and wording of questions.

Live consultation

Live consultation has, historically, been a hallmark of family therapy, and remains a central component of supervision and training, as well as clinical practice. There are a number of ways of conducting this, and while the one-way screen is often involved, it is by no means essential. When appropriately negotiated with family members, it is possible to arrange that a colleague act as an observer, with or without a screen.

The process of the colleague reflecting on their observations can be organised in a number of ways, according to the task, with the main distinction being whether this happens in the presence of family members. For example, the observer can share the experience of the meeting with the family, thus offering alternative feedback and explanations for them to consider. The presence of two or more colleagues observing opens the possibility of conducting the feedback in the format of a reflecting team, as described earlier.

One of the great strengths of live consultation is its utility in training. The observing team can often help with early identification of dilemmas emerging in the session; accordingly many practitioners in training soon find live supervision more valuable than daunting. The supervisor, meanwhile, is able to ensure that the family's need of a good service and the trainee's need to learn are balanced.

Family therapy training

The nationally recognised family therapy training is an academic and clinical course, typically approved at Masters level, usually taken over 4 years. Graduates of courses accredited by the professional body, the Association for Family Therapy and Systemic Practice (for further information see http://www.aft.org.uk), become eligible for professional registration with the UK Council of Psychotherapy. Most graduates go on to work as professional family therapists, with a growing number employed in the public sector. There are, however, those, such as psychiatrists, who retain their primary professional identity, with their systemic psychotherapy training serving as an important additional context.

Many more practitioners undertake part-time courses over 1 or 2 years, which allows them to add a systemic dimension to their practice.

Systemic training has attained more prominence within psychiatric training over recent years. In particular, higher trainees in psychotherapy now study systemic psychotherapy and have the option of choosing this as their 'major' subject.

Conclusion

This chapter has offered an account of systemic theory, proposing its usefulness both in the particular setting of family therapy, and more widely within the fields of health, mental health and psychotherapy practice.

It proposes that practitioners investigating systemic ideas have an opportunity to enhance their practice, but equally importantly, to engage with a body of knowledge and practice that offers significant opportunities for professional development.

References

Ainsworth, M. D. S. (1967) *Infancy in Uganda. Infant Care and the Growth of Love*. Baltimore: John Hopkins University Press.

Andersen, T. (1987) The reflecting team: dialogue and meta-dialogue in clinical work. *Family Process*, **26**, 415–428.

Anderson, H. & Goolishian, H. (1988) Human systems as linguistic systems: preliminary and evolving ideas about the implications for clinical theory. *Family Process*, **27**, 371–393.

Bateson, G. (1972) *Steps to an Ecology of Mind*. London: Paladin.

Bateson, G., Jackson, D., Haley, J., *et al* (1956) Towards a theory of schizophrenia. *Behavioral Science*, **1**, 251–264.

Bentovim, A. (1992) *Trauma Organised Systems*. London: Karnac.

Burck, C. (1997) Language and narrative: learning from bilingualism. In *Multiple Voices: Narrative in Systemic Family Psychotherapy* (eds R. Papadopoulos & J. Byng-Hall), pp. 64–85. London: Duckworth.

Burck, C. (2004) Living in several languages: implications for therapy. *Journal of Family Therapy*, **26**, 314–339.

Byng-Hall, J. (1995) Creating a secure family base: some implications of attachment theory for family therapy. *Family Process*, **34**, 45–58.

Byrne, M., Carr, A. & Clark, M. (2004) Power and relationships of women with depression. *Journal of Family Therapy*, **26**, 407–430.

Campbell, D. (1997) The other side of the picture. In *Multiple Voices: Narrative in Systemic Psychotherapy* (eds R. Papadopoulos & J. Byng-Hall), pp. 15–40. London: Duckworth.

Carr, A. (2000) *Family Therapy: Concepts, Process and Practice*. London: Wiley.

Carr, A. (2004) Thematic review of family therapy journals in 2003. *Journal of Family Therapy*, **26**, 430–445.

Cecchin, G. (1987) Hypothesising, circularity, neutrality revisited: an invitation to curiosity. *Family Process*, **26**, 405–413.

Cecchin, G. (1992) *Irreverence: A Strategy for Therapists' Survival*. London: Karnac.

Dallos, R. (2004) Attachment narrative therapy: integrating ideas from narrative and attachment theory in systemic family therapy with eating disorders. *Journal of Family Therapy*, **26**, 40–65.

Dallos, R. & Draper, R. (2000) *An Introduction to Family Therapy*. Buckingham: Open University Press.

deShazer, S. (1994) *Words Were Originally Magic*. New York: Norton.

Donovan, M. (2003) Mind the gap: the need for a generic bridge between psychoanalytic and systemic approaches. *Journal of Family Therapy*, **25**, 115–131.

Eisler, I. (2003) Why talking (and listening) is better than trying to build bridges. *Journal of Family Therapy*, **25**, 436–442.

Eisler, I., Dare, C., Hodes, M., *et al* (2000) Family therapy for adolescent anorexia nervosa: the results of a controlled comparison of two family interventions. *Journal of Child Psychology and Psychiatry*, **41**, 727–736.

Fiese, B. & Wamboldt, F. (2003) Use of attachment theory to inform a study of coherence of accounts of coping with chronic illness. *Family Process*, **42**, 439–457.

Flaskas, C. & Perlesz, A. (1996) *The Therapeutic Relationship in Systemic Therapy*. London: Karnac.

Haley, J. (1976) *Problem Solving Therapy*. New York: Jossey Bass.

Hardy, K. & Laszloffy, T. (1995). The cultural genogram: key to training culturally competent family therapists. *Journal of Marital and Family Therapy*, **21**, 227–237.

Hawley, D. & De Haan, L. (1996) Towards a definition of family resilience: integrating life-span and family perspectives. *Family Process*, **35**, 283–298.

Hedges, F. & Lang, S. (1993) Mapping personal and professional stories. The personal development of psychotherapy trainees: contributions from within a social constructionist discourse. *Human Systems*, **4**, 277–298.

Henggeler, S. & Sheidow, A. (2003) Conduct disorder and delinquency. *Journal of Marital and Family Therapy*, **29**, 505–522.

Hoffmann, L. (1990) *Exchanging Voices: A Collaborative Approach to Family Therapy*. London: Karnac.

Inger, I. & Inger, J. (1994) *Creating an Ethical Position in Family Therapy*. London: Karnac.

Jones, E. & Asen, E. (2000) *Systemic Couple Therapy and Depression*. London and New York: Karnac.

Kuipers, L., Leff, J. & Lam, D. (2002) *Family Work for Schizophrenia: A Practical Guide*. London: Gaskell.

Larner, G. (2004) Family therapy and the politics of evidence. *Journal of Family Therapy*, **26**, 17–39.

Larner, G. (1995) The real as illusion: deconstructing power in therapy. *Journal of Family Therapy*, **17**, 191–218.

Leff, J., Vearnals, S., Brewin, C. R., *et al* (2000) The London Depression Intervention Trial. Randomised controlled trial of antidepressants v. couple therapy in the treatment and maintenance of people with depression living with a partner: Clinical outcome and costs. *British Journal of Psychiatry*, **177**, 95–100.

Leff, J., Alexander, B., Asen, E., *et al* (2003) Modes of action of family interventions in depression and schizophrenia: the same or different? *Journal of Family Therapy*, **25**, 357–370.

Mason, B. (1993) Towards positions of safe uncertainty. *Human Systems*, **4**, 189–200.

McGoldrick, M., Gerson, R., Shellenberger, S., *et al* (1999) *Genograms: Assessment and Interventions* (2nd edn). New York: Norton.

Minuchin, S. (1974) *Families and Family Therapy*. London: Tavistock.

Phillips, A. (1997) *Terrors and Experts*. London: Faber & Faber.

Pocock, D. (1995) Searching for a better story: harnessing modern and postmodern positions in family therapy. *Journal of Family Therapy*, **17**, 149–174.

Rowe, C. & Liddle, H. (2003) Substance abuse. *Journal of Marital and Family Therapy*, **29**, 86–120.

Sackett, D. L., Rosenberg, W. M., Gray, J. A., *et al* (1996) Evidence-based medicine: what it is and what it isn't. *BMJ*, **312**, 71–72.

Selvini, M. P., Boscolo, L., Cecchin, G., *et al* (1980) Hypothesizing, circularity, neutrality: three guidelines for the conductor of the session. *Family Process*, **19**, 3–12.

Speed, B. (1996) You cannot not relate. In *The Therapeutic Relationship in Systemic Therapy* (eds C. Flaskas & A. Perlesz), pp.108–124. London: Karnac.

Stratton, P. (2003) Causal attributions during therapy I: responsibility and blame. *Journal of Family Therapy*, **25**, 136–160.

Taylor, C. & White, S. (2000) *Practising Reflexivity in Health and Welfare*. Guildford: Open University Press.

Vetere, A. & Cooper, J. (2003) Setting up a domestic violence service. *Child and Adolescent Mental Health*, **8**, 61–67.

Walsh, F. (1993) Conceptualisations of normal family processes. In *Normal Family Processes* (2nd edn), (ed. F. Walsh), pp. 3–69. London: Guilford Press.

Walsh, F. (2002) A family resilience approach: innovative practice applications. *Family Relations*, **51**, 130–137.

Walsh, F. (2003) Family resilience: a framework for clinical practice. *Family Process*, **42**, 1–18.

Webster Stratton, C. & Hammond, M. (1997) Treating children with early onset conduct problems. *Journal of Consulting and Child Psychology*, **65**, 93–109.

White, M. & Epston, D. (1990) *Narrative Means to Therapeutic Ends*. London: Norton.

Wilson, J. (1998) *Child-Focused Practice: A Collaborative Systemic Approach*. London: Karnac.

CHAPTER 12

Research in psychotherapy*

Anthony Bateman

Many people believe that psychotherapy is inherently 'unresearchable' and that there is little evidence-base for its efficacy. The primary aim of this chapter is to refute such assumptions and to illustrate Howard *et al*'s (1995: p. 4) statement that psychotherapy 'is the best documented medical intervention in history'. It is not possible in a brief chapter to cover comprehensively all the research on the different models of psychotherapy. Roth & Fonagy (1996) have ably done this in terms of the evidence-base for effectiveness of different models in various psychiatric disorders. The secondary aim here is to steer the reader through the complexities of psychotherapy research and to demonstrate that psychotherapy is not only eminently researchable but also well advanced in its methods. In fact, it is more advanced and takes more care of the detail of research than many other areas of medicine, including biological psychiatry.

There is a tension in psychotherapy research between quantification of change on the one hand and meaning of psychotherapeutic process on the other. Some psychotherapies, for example cognitive–behavioural therapy (CBT) and interpersonal therapy, have embraced quantification with enthusiasm, while others, such as psychoanalytic psychotherapy, have clung steadfastly to establishing the meaning of change. Some psychoanalytic psychotherapists have even argued that 'scientific' research is either not an appropriate paradigm with which to investigate psychoanalytic psychotherapy or that it is so intrusive that the therapy itself is compromised (Steiner, 1985). This has led to a reliance on single case studies as evidence of efficacy for psychoanalytic therapy, although this situation is rapidly changing. Whatever the type of psychotherapy, the task of good research is to steer a course between quantification and meaning, ensuring that aspects of treatment that really matter to practitioners are taken into account while remaining true to the scientific endeavour.

---

*Part of this chapter is adapted from Margison & Bateman (2006) by permission of Oxford University Press.

An evidence-based approach

Fundamentally an evidence-base implies that the value of an intervention can be judged by its consequences. Therapy is only any good if a patient gets better. But such a stark and unrefined approach has a number of problems for psychotherapy research.

First, it tells us nothing about how a patient gets better. Only process and process–outcome research can answer this question in any detail. Process research is designed to identify the critical ingredients of therapy and the mechanisms of change in order to increase our understanding of human change processes, improve the delivery of therapy, and to maximise treatment efficacy. In addition, process–outcome research yields data that is meaningful to practitioners and may influence how therapists practice.

Second, there is difficulty in agreeing meaningful measures of outcome that accurately reflect improvement. Psychotherapy is an elaborate intervention and is rarely used to target symptoms alone, although this may be the case in some behavioural treatments. The tendency can be to over-simplify problems. For example depression is reduced to a score on the Beck Depression Inventory (BDI) (Beck *et al*, 1961) or the Hamilton Rating Scale (Hamilton, 1960) and these measures are conflated with the illness itself. Improvement on the scales then equates with good outcome. But the measures are not the illness and neither represent the complexity and heterogeneity of depression nor give any indication of change in an individual's life. To circumvent this problem researchers have, more recently, used batteries of measures looking at different domains such as interpersonal function and social adjustment, as well as at symptoms.

Third, symptomatic improvement alone may be a poor measure of the benefit of a treatment. A good outcome may be illustrated by the fact that the patient did not commit suicide or can manage more complex social situations. These may be important effects of therapy albeit difficult to measure.

Finally it needs to be decided who is the arbiter of outcome. Is it the therapist, the patient, or an independent observer, for example, or is it all three? Most research introduces an independent researcher but this in itself is not a neutral phenomenon. Such an 'Oedipal' procedure may have both conscious and unconscious reverberations. Some patients may like seeing the researcher and do their best to please him; others may want to spoil the research and so deliberately mark questionnaires negatively and so on. Patient satisfaction as outcome has become increasingly important. Long-term therapy does well in this regard. The Consumer Reports study (Seligman, 1995), based on self-report, concluded that long-term therapy worked better than short-term therapy, and that treatment satisfaction was high. But patient satisfaction alone is not an acceptable measure of outcome even though it may be superficially attractive. Patients may like all sorts of inappropriate treatments for a variety of reasons or simply because they are pleasurable.

Methodology

A major problem for evaluating evidence for the usefulness of psychotherapy is the gap between 'efficacy' and 'effectiveness'. Efficacy of treatment refers to the results that are achieved in carefully designed trials. Efficacy trials are designed to maintain internal validity so that causal inferences can be made. As many factors as possible are controlled so that the major variable is the intervention itself. In this way any measured change is likely to be a consequence of the treatment rather than a result of another factor such as passage of time. But too great an emphasis on internal validity compromises external validity and treatment found to be efficacious in carefully defined conditions may not generalise to everyday clinical practice. In general, interventions that are found to be efficacious in research trials are less effective when studied in normal clinical populations. This has led to calls for more 'effectiveness' research, i.e. how therapy performs within hard-pressed clinical services with few fully trained staff. It is probably true to say that the schism between efficacy and effectiveness studies and internal and external validity respectively is overstated; all research is a compromise.

In fact all research goes through different stages, conceptualised as an 'hourglass' model by Salkovskis (1995). Initially clinicians work with individual patients conducting 'messy' research, refining theoretical views and trying out different strategies. This gradually becomes more refined. Patients are more carefully selected, protocols defining interventions are developed, and the culture becomes purer. Carefully conducted trials are implemented and used to inform further strategies and there may even be a need to return to the beginning to refine further the treatment. The model is not sequential but dynamic with each area informing others. In essence different psychotherapies are at different stages and psychodynamic therapy is working hard to catch up in some areas even though it is quite refined in process research (see later).

Single case studies

Single case studies may be descriptive or quantitative. While descriptive cases help an understanding of complex unconscious processes, any interpretation and generalisation of the findings is limited since interventions have a range of specific and non-specific effects and there is no contrasting intervention. However, quantitative single case studies do not suffer from these problems. Appropriate baseline measures may be taken and interventions given or withdrawn in an organised manner and the effects monitored. The patient acts as his own control. This has been used both in CBT and in psychoanalytic therapy. An example of the process in CBT is summarised by Salkovskis (1995) who developed a theoretically driven approach for treatment of panic disorder. In psychoanalytic research, Moran and Fonagy (Fonagy *et al*, 1987) followed the progress of an analysis in a 13-year-old diabetic girl, using blood sugar readings as a marker of the state of her internal world and relating these to the analyst's detailed session recordings. Using the statistical technique of 'lag correlation', they showed that there was a temporal relationship between the interpretation of Oedipal conflicts and the emergence of better diabetic control. They argue that findings such as these help to counter Grunbaum's (Grunbaum, 1986) claim that psychoanalysis is based on 'suggestion', since the analyst was ignorant of, and made no reference to, the state of the patient's diabetic control.

Such single case designs are important and should not be dismissed. When replicated across randomly sampled cases they have excellent generalisability, particularly about the effectiveness of an intervention on specific symptoms. However, until recently psychodynamic psychotherapy was reliant on descriptive single case studies that have been rich in clinical detail but of limited use in terms of understanding how effective the treatment is. Psychodynamic therapists have been severely criticised for this on the basis that knowledge gleaned from single case studies is less valid and less generalisable than that obtained from groups of individuals. There is some truth in this criticism.

Cohort studies

Cohort studies reflect a naturalistic approach to a group of patients undergoing treatment and have been used more commonly to investigate dynamic therapies than cognitive, systemic or other treatments, partly because dynamic therapies have tended to be longer-term. Patients may have to fit strict criteria to enter the trial but there is no control group, although some studies use a comparison group. As a result any change may be an effect of other factors such as passage of time. However if a cohort of patients is large enough, it is possible to draw conclusions about the relative value of a treatment. This method has been used particularly in the study of effectiveness of services treating individuals with personality disorder over the longer-term (Rosser et al, 1987; Najavits & Gunderson, 1995; Blatt, 1996, 1998; Dolan et al, 1997).

A mixed approach has been taken more recently using cohorts of patients who are allocated to different psychotherapeutic treatments non-randomly but on another basis such as domicile. The relative effectiveness of three psychodynamically-oriented treatment models for a mixed group of personality disorders was studied in this way:

- long-term residential treatment using a therapeutic community approach
- briefer in-patient treatment followed by community-based dynamic therapy (step-down programme)
- general community psychiatric treatment.

Results suggest that the brief in-patient therapeutic community treatment followed by out-patient dynamic therapy is more effective than both long-term residential therapeutic community treatment and general psychiatric treatment in the community on most measures including self-harm, attempted suicide, and readmission rates to general psychiatric admission wards and more cost-effective (Chiesa *et al*, 2002). Follow-up at 36 months has confirmed that patients in the step-down programme continued to show significantly greater improvement than the in-patient group on social adjustment and global assessment of mental health. In addition they were found to self-mutilate, attempt suicide, and be readmitted significantly less at 24- and 36-month follow-up (Chiesa & Fonagy, 2003).

In another interesting field study, the Stockholm Outcome of Psychotherapy and Psychoanalysis Project (Blomberg *et al*, 2001; Sandell *et al*, 2002), 405 patients in psychoanalysis or psychoanalytic psychotherapy were compared. The groups were matched on many clinical variables and followed for up to 3 years after treatment. Outcome was similar at the end of treatment irrespective of whether the patient received sessions 4 or 5 times or once or twice a week. But at 3-year follow-up of 156 patients, psychotherapy patients did not change further; yet those who received psychoanalysis continued to improve almost to the point at which their scores were indistinguishable from a non-clinical sample. This suggests that rehabilitative changes were stimulated in patients who received high-duration/high frequency treatment. Few other therapies can boast either such long-term follow-up or evidence for increasingly positive effects over time and there is increasing evidence that dynamic therapies are associated with rehabilitative change.

Despite the useful information that may be derived from both single case and cohort studies and their ease of implementation, greater emphasis has been given to the randomised controlled trial (RCT) which, in some ways but not others, is a more refined element of the 'hourglass'.

Randomised controlled trial

The application of the RCT to psychotherapy research is deceptively simple if the paradigm of biological research is followed. This is known as the 'drug metaphor'. A homogeneous group of patients with a specific problem are allocated randomly to different treatments. Skilled therapists deliver interventions in a pure and measurable form and in a specific dose (for example, 16 sessions) and outcome is reliably measured. This is seen as the gold standard for assessment of a treatment and has been more widely used in CBT and interpersonal therapy than dynamic and other therapies.

The other important distinction in determining the value of an intervention is whether its value has been demonstrated in standard practice rather than under strict experimental conditions. This distinction was first highlighted by Schwarz & Lellouch (1967) in discussing differences between randomised trials and is commonly described as the difference between an explanatory trial, i.e. a trial in which treatments are compared under ideal (experimentally manipulated) conditions, and a pragmatic trial. In a pragmatic trial the study is carried out under the conditions normally appertaining to ordinary practice in which possible confounders to the intervention may be present and which, although they can be removed, doing so creates an artificial environment that does not allow the results to be transferred to ordinary practice. Schwarz & Lellouch showed that the results of these trials could be very different even though the treatments under test were the same. In evidence-based psychiatry, as previously mentioned, these are sometimes described as trials of efficacy (explanatory) and effectiveness (pragmatic). Each has its advantages and disadvantages but in general it is common to establish efficacy under controlled conditions first before testing an intervention in conditions of ordinary practice.

Perfect implementation of an RCT may not be necessary to determine adequately the outcome of treatment and randomisation should not be conflated with efficacy. It is possible to randomise within a clinical setting thereby gaining the advantage of treatment being given within a context in which it will be applied in normal practice.

Despite the present popularity of RCTs as the gold standard by which treatments are assessed, there are a number of problems:

- Randomisation of patients to different therapies does not represent normal patient entry into, and continuation with, treatment. Strict randomisation may lead to patients being allocated to treatments they would otherwise not normally accept.
- There is increasing evidence that patient expectation of therapy is important for outcome (Horowitz *et al*, 1993).
- Sample size is often small and attrition of patients may be significant leading to a situation in which those patients remaining in a trial are far from random. Different patients respond differently to the same treatment leading to variation in outcome within the same group which may distort the outcome (see SPP–1 below).
- The 'named' treatment is often delivered by different therapists so, even if a manual is followed, patients may well be getting treatment that differs in significant respects. Therapists show considerable flexibility in interpreting manuals even after training (Gibbons *et al*, 2003). Fidelity of application is commonly measured by recording sessions, although few studies record all sessions, and randomly transcribe them, to ensure therapists keep to the model of therapy. Anyway, manualisation of therapies has been found wanting empirically. Henry *et al* (1993) demonstrated that adherence to treatment protocols obtained by additional training results in decreases in quality of generic therapist functioning. This may either reduce the effectiveness of a therapy or, at least, not improve it (Bein *et al*, 2000).
- Therapists themselves are rarely matched to patients even though patient–therapist fit may influence outcome (Rubino *et al*, 2000 or Lambert, 2004 for a review).
- Non-specific factors powerfully influence outcome and masked evaluations are hard to achieve.

- Possibly most importantly, investigator allegiance affects outcome (Gaffan, 1995). Professionals heavily identified with a therapy are more likely to show a better outcome for that therapy than an alternate control. Luborsky & colleagues (Luborsky *et al*, 1999) suggest that the allegiance of the researcher accounts for 70% of the variance in outcome studies, suggesting that most of the time we can predict which treatment is likely to be most effective merely based on the loyalty of the researcher.

Randomised controlled trials favour short-term treatments since they are difficult to maintain over a prolonged period of time. In long-term treatment patients tend to drop out or begin to resent the intrusion on treatment and decline to take part, leading to holes in the data. This disadvantages research in longer-term therapy, which until recently has been underrepresented in the literature other than through the 'open trial' or cohort study. There are, however, some notable exceptions and there are some RCTs of longer-term treatment of personality disorder with reasonable follow-up (Linehan *et al*, 1991, 1993; Bateman & Fonagy, 1999, 2001).

Comparative outcome studies

Eysenck (1952) in his often-quoted review of evidence then available, asserted that two-thirds of patients with neurosis improve whether they are treated or not, but his view has been sharply criticised. He compared out-patients who improved in analysis with in-patients considered well enough to be discharged from state mental hospitals within a year; the groups were scarcely comparable in terms of type and severity of illness, social background, or criteria of change. Re-analysis of Eysenck's data (McNeilly & Howard, 1991) showed that the impact of a few months of psychotherapy was equal to the impact of 2 years of all other forms of help available to an individual, confirming the potency of psychotherapy. Nevertheless Eysenck's remarks challenged the complacency of psychotherapy and stimulated more detailed research on outcome.

A notable example of an outcome study conducted by the National Institute of Mental Health (NIMH) in the USA was called the Treatment of Depression Collaborative Research Program (TDCRP) (Elkin *et al*, 1989). The study had two major aims: the first was to see if collaborative clinical trials of psychotherapy on a large scale were feasible; and the second was to compare the effectiveness of two brief psychotherapies for the treatment of depression with standard medical treatment using antidepressants.

The study comprised 250 people with depression who were randomly assigned to four treatment conditions; CBT, interpersonal psychotherapy, imipramine as a standard antidepressant plus clinical management (imipramine), and placebo plus clinical management (placebo). Therapists were trained in their model, supervised regularly, sessions were tape-recorded to ensure that therapy was given according to the model and adherence was carefully checked. Patients were assessed for levels of depression and social function before treatment and at 4, 8, 12 and 16 weeks and followed up at 6, 12 and 18 months.

Inevitably the results are complicated but in essence there was little difference in outcome between all the groups. Those patients receiving imipramine were least symptomatic and those receiving placebo the most symptomatic at the end of treatment. Comparison of relative scores representing recovery rates showed some differences although these were not marked. Patients receiving imipramine or interpersonal psychotherapy were most likely to recover. This was upsetting to those vociferously supporting CBT, who have argued that the CBT was inadequately given on one site, although there is little data to support this (Hollon & Beck, 2004); and so the results have been criticised and the data re-analysed. But re-analysis (Elkin *et al*, 1995) confirmed the equivalence of treatment options for patients who were less depressed. However, there was greater differentiation among therapies for the more depressed sample. On measures of depression imipramine (plus clinical management) and interpersonal psychotherapy were equally effective. Imipramine (plus clinical management) was more effective than CBT or placebo.

Follow-up of individuals studied suggested that relapse rates were similar across groups, although there was a trend towards fewer relapses in those individuals receiving psychotherapy suggesting some delayed effects for those given a psychological treatment. Patients in interpersonal psycho-therapy reported greater satisfaction with treatment, and individuals in both interpersonal psychotherapy and CBT reported significantly greater effects of treatment on their capacity to establish and maintain interpersonal relation-ships and to recognise and understand sources of their depression than did patients in the imipramine or placebo groups (Blatt *et al*, 2000). Overall the results were disappointing to those adherents of brand-named therapies who had hoped to prove once and for all that their therapy was the best.

Similar results were found in three studies conducted in England, which looked at the outcome of depression treated with either CBT or psychodynamic–interpersonal therapy. The latter is a manualised therapy theoretically derived from psychodynamic principles with some humanistic and interpersonal elements. The studies were the Sheffield Psychotherapy Project (SPP–1) (Shapiro & Firth-Cozens, 1987), the Second Sheffield Psychotherapy Project (SPP–2) (Shapiro *et al*, 1994; 1995) and the Collaborative Psychotherapy Project (CPP) (Barkham, 1996).

All three studies were rigorously designed trying to take into account the problems of RCTs discussed above, conducted with independent assessors, used operationalised therapy that was monitored for adherence, and included careful follow-up. Subjects for all three studies had to have symptoms of depression and, in the SPP–2 and the CPP, individuals were stratified into mild, moderate or severe according to level of depression. In essence SPP–1 and SPP–2 were efficacy studies in that they involved the recruitment of white-collar workers with depression who were then treated within a research clinic. The CPP was different and was designed to assess the effectiveness of and the generalisability of the treatments and so took place within a clinical setting.

The SPP–1 was a crossover study. Individuals were treated by the same therapists with CBT plus psychodynamic–interpersonal therapy (8 sessions of each) or psychodynamic–interpersonal therapy plus CBT (8 sessions of each) in order to mimic eclectic but professionally delivered therapy. There was no difference in outcome between the two groups and the order of therapy had no impact on outcome. Small differences on some measures were attributable to differential effects of therapists rather than therapy model.

The Second Sheffield Psychotherapy Project was an RCT designed not only to assess overall outcome of CBT and psychodynamic–interpersonal therapy in the treatment of depression but also to explore the impact of investigator allegiance, the importance of symptom severity, and the speed of recovery or 'dose–response'. Therapists were considered as being in 'equipoise' for CBT and psychodynamic–interpersonal therapy, having no specific allegiance, and all delivered both treatments. Treatments were given for either 8 weeks or 16 weeks, and individuals stratified according to level of depression. All the subjects who received CBT or psychodynamic–interpersonal therapy showed substantial, and broadly equivalent, improvement. The effects of both psychotherapies were exerted with equal rapidity and were the same at all three levels of symptom severity. An interaction was found between initial symptom severity and duration of therapy, with those patients who were more severely depressed showing significantly better outcomes with 16 sessions compared with those receiving only 8 sessions. Although there were improvements following 8 sessions of psychodynamic–interpersonal therapy, it was not as effective as the other 3 treatments (8 sessions CBT, 16 sessions CBT, 16 sessions psychodynamic–interpersonal therapy). Follow-up at 1 year found no differences in outcome or in maintenance of gains between CBT and psychodynamic–interpersonal therapy, although those receiving only 8 sessions of psychodynamic–interpersonal therapy continued to do less well.

It has already been mentioned that it is all very well for treatments to work within a research setting when they are applied by well-trained workers, but this is not the same as them working within a clinical setting (the efficacy versus effectiveness debate). The CPP was designed to test this; subjects were recruited from National Health Service clinics and once again stratified according to severity of symptoms and given either 8 or 16 sessions of either CBT or psychodynamic–interpersonal therapy.

Not surprisingly the results were less good than those found in the SPP–2, although all subjects did show substantial gains. There were two main effects. First, individuals did better with 16 sessions of treatment and second, the immediate post-therapy gains were not maintained at 3 months and at 1-year.

Many other comparative studies have found little difference between treatments for a number of conditions. Sloane *et al* (1975) studied individuals suffering from a variety of moderately severe neuroses and personality disorders, who, after a lengthy initial assessment (which could itself be therapeutic), were randomly allocated to one of three groups for 4 months. One group was treated by behaviour therapists, one by analytically orientated psychotherapists, and the third remained on a waiting list with the promise of eventual treatment (and were kept in telephone contact). Within 4 months, the severity of target symptoms had declined significantly in all three groups, but in both treated groups more than in the waiting-list group; and in both treatment groups outcome was related to the quality of the relationship between the individual and therapist. However, while only the behaviour therapy group had improved in 4 months on both work and social adjustment ratings, during the subsequent 8-month follow-up, after treatment had stopped, the analytical psychotherapy group continued to improve with regard to social adjustment, indicating a need for follow-up of individuals after the end of therapy.

Snyder & Willis (1989) conducted another carefully crafted study looking at differential effectiveness of therapies and including long-term follow-up. They compared behavioural marital therapy (BMT) to insight-orientated marital therapy (IOMT) and found both treatments more effective than no treatment but generally equivalent to each other at the end of the trial and at 6-month follow-up. Couples were then followed-up 4 years later (Snyder *et al*,1991). There was a marked difference in divorce rates between the two groups; 38% of the BMT group were divorced compared with only 3% of the IOMT group. It seems that there was something particular about IOMT that had a continuing effect over time, which was absent in BMT. There are of course other possible explanations but therapist adherence to treatment was carefully monitored and it was established that both treatments, designed to have clear difference, had been given appropriately. This study underscores the need for long follow-up in psychotherapy research, which is sadly lacking.

The consistent finding of equivalence of different therapies in a number of disorders is known as the 'dodo verdict' (Luborsky *et al*, 1975) after the story in *Alice's Adventures in Wonderland* (Carroll, 2003) in which a prolonged discussion occurs about the winner of a race in which all the competitors run around and round; 'everybody has won and all must have prizes'. Certainly the dodo verdict remains a plausible summary of the research, and difference in outcome between therapies needs more careful consideration than discovering similarity. It may be that we just do not yet have the research capability to detect difference, but it remains possible that all therapies have many factors in common and that these factors in themselves are potent agents of change. They are often subsumed under the rubric of the therapeutic alliance or working alliance (see below).

Meta-analytic studies

Meta-analytic studies collect data from separate studies allowing the calculation of an effect size. The effect size refers to group differences in standard deviation units on the normal distribution. Basically this is the degree to which the average treated client is better off than a control individual. This technique has been used to investigate outcome and cost-effectiveness. Effect sizes found in meta-analyses (Wampold *et al*, 1997) show that psychotherapy is better than placebo (effect size = 0.46) and substantially better than no psychotherapy (effect size = 0.82). The small differences reported among the mainstream therapies suggest that they are more or less equivalent, although some would argue that this is not the case and simply obfuscates the problem of comparing therapies by generalising. Some therapies show superior effect sizes to others in specific conditions. Cognitive–behaviour therapy shows a greater effect size for the treatment of anxiety than other therapies (Andrews *et al*, 1994). Psychodynamic therapy appears to have a greater effect in personality disorder (Leichsenring & Leibing, 2003). Leichsenring & Leibing found that psychodynamic therapy yielded a large overall effect size of 1.46, with effect sizes of 1.08 for self-report measures and 1.79 for observer-rated measures. This contrasts with CBT in which the corresponding values were 1.00, 1.20, and 0.87. In addition the psychodynamic studies had a mean follow-up period of 1.5 years compared with only 13 weeks for CBT.

There is a limited literature on cost-effectiveness of psychotherapy but meta-analysis suggests that considerable savings can be made in health service utilisation and other costs (Gabbard *et al*, 1997).

Therapeutic alliance

The importance of the relationship between therapist and patient as a contributor to the success of any therapy is without doubt. In a meta-analytic study, Horvath & Simmonds (1991) concluded that there was a 26% difference in level of therapeutic success dependent on the therapeutic alliance. Thus although most studies show little if any difference in outcome between therapies, when there is a difference this may simply be a reflection of the alliance between patient and therapist and not a differential effect of a therapy. In general the early alliance between patient and therapist is a better predictor of success than the strength of the alliance later in therapy, although this pattern is less evident in more recent studies.

It may be thought that the alliance is likely to be of most importance in dynamic therapies since psychoanalytic therapy uses the relationship between patient and therapist as a mediator of change. However the alliance seems equally important in other therapies. Castonguay *et al* (1996) reported significant associations between the alliance and outcome measures at mid- and post-treatment for patients receiving CBT and CBT plus an antidepressant. However a study by DuRubeis & Feeley (1990) implies that the alliance is less predictive in more highly structured interventions.

The impact of the alliance on outcome has been reported both for the NIMH and the Sheffield project discussed earlier. Krupnick *et al* (Krupnick, 1996) reported that the alliance level averaged over all the treatment sessions accounted for 21% of the variance in outcome in the

NIMH trial. Interestingly this factor showed importance across all the treatments including pharmacotherapy. But this group was also given clinical management, which may itself be another name for therapeutic alliance. Detailed work suggested that the alliance was greater for the most improved cases particularly in interpersonal psychotherapy. In the Sheffield study the results are more complex but Stiles et al (1998) also found a statistically significant association between a number of outcome measures and the alliance.

There seems little doubt that the alliance, when positive, makes a substantial contribution to the outcome of all forms of therapy. Of course this could be a self-fulfilling prophecy, with individuals reporting a positive alliance if their treatment is going well. But those studies that have looked at this possibility suggest that this is not the case. There is no evidence that those individuals with a good outcome view their therapy in a more positive frame than those individuals whose treatment goes less well.

Process research and the quantification of meaning

It could be argued that a large amount of effort has been expended in chasing relatively little difference, especially in the arena of comparative outcome research. This has led to more attention being paid to process research, which is likely to yield useful information relevant to the practice of therapy. Research looking at the detail of psychotherapeutic process represents an attempt to understand the complexity of the endeavour and to that extent moves research away from quantification towards meaning.

While there may be equivalence in outcome between therapies there is a notable non-equivalence in process. Stiles (1979) coded sessions given by expert practitioners and found evidence of technical non-equivalence. Therapists of different persuasions were actually giving interventions consistent with their model. Psychoanalytic therapists restricted themselves to interpretations, clarifications, acknowledgements, and reflections. Gestalt therapists stayed in the 'now' and client-centred therapists used reflections and acknowledgement as their primary interventions.

But it remains unclear whether the theoretically derived interventions are actually the active ingredients of therapy leading to change. Researchers have therefore tried to identify the potent factors of therapies in the hope that more of what is effective will improve outcome. This is a rather simplistic notion that follows the 'drug metaphor' of therapy. If a little aspirin is good for a headache then increasing the dose may be more effective. While this is true to an extent in pharmacotherapy, there may of course be a therapeutic window, a dose–response curve and so on. The same applies to psychotherapy. It is possible either to overdose or to underdose and the dose may be dependent on the underlying condition. Howard et al (1986) reported a meta-analysis on 2431 patients from psychotherapy research covering a 30-year period. They found that there was a stable pattern across studies indicating that by the 8th session approximately 50% of individuals are measurably improved and that by the end of 6 months 75% are improved. Those with comorbidity require the 'biggest dose'.

Psychotherapy research has begun to unravel the complex process of psychological treatment, looking at what makes people better. Piper *et al* (1991; 1993) explored the relationship between number (concentration) and accuracy of transference interpretation and outcome of therapy. The results are complex and tentative. Those individuals with the most psychological-mindedness as measured on the Quality of Object Relations (QOR) scale (Azim *et al*, 1991) had the best outcomes if interpretation was both accurate and of low concentration. Those patients with low quality of object relations did not do well, particularly if interpretations were inaccurate and of high concentration. Simply increasing the number of transference interpretations may represent desperation on the part of the therapist and so be negatively correlated with improvement.

In a study by Horowitz & Marmac (1984), improvement for individuals who were bereaved and were given short-term psychotherapy was related to psychological maturity at the beginning of treatment and not to intervention. Those individuals with good motivation and a stable, coherent sense of themselves did best with psychodynamic exploration of their difficulties. Those with a poor sense of self responded better to supportive therapy. In later studies Horowitz *et al* (Horowitz, 1988; Horowitz *et al*, 1993) suggested that individuals who viewed their difficulties in interpersonal terms do best with psychodynamic therapy.

Similar effects may occur in cognitive therapy since all interventions need to be given at the right time, in the right way and within the right patient–therapist context if they are to be effective. The number of cognitive interventions does not correlate with outcome. Cognitive therapy itself is not unique in its ability to diminish or change cognition and individuals may improve, while dysfunctional attitudes and assumptions remain unchanged. Stiles & Shapiro (1994) analysed tapes of cognitive and psychodynamic treatments given in the Sheffield Psychotherapy Project using a large number of process measures and found outcome did not correlate with theoretically important process components.

Other studies have had similar difficulty in linking process measures to outcome. In other words the 'dodo verdict' seems to hold even when we look carefully at the process of different psychotherapies. Although the process looks different it does not seem to matter. It may be that we have not yet considered the true active ingredients or that we are not measuring them. But if this is the case then it suggests that the theories underpinning different therapies are themselves flawed.

There are two detailed lines of study that inform this interesting picture. First, there is the therapeutic alliance research discussed above. Second, there is the most widely known attempt to put psychotherapeutic insights on a reliable, replicable, and scientifically reputable basis. This is the Core Conflictual Relationship Theme (CCRT) method (Luborsky & Crits-Christoph, 1990) used to study psychodynamic therapy. The method is laborious, but it yields psychodynamically meaningful data about the inner world. It starts from the idea that every therapy session contains a number of unconscious personal themes that can be identified through studying transcripts of the sessions.

Identifying CCRTs is a two-stage process; first, pairs of trained judges extract from the transcript a number of 'relationship episodes' which have been described or enacted by the individual in the session (i.e. a story about work, home or the individual's reactions to the therapist). Most individuals generate about four such relationship episodes per session. The list of these episodes is then passed on to a second set of judges who analyse them into three components:

- the individual's wishes, needs, or intentions
- the response elicited from others, either positive or negative
- the reactions of the self to these other reactions, again positive or negative.

Common examples of wishes are for closeness, dominance or autonomy; of responses are those of being rejected, controlled or dominated; and of self-responses are anger, withdrawal, and disappointment. These categories are initially made freehand by the judges so as to produce 'tailor-made' categories, which are then translated into a predetermined list of standard categories that allow for more reliable comparisons. From these there emerges a CCRT or set of CCRTs that characterise the individual's core state; a typical example would be the wish for closeness, feeling rejected, and responding with withdrawal.

The CCRTs formulations are clinically derived and do not use sophisticated psychoanalytic concepts or terminology, but are highly reliable (Crits -Cristoph et al,1988), and thus have considerable flexibility as a research tool. They can be modified into a set of statements that the individual can then use to think about himself. CCRTs correspond with the 'core beliefs' found to be important in cognitive therapy.

Luborsky has used CCRTs to research a number of important psycho-analytic issues. CCRT 'pervasiveness' decreases in the course of successful therapy, so that by the end of therapy individuals are less dominated by their core themes. Wishes change less than responses, therapeutic change being associated particularly with the capacity to cope with negative responses and to elicit more positive ones from others, rather than some idealised 'resolution of underlying conflict'. Another study used CCRTs to look at the relationship between the 'accuracy' of interpretations, as measured by their closeness to CCRTs. In general the more skilful the therapist, the better the outcome, especially in so far as they were able accurately to identify wishes, responses elicited and reactions. In this study, while accuracy of interpretation is related to good outcome, the type of interpretation was not, i.e. non-transference interpretations were just as effective as transference ones (Fretter et al, 1994).

Luborsky *et al* (1993) believe that the CCRT approach provides the first scientific confirmation and objective measure of the concept of transference.

By comparing the features of CCRT with Freud's statements about transference they confirm that:

- individuals have only a few basic transference patterns
- these are manifest both in their relationships generally and with the therapist
- they seem to derive from early parental relationship patterns
- transference patterns are as evident outside therapy as in it
- these patterns are susceptible to gradual change in the course of treatment.

An important feature of any research method is its capacity to be used by all workers in the field, not just by those who devised it. This has not perhaps been the case with CCRT, but may be true of a new instrument, the Adult Attachment Interview (AAI), devised by Mary Main and her colleagues (Main & Goldwyn, 1991) based on the principles of attachment theory (Bowlby, 1988; Holmes, 1993; see also Chapter 3), which is being widely used in psychodymamic psychotherapy research. The AAI also starts with interview transcripts, but, unlike most instruments, it is concerned not so much with the content as the form and style of the individual's narrative. Like therapy itself, the AAI tries to 'listen with the third ear' (Reik, 1922), but in a way that can be researched. A psychodynamic-type assessment interview is carried out, concentrating on the subject's past and present attachments and losses. It is assumed that a person's underlying relational dispositions (which may well be unconscious) will be evident in the structure of their narrative, its consistence, coherence, elaboration or restrictedness.

Interviews are assigned to one of four major categories: autonomous-free, in which the subject can talk openly and coherently about his childhood and parents, including painful experiences from the past; dismissive–detached, in which narratives are not elaborated and subjects have few childhood memories and tend to deny difficulty or devalue relationships in a grandiose way; and preoccupied–enmeshed, in which the narrative style is muddled and confusing and the individual appears to be dominated by affects from the past such as anger or overwhelming sadness; and unresolved, in which the subject shows lapses of reasoning and gives inconsistent information, particularly when discussing traumatic events such as physical or sexual abuse. The AAI also identifies significant 'breaks' or incoherence which may appear in any type of interview, which may reflect past trauma such as sexual abuse that has been repressed but momentarily surfaces during the interview. Many of these interviews may be classified as unresolved although it has become apparent that it is impossible to classify some individuals.

The AAI has been used to track change in psychoanalytic therapy, showing how individuals can move from dismissive or enmeshed to secure narrative styles as therapy progresses (Fonagy *et al*, 1995). It has also been used to trace the intergenerational transmission of attachment patterns, showing how the classification of prospective parents on the AAI before their babies are born correlates well with the subsequent child's attachment status at 1 year. An unexpected but important finding of this study was that infants appear to develop quite independent attachment patterns with each parent, so that they may be secure with father and insecure with mother and vice versa, depending on the parent's AAI. This is consistent with a psychoanalytic view of an inner or representational world containing models or prototypes of relationships that may act independently of one another. Presumably similar internal models of attachment are built up in the course of therapy, which then supersede previous insecure relationship patterns.

A number of studies of psychotherapy process have suggested that therapist behaviour, particularly in flexibility and competence influences outcome even in manualised treatments (Shaw *et al*, 1999) and that the interpersonal skills of the therapist may be a determining factor of patient retention and outcome. The personality of the therapist may interact with that of the patient in a positive or negative way. Data from the Vanderbilt II study in which 67% of patients had an Axis II disorder suggest that both patient and therapist early parental relationships have an effect on therapy process, which in turn has a direct effect on outcome (Hilliard *et al*, 2000). Evidence, albeit limited, suggests that some therapists achieve larger positive effects than others (Blatt *et al*, 1996). In one study of treatment of drug abuse (Project MATCH Research Group, 1998), in which a large number of individuals were likely to have a personality disorder, 4 out of 80 therapists produced substantial therapist effects as a result of poor outcomes, while 1 therapist showed markedly better outcomes (Najavits & Weiss, 1994). This variation may arise from practitioner characteristics and interpersonal function rather than technical skill and is likely to be more pronounced in treatment of personality disorder in which the formation of a therapeutic bond between the psychiatrist, mental health practitioner and patient is essential if the patient is to engage and remain in treatment.

Conclusions

There has been a move away from 'head-to-head' clashes of different psychotherapies and a move towards a better understanding of the subtlety and meaning of psychotherapy. This is one area in which psychodynamic therapy has developed a specific methodology. But we still have limited knowledge of process and outcome and know even less about patient, therapist and therapy characteristics that are important for favourable outcome to treatment. Certainly social class, age, ethnicity, and gender do not predict outcome or guide choice of therapy. There is greater need for research into the interaction between patient characteristics and treatment method than there is for sterile comparisons of outcome between therapies in different conditions. Variance in treatment outcome for most disorders is small in efficacy studies and is likely to be even smaller in clinical practice. We urgently need to understand the mechanisms of change, to identify those that are specific to each method, and to evaluate those that are common to all therapies. Only then will we be able fruitfully to combine process research with outcome research in such a way that the practice of psychotherapy changes.

References

Andrews, G., Crino, R., Hunt, C., *et al* (1994) *The Treatment of Anxiety Disorders*. New York: Cambridge University Press.

Barkham, M., Rees, A., Shapiro, D. A., *et al* (1996) Outcome of time-limited psychotherapy in applied settings: replication the Second Sheffield Psychotherapy Project. *Journal of Consulting and Clinical Psychology*, **64**, 1079–1085.

Bateman, A. & Fonagy, P. (1999) The effectiveness of partial hospitalization in the treatment of borderline personality disorder – a randomized controlled trial. *American Journal of Psychiatry*, **156**, 1563–1569.

Bateman, A. & Fonagy, P. (2001) Treatment of borderline personality disorder with psychoanalytically oriented partial hospitalization: an 18-month follow-up. *American Journal of Psychiatry*, **158**, 36–42.

Beck, A. T., Ward, C. H., Mendelson, M., *et al* (1961) An inventory for measuring depression. *Archives of General Psychiatry*, **4**, 561–571.

Bein, E., Andersen, T., Strupp, H. H., *et al* (2000) The effects of training in time-limited dynamic psychotherapy: changes in therapeutic outcome. *Psychotherapy Research*, **10**, 119–132.

Blatt, S., Berman W, Cook B.P., *et al* (1998) Effectiveness of long-term, intensive, in-patient treatment for seriously disturbed young adults: a reply to Bein. *Psychotherapy Research*, **8**, 42–53.

Blatt, S. J., Sanislow, C. A., Zuroff, D., *et al* (1996) Characteristics of effective therapists: further analysis of data from the National Institute of Mental Health treatment of depression collaborative research programme. *Journal of Consulting and Clinical Psychology*, **64**, 1276–1284.

Blatt, S. J., Stayner, D. A., Auerbach, J. S., *et al* (1996) Change in object and self-representations in long-term, intensive, inpatient treatment of seriously disturbed adolescents and young adults. *Psychiatry*, **59**, 82–107.

Blatt, S. J., Zuroff, D., Bondi, C. M., *et al* (2000) Short- and long-term effects of medication and psychotherapy in the brief treatment of depression: further analyses of data from the NIMH TDRCP. *Psychotherapy Research*, **10**, 215–234.

Blomberg, J., Lazar, A. & Sandell, R. (2001) Long-term outcome of long-term psychoanalytically oriented therapies: first findings of the Stockholm Outcome of Psychotherapy and Psychoanalysis study. *Psychotherapy Research*, **11**, 361–382.

Bowlby, J. (1988) *A Secure Base: Clinical Applications of Attachment Theory*. London: Routledge.

Carroll, L. (2003) *Alice's Adventures in Wonderland and Through the Looking Glass*. Harmondsworth: Penguin Books.

Castonguay, L., Goldfried, M., Wiser, S., *et al* (1996) Predicting the effect of cognitive therapy for depression: a study of unique and common factors. *Journal of Consulting and Clinical Psychology*, **64**, 497–504.

Chiesa, M. & Fonagy, P. (2003) Psychosocial treatment for severe personality disorder: 36-month follow-up. *British Journal of Psychiatry*, **183**, 356–362.

Chiesa, M., Fonagy, P., Holmes, J., *et al* (2002) Health Service use costs by personality disorder following specialist and non-specialist treatment: a comparative study. *Journal of Personality Disorders*, **16**, 160–173.

Dolan, B., Warren, F. & Norton, K. (1997) Change in borderline symptoms one year after therapeutic community treatment for severe personality disorder. *British Journal of Psychiatry*, **171**, 274–279.

DuRubeis, R. J. & Feeley, M. (1990) Determinants of change in cognitive therapy for depression. *Cognitive Therapy Research*, **14**, 469–482.

Elkin, I., Gibbons, R. D., Shea, M. T., *et al* (1995) Initial severity and differential treatment outcome in the National Institute of Mental Health Treatment of Depression Collaborative Research Program. *Journal of Consulting and Clinical Psychology*, **63**, 841–847.

Elkin, I., Shea, M. T., Watkins, J. T., *et al* (1989) National Institute of Mental Health Treatment of Depression Collaborative Research Program: general effectiveness of treatments. *Archives of General Psychiatry*, **46**, 971–982.

Eysenck, H. J. (1952) The effects of psychotherapy: an evaluation. *Journal of Consulting Psychology*, **16**, 319–324.

Fonagy, P., Moran, G. S., Lindsay, M. K. M., *et al* (1987) Psychological adjustment and diabetic control. *Archives of Disease in Childhood*, **62**, 10009–11013.

Fonagy, P., Target, M., Steele, M., *et al* (1995) Psychoanalytic perspectives on developmental psychopathology. In *Developmental Psychopathology: Theory and Methods* (eds D. Cicchetti & D. J. Cohen), pp. 504–554. New York: John Wiley & Sons, Inc.

Fretter, P., Bucci, W., Broitman, J., *et al* (1994) How the patient's plan relates to the concept of transference. *Psychotherapy Research*, 4, 58–71.

Gabbard, G. O., Lazar, S. G., Hornberger, J., *et al* (1997) The economic impact of psychotherapy: a review. *American Journal of Psychiatry*, **154**, 147–155.

Gaffan, E. A., Tsaousis, I. & Kemp-Wheeler, S.M. (1995) Researcher allegiance and meta-analysis: the case of cognitive therapy for depression. *Journal of Consulting and Clinical Psychology*, **63**, 966–980.

Gibbons, M. C., Crits-Christoph, P., Levinson, J., *et al* (2003) Flexibility in manual-based psychotherapies: predictors of therapist interventions in interpersonal and cognitive–behavioural therapy. *Psychotherapy Research*, **13**, 169–185.

Grunbaum, A. (1986) Precis of the foundations of psychoanalysis: a philosophical critique, with commentary. *Behavioural and Brain Sciences*, **9**, 217–284.

Hamilton, M. (1960) A rating scale for depression. *Journal of Neurology, Neurosurgery and Psychiatry*, 23, 56–62.

Henry, W. P., Strupp, H. H., Butler, S. F., *et al* (1993) The effects of training in time-limited psychotherapy: changes in therapists' behaviour. *Journal of Consulting and Clinical Psychology*, **61**, 434–440.

Hilliard, R. B., Henry, W. P. & Strupp, H. H. (2000) An interpersonal model of psychotherapy: linking patient and therapist developmental history, therapeutic process, and types of outcome. *Journal of Consulting and Clinical Psychology*, **68**, 125–133.

Hollon, S. D. & Beck A. T. (2004) Cognitive and cognitive behavioural therapies. In *Handbook of Psychotherapy and Behaviour Change* (ed M. J. Lambert), pp: 447–492. New York: Wiley.

Holmes, J. (1993) *John Bowlby and Attachment Theory*. London: Routledge.

Horowitz, L. M., Rosenberg, S. E. & Bartholomew, K. (1993) Interpersonal problems, attachment styles and outcome in brief dynamic therapy. *Journal of Consulting and Clinical Psychology*, **61**, 549–560.

Horowitz, M. & Marmac, C. (1984) Brief psychotherapy of bereavement reactions: the relationship of process to outcome. *Archives of General Psychiatry*, **41**, 438–448.

Horowitz, M. J. (1988) Psychodynamic phenomena and their explanation. In *Psychodynamics and Cognition* (ed. M. J. Horowitz), pp. 3-20. University of Chicago Press.

Horvath, A. O. & Simmonds, B. D. (1991) Relation between working alliance and outcome in psychotherapy: a meta-analysis. *Journal of Consulting and Clinical Psychology*, **38**, 139–149.

Howard, K. I., Kopta, S. M., Krause, M. S., *et al* (1986) The dose–effect relationship in psychotherapy. Special issue: psychotherapy research. *American Psychologist*, **41**, 159–164.

Howard, K. I., Orlinsky, D. E. & Lueger, R. J. (1995) The design of clinically relevant outcome research: some considerations and an example. In *Research Foundations for Psychotherapy Practice* (eds M. Aveline & D. A. Shapiro), pp. 3–47. Chichester: Wiley.

Krupnick, J. L., Sotsky, S. M., Simmons, S., *et al* (1996) The role of the therapeutic alliance in psychotherapy and pharmacotherapy outcome: findings in the NIMH Collaborative Research Program. *Journal of Consulting and Clinical Psychology*, **64**, 532–539.

Lambert, M. J. (2004) *Bergin and Garfield's Handbook of Psychotherapy and Behavior Change.* New York: John Wiley.

Leichsenring, F. & Leibing, E. (2003) The effectiveness of psychodynamic therapy and cognitive behavior therapy in the treatment of personality disorders: a meta-analysis. *American Journal of Psychiatry*, **160**, 1223–1232.

Linehan, M. M., Armstrong, H., Suarez, A., *et al* (1991) Cognitive–behavioural treatment of chronically parasuicidal borderline patients. *Archives of General Psychiatry*, **48**, 1060–1064.

Linehan, M. M., Heard, H. L. & Armstrong, H. E. (1993) Naturalistic follow-up of a behavioral treatment for chronically parasuicidal borderline patients. *Archives of General Psychiatry*, **50**, 971–974.

Luborsky, L. & Crits-Christoph, P. (1990) *Understanding Transference: The CCRT Method.* New York: Basic Books.

Luborsky, L., Barber, J. P., Binder, J., *et al* (1993) Transference-related measures: a new class based on psychotherapy sessions. In *Psychodynamic Treatment research: A Handbook for Clinical Practice* (eds N. E. Miller, *et al*), pp. 326–341. New York: Basic Books.

Luborsky, L., Diguer, L., Seligman, D. A., *et al* (1999) The researcher's own therapy allegiances: a 'wild card' in comparisons of treatment efficacy. *Clinical Psychology: Science and Practice*, **6**, 95–106.

Luborsky, L., Singer, B. & Luborsky, L. (1975) Comparative studies of psychotherapies: is it true that 'everybody has won and all must have prizes'? *Archives of General Psychiatry*, **37**, 471–481.

Main, M. & Goldwyn, R. (1991) *Adult Attachment Classification System. Version 5.* University of California, Berkeley.

Margison, F. & Bateman, A. (2006) Research in Psychotherapy. In *Introduction to the Psychotherapies* (ed. S. Bloch). Oxford University Press.

McNeilly, C. L. & Howard, K. I. (1991) The effects of psychotherapy: a re-evaluation based on dosage. *Psychotherapy Research*, **1**, 74–78.

Najavits, L. & Weiss, R. (1994) Variations in therapist effectiveness in the treatment of patients with substance use disorders: an empirical review. *Addiction*, **89**, 679–688.

Najavits, L. M. & Gunderson, J. G. (1995) Improvements in borderline personality disorder in a 3-year prospective outcome study. *Comprehensive Psychiatry*, **36**, 296–302.

Piper, W. E., Azim, H. F. A., Joyce, A. S., *et al* (1991) Transference interpretations, therapeutic alliance, and outcome in short-term individual psychotherapy. *Archives of General Psychiatry*, **48**, 946–953.

Piper, W. E., Joyce, A. S., McCallum, M., *et al* (1993) Concentration and correspondence of transference interpretation in short-term psychotherapy. *Journal of Consulting and Clinical Psychology*, **61**, 586–610.

Project MATCH Research Group (1998) Therapist effects in three treatments for alcohol problems. *Psychotherapy Research*, **8**, 455–474.

Reik, T. (1922) *The Inner Eye of a Psychoanalyst.* London: Allen Unwin.

Rosser, R., Birch, S., Bond, H., *et al* (1987) Five-year follow-up of patients treated with in-patient psychotherapy at the Cassel Hospital for Nervous Diseases. *Journal of the Royal Society of Medicine*, **80**, 549–555.

Roth, A. & Fonagy, P. (1996) *What Works for Whom? A Critical Review of Psychotherapy Research.* New York: Guilford Press.

Rubino, G., Barker, C., Roth, T., *et al* (2000) Therapist empathy and depth of interpretation in response to potential alliance ruptures: the role of therapist and patient attachment styles. *Psychotherapy Research*, **10**, 408–420.

Salkovskis, P. (1995) Demonstrating specific effects in cognitive and behavioural therapy. In *Research Foundations in Psychotherapy Practice* (eds M. Aveline & D. A. Shapiro), pp. 191–228. Chichester: Wiley.

Sandell, R., Blomberg, J. & Lazar, A. (2002) Time matters: on temporal interactions in long-term follow-up of long-term psychotherapies. *Psychotherapy Research*, **12**, 39–58.

Schwarz, D. & Lellouch, J. (1967) Explanatory and pragmatic attitudes in therapeutic trials. *Journal of Chronic Diseases*, **20**, 637–648.

Seligman, M. E. P. (1995) The effectiveness of psychotherapy. *American Psychologist*, **50**, **20**, 965–974.

Shapiro, D. & Firth-Cozens, J. (1987) Prescriptive v. exploratory therapy. Outcomes of the Sheffield Psychotherapy Project. *British Journal of Psychiatry*, **151**, 790–799.

Shapiro, D. A., Barkham, M., Rees, A., *et al* (1994) Special feature. Effects of treatment duration and severity of depression on the effectiveness of cognitive–behavioral and psychodynamic–interpersonal psychotherapy. *Journal of Consulting and Clinical Psychology*, **62**, 522–534.

Shapiro, D. A., Rees, A., Barkham, M., *et al* (1995) Effects of treatment duration and severity of depression on the maintenance of gains after cognitive–behavioral and psychodynamic–interpersonal psychotherapy. *Journal of Consulting and Clinical Psychology*, **63**, 378–387.

Shaw, B. F., Elkin, I., Yamaguchi, J., *et al* (1999) Therapist competence ratings in relation to clinical outcome in cognitive therapy of depression. *Journal of Consulting and Clinical Psychology*, **67**, 837–846.

Sloane, R. B., Staples, F. R., Cristol, A. H., *et al* (1975) Short-term analytically oriented psychotherapy versus behaviour therapy. *American Journal of Psychiatry*, **132**, 373–377.

Snyder, D. & Willis, R. (1989) Behavioural versus insight-oriented marital therapy: effects on individual and interspousal functioning. *Journal of Consulting and Clinical Psychology*, **57**, 39–46.

Snyder, D. K., Willis, R. M. & Grady-Fletcher, A. (1991) Long-term effectiveness of behavioral versus insight-oriented marital therapy: a 4-year follow-up study. *Journal of Consulting and Clinical Psychology*, **59**, 138–141.

Steiner, J. (1985) Psychotherapy under attack. *Lancet*, **i**, 266–267.

Stiles, W. (1979) Verbal response modes and psychotherapeutic technique. *Psychiatry*, **42**, 49–62.

Stiles, W. B. & Shapiro, D. A. (1994) Disabuse of the drug metaphor: psychotherapy process–outcome correlations. *Journal of Consulting and Clinical Psychology*, **62**, 942–948.

Stiles, W. B., Agnew-Davies, R., Hardy, G.E., *et al* (1998) Relations of the alliance with psychotherapy outcome: findings in the second Sheffield Psychotherapy Project. *Journal of Consulting and Clinical Psychology*, **66**, 791–802.

Wampold, B. E., Mondin, G. W., Moody, M., *et al* (1997) A meta-analysis of outcome studies comparing bona fide psychotherapies: empirically, 'all must have prizes'. *Psychological Bulletin*, **122**, 203–215.

Index

Compiled by Caroline Sheard

LIBRARY & INFORMATION SERVICE
TEES, ESK & WEAR VALLEYS
NHS FOUNDATION TRUST
COUNTY HOSPITAL